Mobilisation
WITH
Movement
The art and the science

Mobilisation
WITH
Movement
The art and the science

Bill Vicenzino   Wayne Hing   Darren Rivett   Toby Hall

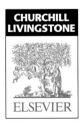

CHURCHILL LIVINGSTONE

ELSEVIER

Edinburgh   London   New York   Philadelphia   St Louis   Toronto

Churchill Livingstone
is an imprint of Elsevier

Elsevier Australia. ACN 001 002 357
(a division of Reed International Books Australia Pty Ltd)
Tower 1, 475 Victoria Avenue, Chatswood, NSW 2067

ELSEVIER

National Library of Australia Cataloguing-in-Publication Data

---

Title: Mobilisation with movement : the art and the science / Bill Vicenzino ... [et al.]

ISBN: 9780729538954 (pbk.)

Subjects: Physical therapy--Australia.

    Movement therapy--Australia.

    Physical therapy--Handbooks, manuals, etc

    Movement therapy--Handbooks, manuals, etc

Other Authors/Contributors: Vicenzino, Bill.

Dewey Number: 615.82

Publisher: Melinda McEvoy
Developmental Editors: Sam McCulloch and Rebecca Cornell
Publishing Services Manager: Helena Klijn
Project Coordinator: Geraldine Minto
Edited and indexed by Forsyth Publishing Services
Proofread by Gabrielle Challis
Cover and internal design by Lisa Petroff
Photography by Porfyri Photography
Illustrated by Lorenzo Lucia of Galaxy Studios
Typeset by TNQ Books and Journals Pvt. Ltd.
Printed by China Translation & Printing Services Ltd

CONTENTS

FOREWORD BY BRIAN MULLIGAN

The need for an appropriate textbook on my concepts has at last been met. Mobilisation with Movement (MWM) has been developing for nearly three decades and the evidence base for its use is mounting. Justification for its use based on such evidence, clinical reasoning and reflection is within these pages making this volume an excellent reference for the researcher, teacher and clinician, and it will become a worthy standard text on my concepts.

What has enabled the successful teaching of the concepts to date, without the much needed scientific backing, has been the fact that MWMs are only to be used as a treatment when, on assessment, they have a **'PILL'** effect. The acronym stands for **p**ain-free, **i**nstant result and **l**ong **l**asting.

Pain-free refers to both the mobilisation and movement components.

Instant result means that at the time of delivery there is an immediate pain-free improvement in function. This is not true of many manual therapy techniques taught.

Long **l**asting means that all or most of the improvement gained is maintained. If the patient regresses between visits and there is no obvious correctable reason for this, after three visits you can say that MWMs are not indicated.

On this basis MWMs should be used as an assessment tool by all those involved in the field of musculoskeletal therapy to ascertain if they are a valuable and appropriate treatment tool.

Another important acronym we use when teaching MWMs is **'CROCKS'**, which deals with their application.

C stands for the contraindications to manual therapy which, of course, will be known by all manual therapists.

R stands for repetitions. With an extremity joint that has been dysfunctional for weeks or even longer, up to three sets of 10 MWMs can be used. With acute injuries, on day one, it is wise because of irritability to apply the techniques three to six times. With the spine we have 'the rule of three'. On day one only use MWMs three times. This is because some patients following any form of manual therapy get a latent reaction to their treatment. This is minimised by the rule of three. Even when they get this reaction it is of short duration and when it settles they are still much better and further treatment can be given.

O stands for overpressure. Basically, the mobilisation component of MWM is really a sustained repositioning of the joint surfaces. This, when indicated, enables pain-free function to occur and, when restricted joints are treated, passive overpressure must be given. While painless, maximum movement must be gained and this can only be attained by applying overpressure. With longstanding restrictions the movement gained on day one is usually all passive. If overpressure is not applied the results will not be long lasting.

C stands for communication and cooperation. You must explain in detail to the patient what you are about to do. They must know to tell you immediately if there is any discomfort. Without their feedback you will not succeed.

K stands for knowledge. Manual therapists must have an excellent knowledge of musculoskeletal medicine. They must know their anatomy and it is critical that they know all joint configurations and, in particular, joint planes.

S stands for many things. Sustain your mobilisation throughout the movement. Sustain the repositioning until you return to the starting position.

Skill is required. Handling skills when dealing with sensitive painful structures are important. You need a sensibility in your fingertips to locate accurately and firmly without squeezing. Sometimes a plastic sponge can be used for patient comfort. Handling skills determine how much force you use. With some structures the movement taking place may be less than 1 mm.

Sense — commonsense and sometimes a sixth sense are invaluable.

Subtle changes in direction are required when repositioning joint surfaces to completely eliminate any discomfort. This ties in with handling skills.

To now have this reference book, *Mobilisation with Movement: the art and the science,* is wonderful. I feel humble and I am personally indebted to Bill Vicenzino, Wayne Hing, Darren Rivett and Toby Hall and all the individual contributors for the immense time and effort that has gone into its creation. I cannot thank them enough.

Brian Mulligan 2010

FOREWORD BY PROFESSOR GWENDOLEN JULL

The term Mobilisation with Movement, or MWM, is in common usage in the vocabulary of manual therapy practitioners worldwide. MWM is a method of manual therapy that is being increasingly incorporated into management regimes for patients with musculoskeletal disorders. The term is also synonymous with New Zealand physiotherapist Brian Mulligan, a gifted and innovative clinician and manual therapist who has developed the approach over several decades, with the assistance of his patients. Brian Mulligan has made a major contribution to the field of manual therapy. He has generously shared his knowledge, clinical expertise and experience. He has taught the MWM approach widely, nationally and internationally, and importantly he has trained others to teach the approach. Brian Mulligan has also published books and DVDs which detail the indications and applications of techniques for clinicians and patients alike.

The therapeutic approach to MWM has undoubtedly gained the attention of clinicians because of its effectiveness in the management of patients with musculoskeletal pain and movement disorders. There has been some research investigating its efficacy and the hypotheses for its mechanisms of effect. However, to date the MWM approach has had its seminal basis in clinical observation of responsiveness to the clinically reasoned application of passive movement/positioning in combination with active movement. While the primacy of high level clinical reasoning and practical skills can never be underestimated, there is a current desire by clinicians, researchers and healthcare agencies alike for delivery of practice which is also research informed and evidence based. This text, *Mobilisation with Movement: the art and the science,* embarks upon the process of providing the nexus between a seemingly successful clinical approach and its clinical science base.

The text's authors, Bill Vicenzino, Wayne Hing, Toby Hall and Darren Rivett are all highly regarded clinical researchers and teachers, well versed in the MWM approach. They have all been involved in research into the efficacy and effectiveness of MWM and thus have a strong and authoritative clinical and research base to explore both the art and science of Brian Mulligan's approach.

A treatment method has a risk of 'non survival' without clinical and research paradigms that can be tested and advanced. The authors are to be congratulated on the scholarship evident in this text. They have constructed and presented novel paradigms which stand to advance the understanding and applications of MWM. To advance the field, they have developed a well reasoned clinical paradigm for MWM (Chapter 2) and have introduced a model incorporating what they have named the Client Specific Impairment Measure (CSIM) which acts as a key and central feature of the approach to patient assessment and management. This model is well conceived, comprehensive and stands to guide the clinician's clinical reasoning in patient assessment and management. Importantly, use of such a model can guide design of future research ranging from, for example, Phase I to Phase III trials.

It is easy for the enthusiast to laud uncritically a management approach and 'spread the doctrine'. What is appreciated and valuable in this text, is the authors' balanced approach between the science and the art and their determination to advance the field. The available evidence of benefit of MWM has been presented in an unbiased way using the rigorous methodology of a systematic review. While some preliminary evidence of benefit is emerging, the need for further high quality trials is noted. In relation to mechanisms of action to explain the effects of MWM, the historical positional fault hypothesis of MWM is critically reviewed. While appreciating the available evidence, the authors forge ahead and present a new model for consideration of the mechanisms of action of MWM to advance the field both clinically and in research. Importantly and realistically, there is an expansion of the hypothesis for MWM mechanisms from a previously predominantly biomechanical one, to one which also incorporates the neurosciences (the sensory and motor systems) and the behavioural sciences, and expert input into the field has been provided.

It is often difficult in a theoretical construct, such as a book, to 'bring to life' the clinical reasoning and methodologies of the approach together with the nuances of patients, especially when dealing with the heterogeneity in presentation of musculoskeletal disorders. The authors have successfully addressed this challenge by providing several well crafted chapters of patient cases presented by leading clinicians in the field, as well as the authors themselves. What is of enormous value in these chapters for clinicians is the inclusion of the clinical reasoning process that is integrated with the description of the technical aspects of patient management. In addition, the cases serve to display the wide application of the principles and practice of the MWM approach in the musculoskeletal field.

As mentioned, the MWM approach has generated considerable interest and enthusiasm in the field of manual therapy. From a clinical standpoint, it has, over the past two or more decades, provided an advance to the art of manual therapy and assisted many patients with painful musculoskeletal disorders. However, as is commonly encountered, the clinical art of MWM is to date well in advance of its science and evidence base, which is essentially at the beginning of its journey. This text provides a vital basis on which the science can be developed further to ensure that the Mulligan MWM approach will grow and thrive for the benefit of future patients and manual therapists. The authors are to be congratulated on the eloquent way they have brought the art and science of MWM together in this text with due scientific and clinical rigour. It will be appreciated by clinicians and researchers alike.

Gwendolen Jull MPhty, PhD, FACP
Professor of Physiotherapy
The University of Queensland
Australia

PREFACE

We aimed to make this book a comprehensive and unique exposition of the state of the scientific evidence for a relatively new form of manual therapy, Mobilisation with Movement (MWM). When Brian Mulligan first described MWM in 1984 the only evidence base was his expert opinion and a small number of his case reports. In the intervening period the empirical evidence has steadily grown to now include randomised controlled trials and systematic reviews. Moreover, the biological understanding of MWM has evolved from Mulligan's self-admitted simplistic 'positional fault hypothesis' to the testing of scientific hypotheses in sophisticated studies involving MRI and controlled laboratory conditions. It is now timely to review and present the evidence for all forms of MWM (including sustained natural apophyseal glides of the spine) from the past quarter of a century in one volume.

In addition to the science underpinning MWM, this text also describes 'the art' inherent in its successful implementation. Basic principles are outlined and more advanced aspects of its clinical application are developed and critiqued, including guidelines on dosage and troubleshooting. Most importantly, the practical art of MWM is illustrated in a series of case studies in which real life clinical presentations elucidate the clinical reasoning underlying its effective application, including consideration of the evidence base, and provide detailed descriptions of selected techniques and home exercises. These cases help bridge the divide that typically separates the science and the art of various approaches in manual therapy.

Although the primary focus of the book is MWM, much of its content is applicable to manual therapy in general. In particular, the chapters describing the current understanding of potential mechanisms of action provide a summary of the contemporary theories explaining the clinical benefits of manual therapy. Similarly, the case reports stand alone as a resource to foster the development of skills in clinical reasoning as they relate to the management of musculoskeletal disorders.

The book is essentially in five parts. The first part introduces the concept of MWM and its principles of application. Part two provides a systematic review of the evidence for its efficacy. The third part focuses on possible underlying mechanisms of action, an examination of potential sensory and motor effects, and an evaluation of Mulligan's positional fault hypothesis. Part four is comprised of twelve case reports in which the authors and other expert case contributors describe the application (with underpinning clinical reasoning) of MWM for a wide range of musculoskeletal disorders of varying complexity. The reader will get most value from these case reports if the preceding chapters have been first digested, as the cases incorporate discussion and commentary integrating the scientific evidence with the clinical guidelines in the context of the patient's unique presentation. The book concludes with the fifth part; a troubleshooting section that aims to guide practitioners in optimising their application of MWM.

This book has been written for the clinician, teacher and post-graduate student interested in furthering their understanding and skill in MWM, and indeed manual therapy more broadly. It builds on but does not replace Mulligan's texts as it is not intended to be a catalogue of techniques. We have also provided the undergraduate student with information that will benefit them in their studies of manual therapy and evidence-based management of musculoskeletal disorders.

Professor Bill Vicenzino
Brisbane, Australia, 2010
Associate Professor Wayne Hing
Auckland, New Zealand, 2010
Professor Darren Rivett
Newcastle, Australia, 2010
Dr Toby Hall
Perth, Australia, 2010

AUTHORS

Bill Vicenzino PhD, MSc, BPhty, Grad Dip Sports Phty
Professor of Sports Physiotherapy,
Head of Physiotherapy, School of Health and
Rehabilitation Sciences, University of Queensland

Wayne Hing PhD, MSc(Hons), ADP(OMT), DipMT,
DipPhys, FNZCP
Associate Professor, Head of Research,
School of Rehabilitation and Occupation Studies,
Auckland University of Technology, New Zealand

Darren Rivett PhD, MAppSc (ManipPhty),
BAppSc(Phty), Grad Dip Manip Ther
Professor of Physiotherapy, Head of School,
School of Health Sciences, Faculty of Health,
The University of Newcastle

Toby Hall PhD, MSc, Post Grad Dip Manip, FACP
Specialist Musculoskeletal Physiotherapist,
Adjunct Senior Teaching Fellow (Curtin University),
Senior Teaching Fellow, The University of Western
Australia, Director Manual Concepts

CONTRIBUTORS

Leanne Bisset PhD, MPhty (Sports Phty), MPhty
(Musculoskeletal Phty), BPhty
APA Titled Sports Physiotherapist
APA Titled Musculoskeletal Physiotherapist
Senior Lecturer, Griffith University

Stephen Edmonston PhD, A/Prof.
Director, Postgraduate Coursework Programs, School
of Physiotherapy, Curtin University of Technology

Paul Hodges PhD, MedDr (Neurosci), BPhty (Hons)
Professor and NHMRC Principal Research Fellow
Director, NHMRC Centre of Clinical Research
Excellence in Spinal Pain, Injury and Health
University of Queensland

C Hsieh MS, PT, DC, CA
Private practice, Owner of John Hsieh

M Hu
Associate Professor, School and Graduate Institute of
Physical Therapy, National Taiwan University, Taipei,
Taiwan, Republic of China

Kika Konstantinou MSc, MMACP, MCSP
Spinal Physiotherapy Specialist/Physiotherapy
Researcher, Primary Care Musculoskeletal Research
Centre, Primary Care Sciences, Keele University

Brian Mulligan FNZSP (Hon), Diploma M.T
Registered Physical Therapist
Developer of the concept of Mobilisation with
Movement

Tracey O'Brien MPhty (Sports Phty), BPhty
Former executive member SMA Qld Board of
Directors (2000–2007), Associate lecturer in
Physiotherapy at the University of Queensland

Mark Oliver MSc
Private Practitioner

Sue Reid MMedSc (Phty), Grad Dip Manip Phty,
BAppSc (Phty), BPharm
Faculty of Health Science, The University of
Newcastle, Callaghan

Kim Robinson BSc, FACP
Specialist Musculoskeletal Physiotherapist
Adjunct Senior Teaching Fellow, Curtin University
Senior Teaching Fellow, The University of Western
Australia
Director Manual Concepts

Michele Sterling PhD, MPhty, BPhty, Grad Dip
Manip Physio (distinction)
Associate Director, Centre for National Research on
Disability and Rehabilitation Medicine (CONROD)
and Director Rehabilitation Research Program
(CONROD)
Senior Lecturer, Division of Physiotherapy, School
of Health and Rehabilitation Sciences, University of
Queensland

Pam Teys MPhty (Sports Phty), BPhty, Grad Cert
Higher Ed
School of Physiotherapy, Bond University

C Yang
President, Calvin Yang MD Medical Imaging

CH Yang
Department of Physical Therapy,
Tzu-Chi University, Hualien, Taiwan, Republic of
China

REVIEWERS

Dr Nikki Petty
Principal Lecturer, Programme Leader Professional
Doctorate in Health and Social Care
Clinical Research Centre for Health Professions,
School of Health Professions
University of Brighton, UK

Dr Alison Rushton
Senior Lecturer in Physiotherapy, School of Health and
Population Sciences
College of Medical and Dental Sciences, University of
Birmingham, UK

Ken Niere
Senior Lecturer, School of Physiotherapy, LaTrobe
University, Melbourne, Australia

ACKNOWLEDGMENTS

To my wife Dorothy and children Michelle, Louise and Selina.

As testament to my father Romeo's belief in the benefits of study and also the support of Mary Vicenzino and Dorothy-May Ritchie.

Bill Vicenzino

Firstly to the centre of my world and love of my life, my little twins Matthew and Philippa. Also to my parents and family who have always been there and supported me through my journeys. Special mention to my extended friends and colleagues of the Mulligan Concept Teachers Association and in particular Brian Mulligan for your enormous contribution to my manual therapy journey. Lastly a big thanks to the numerous friends and work colleagues at AUT University and New Zealand physiotherapy fraternity who have shaped and steered my career.

Wayne Hing

To my children Cameron and Karina, and to my mentor in manual therapy and father Dr Howard Rivett.

Darren Rivett

Many people unknowingly helped steer my career, which ultimately enabled me to contribute to this book. Notable are Bob Elvey, Kim Robinson, Brian Mulligan and Kate Sheehy, but there are many others. Thanks to you all. Special thanks go to my family: my parents Christine and Douglas, wife Liz, son Sam and daughter Amy for putting up with me during the writing process. The support of all my family truly means more to me than anything else.

Toby Hall

Collectively, the authors acknowledge the valuable contributions of:

Brian Mulligan for overseeing the filming of the techniques for the DVD and for performing many of them. He continues to be an inspiration for the correct application of his MWM techniques.

Mark Oliver for performing the MWM techniques for the SIJ and TMJ, his areas of speciality.

The models who volunteered to participate in the filming for the DVD: Simon Beagley, Nadia Brandon-Black, Wolly van den Hoorn, Christopher Newman, Ben Soon and Jeffrey Szeto.

The models who volunteered to participate in the photography sessions for the figures showing MWM techniques: Hans Giebeler, Honi Mansell, Katrina Mercer and Katherine Taylor.

Assistance from the following was also greatly appreciated: Renee Bigalow, Toni Bremner, Marion Duerr, Robin Haskins and Kerry Melifont.

We are grateful for the specialist assistance provided by Dr Natalie Collins in the conduct of the systematic review and quality analyses in Chapter 3.

Mobilisation with Movement: its application

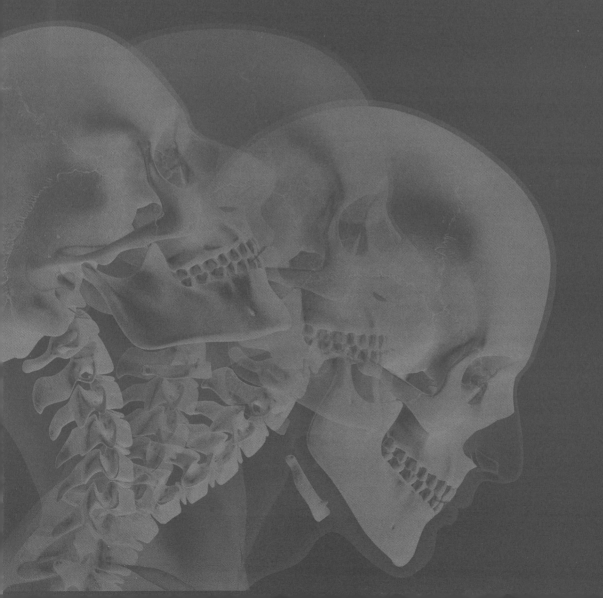

Chapter 1
Introduction

Darren Rivett, Bill Vicenzino, Wayne Hing and Toby Hall

In the history of manual therapy revolutionary changes in clinical practice have appeared from time to time. The individuals responsible for such impacting changes have each contributed innovative and original insights, and developed novel manual therapeutic approaches and techniques. Maitland, McKenzie, Kaltenborn, Paris, Jull and Elvey are just a few of the leading practitioners who, utilising their sophisticated skills in clinical observation, palpation and reasoning, opened new fields in manual therapy which effectively shifted practice paradigms and transcended professional boundaries. Indeed, their names have over time become synonymous with manual therapy itself. Almost without exception, these outliers of manual therapy exhibited self-deprecation and a continual drive to share their ideas, techniques and experiences with other practitioners. Brian Mulligan (Figure 1.1) is a recent addition to this pantheon of leading manual therapy practitioners, with his unique 'Mobilisation with Movement' (MWM) concept significantly impacting on manual therapy practice worldwide over the last two decades.

In Chapter 2 we explain in detail the nuances of MWM, however, simply, MWM can be described as a combination of a sustained passive accessory joint *mobilisation with* an active or functional *movement*. This book is a complete and comprehensive presentation and exploration of the principles of application, potential underpinning mechanisms and evidence base for Mulligan's MWM. Since the early 1990s when MWMs first come to prominence, there has been a rapid expansion in the number of techniques described which can be used for differing clinical scenarios, and a steady increase in the quantity and quality of supporting research. Indeed, from Mulligan's early descriptive case reports and videotaped patient treatments from his clinic in New Zealand, scientific investigation into MWM has progressively advanced such that we now have high quality randomised controlled trials being published in top ranked peer-reviewed international journals (see Chapter 3). Similarly, from Mulligan's relatively simple 'positional fault' hypothesis as to the possible mechanistic basis for the clinically observed effects of his techniques, there are in recent

years studies testing this hypothesis using cutting-edge imaging and other research tools. It is timely that this emerging science is linked to the clinical art of MWM; that is, the evidence for MWM should be integrated with its clinical practice.

Bogduk and Mercer[1] contend that any form of treatment can be appraised against three distinct, complementary axes of evidence: convention, biological basis and empirical proof. A substantial part of this text will be concerned with the latter two forms of evidence; that is, the biological mechanisms that may explain the effects of MWM reported by practitioners and increasingly observed in empirical quantitative trials of its efficacy. The remaining axis of convention, albeit the weakest type of evidence, is clearly supported by the widespread uptake of MWM by manual therapists, the increasing number of publications describing the techniques including entry-level professional texts (Petty, for example[2]), and the growing number of Mulligan courses run annually across 25 countries (see www.bmulligan.com for current courses), as well as the incorporation of MWM into undergraduate and postgraduate university curricula. Moreover, there is now a regular international conference on the Mulligan Concept and an international teachers' association, with a hierarchy of practitioner credentialing.

Before further discussing MWM and to truly understand the concept, it is arguably first necessary to appreciate the history of the individual who initiated and developed this original form of manual therapy, Brian Mulligan himself.

BRIAN MULLIGAN
The following historical recount is based on an interview with Brian Mulligan.

Brian Mulligan began his career as a physiotherapist after a chance conversation with a work colleague early in 1951. A friend was about to take up physiotherapy studies in Dunedin on the South Island of New Zealand, when the conversation took place. This life-changing discussion regarding physiotherapy completely changed the course of Mulligan's life and set in place a chain of events that had major implications for manual therapy.

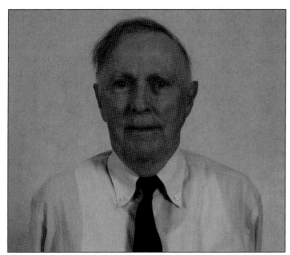

Figure 1.1 Brian Mulligan, creator of Mobilisation with Movement

Mulligan was in his early 20s in 1954 when he graduated from the Otago School of Physiotherapy in Dunedin. This was the same era that two other well known physiotherapists also graduated in Dunedin, Robin McKenzie and Stanley Paris. Mulligan's first job was at Wellington Hospital on the North Island of New Zealand, but he quickly moved out of the public hospital system into private practice. His first private practice work was a two-week private clinic locum position for Robin McKenzie. At that time there were only five private physiotherapy practices in Wellington. Mulligan enjoyed the experience immensely, and decided that this type of physiotherapy practice would be his career path in the future. Accordingly, he started his own private practice in Wellington and was very well supported by the local referring medical practitioners.

Mulligan was very active in the New Zealand Society of Physiotherapists (NZSP). He joined the NZSP after graduation, becoming the secretary of the local Wellington Branch at the end of his first year, and took on the presidency soon after. He attended as many meetings as he could in those early years to increase his clinical knowledge and to develop his skills in practice, being acutely aware of the general lack of understanding in managing patients with musculoskeletal problems at that time.

In the late 1950s, Jennifer Hickling from London gave seminars in New Zealand on Dr James Cyriax's approach to orthopaedic medicine, which included spinal manipulation (high velocity thrust) and passive joint mobilisation techniques.[3] Mulligan attended those seminars and was deeply impressed by Hickling's knowledge and expertise. Mulligan's interest in manual therapy was greatly stimulated by these seminars. About this time, Paris and McKenzie were

similarly developing their interests in manual therapy. Both Paris and McKenzie went to Europe to study with Freddy Kaltenborn and returned to New Zealand to teach this new approach in physiotherapy to Mulligan and other physiotherapists. These were exciting times for young ambitious physiotherapists, but there was still a great deal of frustration with more to be learnt about when to apply these new manual therapy techniques in clinical practice.

The significance of these developments in physiotherapy should be considered in the context of the times. The Otago school and indeed almost all undergraduate programs in physiotherapy in the 1950s did not include any form of manual therapy. Treatments largely consisted of exercise therapy and massage, as well as modalities such as ultraviolet radiation. Faradism, microwave and short-wave diathermy were also common treatments. Ultrasound was a latter addition to the therapeutic armamentarium that required a special licence in New Zealand. In those heady days, manual therapy was a very new and exciting advance in physiotherapy.

Mulligan sought to expand his knowledge in manual therapy and was keen to learn about peripheral joint mobilisation. In 1970 Mulligan was New Zealand's representative at the World Confederation for Physical Therapy (WCPT) conference. Following this he travelled to Helsinki to attend a Kaltenborn peripheral joint mobilisation course. It was the first time he had been exposed to mobilisation techniques for the extremity joints. Shortly after his return to New Zealand he was asked to teach the new skills he had learnt to the local private practitioners' group. He ran his first weekend course on Kaltenborn mobilisation techniques in 1970. Shortly afterwards, in 1972, he was asked to teach a similar course in Perth and Sydney, in Australia. Mulligan then taught regularly in Australia, especially Melbourne, where he visited for 15 consecutive years.

In 1984 Mulligan had his first MWM success, which completely changed his whole approach to manual therapy. The patient was someone he had been treating for some time but could not alter the status of their condition. The patient presented with a grossly swollen finger with painfully limited flexion and extension following a sporting injury. Mulligan used contemporary treatment techniques of the day, which included ultrasound and traction as well as medial and lateral joint glide mobilisations. Nothing appeared to significantly improve the patient's condition.

Mulligan again attempted a medial glide technique but the patient reported this as being painful. He then applied a lateral glide, which the patient stated did not hurt. In a moment of inspired lateral thinking, Mulligan asked the patient to try to flex the injured finger while he sustained the pain-free lateral glide (Figure 1.2). The technique was immediately successful and restored the full range of pain-free movement to the joint in both flexion and extension. Further repetitions rendered the patient symptom-free after only one treatment session. A telephone call several days later revealed that the pain had not returned and the swelling had completely reduced following this single application of MWM. For Mulligan, this was a Louis Pasteur moment: 'Chance favours the prepared mind'.

All MWMs that have since been developed arose from this single observation of a recalcitrant clinical problem. Mulligan thought a great deal about this patient, and soon realised the whole concept of positional faults and MWM. He was keen to apply the same idea to all his patients with finger joint problems, and then to other joints. Medial and lateral glides and rotations with movement were developed first in the fingers, shortly followed by the wrist. The concept of MWM was rapidly evolving. Sustained Natural Apophyseal Glides (SNAGs) were also being developed in the spine at the same time. Mulligan realised that the effects of MWM in the peripheral joints were similar to the effects of SNAGs in the spine. All these techniques essentially involved sustained accessory joint glides together with physiological movement. He rationalised that the techniques somehow restore a positional fault which arose from either trauma or muscle imbalance.

Momentum gathered quickly from this early inception of MWM. Mulligan was very excited by his discovery and knew he had to share it with other physiotherapists. He started to teach these new techniques at courses in New Zealand through the manual therapy special interest group of the NZSP known as the New Zealand Manipulative Therapists Association (NZMTA). At that time Mulligan was teaching a range of techniques from different concepts, including those of Geoff Maitland and Kaltenborn, but gradually his own techniques replaced these other concepts. His first Mulligan Concept course was held in 1986.

Mulligan wrote his first textbook on his concept of manual therapy in 1989.[4] Every few years a new updated version was written as more and more techniques were being developed. Currently the book is in its sixth edition[5] and has sold more than 75 000 copies worldwide. It has also been translated into 10 languages, including Mandarin, Polish, Korean, Portuguese and Spanish. A further publication followed in 2003 based on self-treatment techniques entitled *Self treatments for the back, neck and limbs*, and is currently in its second edition. Techniques from the Mulligan Concept are also now described in CDROM and DVD products (see www.bmulligan.com for a description of these products). Mulligan started to teach his new techniques in many other countries, starting with Australia and the USA. From the beginning, an important focus of these courses has been actual patient treatment demonstrations to clearly show the benefits of the concept.

In 1990 Mulligan lectured at Curtin University of Technology in Perth, Western Australia. Three UK physiotherapists, Toby Hall, Linda Exelby and Sarah Counsel were attending postgraduate courses at the university at the time and were impressed by the approach Mulligan presented. These three physiotherapists took Mulligan's techniques back to the UK and started teaching them to their colleagues. Such interest was generated that this eventually led to invitations for Mulligan to teach in the UK and Europe and to the development of the international Mulligan Concept Teachers Association (MCTA), which had its inaugural meeting in Stevenage, UK in 1998. This teaching group was set up to standardise the teaching of the Mulligan Concept around the world. There are now more than 47 members of MCTA providing courses for physiotherapists all over the world. In addition, due to the demand from clinicians in the USA, and eventually elsewhere, who wished to be acknowledged as competent Mulligan Concept practitioners, Certified

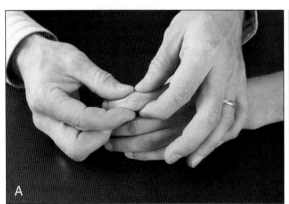 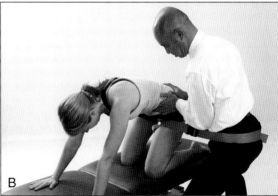

Figure 1.2 (a) Manual application of a lateral glide MWM for a loss of flexion of the proximal inter-phalangeal joint of the index finger
(b) Application of a lateral glide MWM for a loss of hip flexion using a treatment belt

Mulligan Practitioner (CMP) competency examinations were established. To date, there are over 300 clinicians worldwide who have gained this certification.

In recognition of his significant contribution to manual therapy and the physiotherapy profession, Mulligan has received a number of awards. In chronological order of presentation these include: Life Membership of the NZMTA (1988); Honorary Teaching Fellowship from Curtin University of Technology (1991); Honorary Fellowship of the NZSP (1996); Life Membership of the New Zealand College of Physiotherapy (1998); Life Membership of the NZSP (1999); Honorary Teaching Fellowship from the University of Otago (2003); WCPT Award for International Services to the Physiotherapy Profession (2007). The impact that the Mulligan Concept has had on clinical practice was highlighted when Mulligan was named one of 'The Seven Most Influential Persons in Orthopaedic Manual Therapy' as the result of a poll of members of the American Physical Therapy Association.

MOBILISATION WITH MOVEMENT

The fundamental components of the MWM techniques are still as they were when in 1984 Mulligan first observed immediate full restoration of pain-free movement after he sustained a lateral glide mobilisation to an inter-phalangeal joint and asked the patient to actively flex that joint. Furthermore, he observed that it only took one session of this first MWM to bring about long lasting changes. This was especially impressive because the finger joint had not responded to a range of contemporary physical therapies applied over several sessions. This immediate, pain-free and long lasting response has become the key principle guiding MWM application today.

MWM can be defined as the application of a sustained passive accessory force to a joint while the patient actively performs a task that was previously identified as being problematic. A critical aspect of MWM is the identification of a task that the patient has difficulty completing, usually due to pain or joint stiffness (see Chapter 2 for more detail). This task is most frequently a movement or a muscle contraction performed to the onset of pain, or to the end of available range of motion (ROM) or maximum muscle contraction. In this text, we will refer to this as the Client Specific Impairment Measure (CSIM, see Chapter 2 for more detailed description). The passive accessory force usually exerts a translatory or rotatory glide at the joint and as such must be applied close to the joint line to avoid undesirable movements. It may be applied manually or sometimes via a treatment belt (Figure 1.2b).

The direction of the accessory movement that is used is the one that effects the greatest improvement in the CSIM. It is somewhat surprising that a lateral glide is the most commonly cited successful technique used in peripheral joints, but if this direction is not effective then other directions may be tested. Alternate glides may follow the convex–concave rule of joints[6] but in some cases in the opposite direction to the mechanism of injury movement. Sometimes a little trial and error is needed to find the right direction. One distinction with SNAGs, which are effectively the 'MWM of the spine', is that the gliding motion is always in the direction of the facet joint plane. Mulligan generally recommends three sets of 10 repetitions of MWM, or fewer if the impaired task is pain-free on reassessment following the application of a set of MWM or if irritability or acuteness is a factor in the spine when using SNAGs. There are many nuances to the successful application of MWM and these are covered in depth in Chapter 2.

MWM can be easily integrated into the standard manual therapy physical examination to evaluate its potential as an intervention. A seamless integration can be undertaken after examining the active/functional movements, static muscles tests in some cases, and passive accessory movements. They can be readily trialled and implemented in the treatment. Reassessment is generally just a matter of the practitioner taking their hands off the patient and asking them to move (without having to change position), and frequently the treatment and its reassessment can be applied in weight-bearing positions for lower limb and lumbo–pelvic problems. Mulligan recommends discarding the technique immediately if no positive change is evident on initial reassessment.[7]

The indications for MWM in both the physical examination and for treatment are essentially the same as for other 'hands-on' manual therapy approaches, as are the contraindications. This is discussed more comprehensively in Chapter 2. Generally, mobilisation techniques, including MWM have been conceptualised as being indicated for mechanically induced joint pain and joint stiffness limiting ROM. However, MWM has also been proposed by Mulligan to effect what appear to be soft tissue conditions, such as lateral epicondylalgia of the elbow and lateral ankle ligament sprain, and indeed there is growing evidence to support his assertion (see Chapter 3). The various potential mechanisms by which MWM may exert its effects are considered in Chapters 4, 5, 6 and 7.

While innovative and original in nature, the MWM concept has parallels to other 'traditional' mainstream approaches to manual therapy that would facilitate ready adoption by the experienced manual therapist. For example, the consideration of joint mechanics in some MWM techniques is akin to the approach advocated by Kaltenborn,[6] and the strong emphasis on self-management using repeated movements would be familiar to McKenzie practitioners.[8] This is not surprising given that Mulligan was heavily influenced early in his career by both these practitioners through direct mentoring. In common with both the Maitland[9] and McKenzie approaches a change in pain response is used as an indication that the correct technique is being applied, although rather than provoking or localising pain the aim of MWM is its immediate and total elimination. In contrast, there are no 'grades' of mobilisation in MWM as there are in the Maitland approach and some other approaches,[10] and MWM combines both passive and active elements rather than just focusing on one (e.g. passive joint movement as per Kaltenborn) or the other. In regard to the latter, there is some similarity to the combined movement approach described by Brian Edwards[11] in which pain-free joint positioning is used to enable end-range passive mobilisation. The other interesting parallel is the story about how Mulligan 'discovered' MWM, not dissimilar to the account given by McKenzie as to how he chanced upon the therapeutic value of lumbar spine extension for low back pain.[8] These outliers of the manual therapy world appear to share an ability to creatively clinically reason or think outside the box.

MWM AND CLINICAL REASONING

Some approaches to manual therapy have been criticised for fostering 'recipe book' clinical practice. That is, rather than promoting skilled clinical reasoning in autonomous practitioners, some approaches could be considered to relegate the role of the manual therapist to that of a technician, required simply to deliver a predetermined course of therapeutic action. A cursory view of the MWM concept might similarly suggest it simply requires the clinician to routinely follow several basic rules (e.g. the treatment plane rule, convex–concave rule) and therefore is at odds with the development of skilled clinical reasoning. However, on closer inspection it is clear that MWM actually incorporates many of the desirable aspects of contemporary, exemplary clinical reasoning. In particular, these relate to a patient-centred approach to healthcare and promotion of the ongoing development of the practitioner's clinical skills.

MWM promotes patient-centred reasoning

Jones and Rivett[12] have advanced a model of clinical reasoning in manual therapy that places the patient firmly at the centre of the clinical encounter and the associated clinical reasoning processes. Their model is consistent with the patient-centred approach to evidence-based medicine advocated by Sackett et al.[13, 14] Evidence-based medicine has been defined by Sackett et al (p.71)[14] as 'the conscientious, explicit, and judicious use of current best evidence in making decisions about the care of individual patients'. These authors further stress that evidence-based medicine is an integration of the practitioner's clinical expertise with both the best external clinical research evidence and the patient's preferences in making decisions about their care. While for treatment the 'gold standard' for evidence is the randomised clinical trial or a

systematic review of such trials, where this is limited or not available we must use the next best external evidence (see Chapter 3, Table 3.1 for the various levels of evidence), whether it be a case report or from the basic sciences. We therefore prefer the term 'evidence-informed practice', and particularly use this in the case studies which comprise the latter part of the text, as the cases strive to illustrate how expert clinicians apply the external research evidence for MWM within a clinical reasoning framework and without losing the uniqueness and individuality of the patient. The patient is considered an active and equal partner in the clinical problem-solving exercise, as they bring their own beliefs, understandings, expectations and experiences to the unfolding clinical journey. In addition, consistent with the biopsychosocial model of healthcare, the patient is required to actively engage in their treatment and management, as opposed to just passively receiving the 'laying on of hands' implicit in many traditional manual therapy approaches.

The MWM concept arguably promotes patient-centred clinical reasoning in several ways:

- Collaborative clinical reasoning in treatment, as promulgated by Jones and Rivett[12] is central to MWM. First, the patient needs to understand that the technique is completely pain-free and that they must report any pain immediately to the therapist. Second, in most MWM applications, the patient is required to perform an active movement or functional task that is problematic and for which treatment was sought (e.g. a painful or limited movement). Third, many MWM techniques involve the patient applying overpressure at the end of range, and indeed Mulligan[7] considers this component critical in effecting an optimal response. Finally, and perhaps most importantly in this context, some MWMs can be adapted for home exercise as self-MWMs or by using tape to simulate the accessory movement (or mobilisation) component of the technique. Of course, all of the above elements of MWM necessitate that the patient understands the principles of MWM and is willing to actively participate in their own management; thereby rendering the patient a central and necessary factor in successful MWM treatment. The importance of collaboration and patient cooperation to the success of MWM is highlighted in an acronym favoured by Mulligan (personal communication, 2009) in his teaching – **CROCKS**:
  - **C**ontraindications to manual therapy as for any manual therapy techniques
  - **R**epetitions of the technique are required, but with care on initial application and in acute injuries for which three to six repetitions are recommended
  - **O**verpressure to ensure optimal ongoing improvements
  - **C**ommunication and **c**ooperation is essential for safe and effective MWM application with

practitioners informing patients of expected effects and for patients informing practitioners of any discomfort or pain

- **K**nowledge of musculoskeletal medicine, biomechanics and anatomy
- **S**ustain the glide for the entire duration of the repetition. S also stands for **s**kill in the manual handling of the physical application of the MWM, **s**ensibility of the sensing fingertips to accurately locate MWM forces and to detect movement, **s**ubtle changes in glide direction are often required, and common **s**ense.

- The practitioner can facilitate patient compliance with treatment, especially the self-management component, by demonstrating to the patient that application of MWM can produce an immediate pain-free response in their 'worst' movement or activity. Moreover, such a powerful response has significant potential to change any negative beliefs or expectations that the patient may have brought to the clinical encounter. Another of the acronyms that Mulligan (personal communication, 2009) uses when teaching MWM is **PILL**, indicating the desired response from the technique's application:
  - **P**ain-free application of the mobilisation and movement components
  - **I**nstant result at the time of application
  - **L**ong **L**asting effects beyond the technique's application.

- Effective communication is pivotal to the effective application of MWM. The patient must immediately communicate the onset of any pain with either the 'Mobilisation' or the 'Movement' component, or else the technique will be rendered ineffectual. Similarly, the therapist must clearly communicate what is expected of the patient, as outlined in the previous point. Effective communication is also unambiguously the foundation of effective collaborative clinical reasoning.

- Central to the MWM concept is that each patient is an individual and their clinical presentation is unique, although they may share some common features with others. This consideration of individuality and uniqueness is consistent with the 'mature organism model'[15] which proposes that each patient's illness or pain experience is influenced by their own life experiences and immediate contextual circumstances, and therefore their clinical presentation cannot be exactly the same as that of another patient. The 'Movement' component of MWM requires that a movement or functional activity be identified that is most painful or limited for that individual, and which has a significant impact on their daily life. This movement is also used in reassessment as a 'comparable sign' (i.e. a clinical sign that relates to their functional limitation and pain) as described by Maitland et al.[9] Similarly, the use of a CSIM in

relation to MWM recognises the unique clinical presentation of the individual patient.

- Arguably, MWM provides a means by which various types of clinical reasoning hypotheses[12] can be tested, aside from the obvious one of management and treatment. Most notably, the degree of response to MWM can potentially expedite and refine the clinical prognosis.

MWM promotes knowledge organisation

A well-organised knowledge base has been identified as one of the hallmarks of clinical expertise. It is not just the degree of knowledge in its three main types — propositional (essentially basic and applied science), non-propositional (including practical and other professional skills) and personal (an individual's life experiences) — that is important in clinical reasoning, but how these understandings and skills are stored and held together using clinical patterns.[12] A well-organised knowledge base will facilitate the application of advanced clinical reasoning processes, particularly that of pattern recognition which has been shown to be more accurate than hypothetico–deductive processes in manual therapy diagnosis and is typically used by experts.[16]

It can be argued that the MWM concept promotes knowledge organisation by:

- Stimulating research and a growing evidence base which can be used to help guide and inform clinical reasoning. As later chapters demonstrate, there is a burgeoning evidence base, both biological and empirical for MWM.
- Highlighting and integrating key physical examination findings, most notably passive accessory movement findings (the 'Mobilisation') with the 'comparable' active/functional movement findings (the 'Movement').
- Facilitating clinical pattern acquisition through the immediate response to the application of MWM. Effectively this constitutes feedback to the therapist on the accuracy of the related clinical decision(s) and helps to reinforce the association of key clinical findings with correct clinical actions.
- Fostering the development of metacognitive skills through the need to continually adapt the application of MWM on the basis of the patient's initial and changing responses. Metacognitive skills are higher order thinking skills of self-monitoring and reflective appraisal of one's own reasoning, and are a well-recognised characteristic of clinical expertise.[12]

While the Mulligan Concept as it relates to MWM may promote the development of skills in clinical reasoning, there is a risk that an unquestioning inflexibility of thinking may set in if vigilance is not maintained. The writings of Mulligan should be used as a guide to the application of MWM with the techniques adapted for the needs of a particular patient, and not treated as gospel from which heated debates arise over differing interpretations and trivial technical issues. The history of manual therapy is replete with examples where a far-sighted pioneer has been feted like a guru by his followers, who with the fervour of religious zealots then proceed to construct a framework that stifles creativity and the further evolution of the protagonist's approach,[17] and which misdirects future practitioners and advocates of the approach away from the originator's fundamental underpinning concepts.

AIMS AND STRUCTURE OF THIS BOOK

The primary aim of this book is to present a comprehensive and contemporary discourse on Mulligan's MWM management approach for musculoskeletal pain, injury and disability. In particular, it strives to integrate the evidence base for MWM into clinical practice, with an emphasis on explicating the underpinning clinical reasoning.

This book will cover the spectrum of the MWM treatment approach from: (a) the evidence base for its clinical efficacy, clinical and laboratory based effects, and underlying mechanisms; (b) best evidence guidelines for MWM treatment selection and application; and (c) the current state of play with regard to Mulligan's 'positional fault' hypothesis, as well as other impairments/deficits in the pain, sensory, sensorimotor and motor systems that may well be plausibly addressed by the MWM approach; through to (d) a series of case studies (Chapters 8 to 19) that demonstrate how the former considerations can be utilised in the clinical reasoning process. The latter will also demonstrate the framework within which the practitioner is able to design and implement customised MWM techniques for the individual patient, as illustrated by some prominent Mulligan Concept practitioners. By presenting these cases within a clinical reasoning framework it is further intended to demonstrate that the use of MWM is very much dependent on the individual patient's presentation and requires a sophisticated level of thinking by the practitioner. These are not 'recipe book' treatments. Key MWM techniques, particularly those for which evidence is supportive, will be described in detail and depicted. In the event that a practitioner confronts issues in putting into practice the MWM techniques, we have included a technique troubleshooting section (Chapter 20), which is geared towards practitioners self-reflecting and appraising their performances in order to develop strategies and solutions to these issues.

This book will be of benefit for students of manual therapy and for the various health professionals working clinically in this field, and it should provide a valuable resource for instructors and researchers. It is not intended to replace the technical books of Mulligan, but rather is complementary. To make the most of this book, the reader should strive to first understand the principles and evidence underpinning MWM, and to do so with an open but healthily sceptical mind. The case studies comprising the bulk of the chapters will provide the novice reader with the confidence to take the concept of MWM into their clinic, and the experienced clinician with the opportunity to develop their clinical reasoning skill by comparing their reasoning to that of other Mulligan Concept practitioners.

References

1 Bogduk N, Mercer S. Selection and application of treatment. In: Refshauge KM, Gass EM (eds) Musculoskeletal Physiotherapy: Clinical Science and Evidence-Based Practice. Oxford: Butterworth-Heinemann 1995.

2 Petty N. Neuromusculoskeletal Examination and Assessment. Edinburgh: Churchill Livingstone 2005.

3 Cyriax J. Cyriax's Illustrated Manual of Orthopaedic Medicine (2nd edn). Oxford: Butterworth-Heinemann 1993.

4 Mulligan B. Manual Therapy — 'NAGS', 'SNAGS', 'PRPS' etc. Wellington: Plane View Services 1989.

5 Mulligan B. Manual Therapy - 'NAGS', 'SNAGS', 'MWMS' etc. (6th edn). Wellington: Plane View Services 2010.

6 Kaltenborn F. Manual Mobilisation of the Extremity Joints. Basic Examination and Treatment Techniques. Norway: Olaf Norlis Bokhandel 1989.

7 Mulligan B. Manual Therapy - 'NAGS', 'SNAGS', 'MWMS' etc. (5th edn). Wellington: Plane View Services 2003.

8 McKenzie R, May S. The Lumbar Spine Mechanical Diagnosis and Therapy (2nd edn). New Zealand: Spinal Publications 2003.

9 Maitland GD, Hengeveld E, Banks K, English K. Maitland's Vertebral Manipulation (6th edn). Oxford: Butterworth-Heinemann 2001.

10 Boyling J, Jull G. Grieve's Modern Manual Therapy: The Vertebral Column (3rd edn). Edinburgh: Churchill Livingstone 2004.

11 Edwards B. Manual of Combined Movements: Their Use in the Examination and Treatment of Mechanical Vertebral Column Disorders. Edinburgh: Churchill Livingstone 1992.

12 Jones M, Rivett D. Introduction to clinical reasoning. In: Jones M, Rivett D (eds) Clinical Reasoning for Manual Therapists. Edinburgh: Butterworth-Heinemann 2004:3–24.

13 Sackett D, Straus S, Richardson W, Rosenberg W, Haynes R. Evidence-based Medicine: How to Practice and Teach EBM (2nd edn). Edinburgh: Churchill Livingstone 2000.

14 Sackett DL, Rosenberg WM, Gray JA, Haynes RB, Richardson WS. Evidence-based Medicine: What it is and what it isn't. BMJ. 1996;312:71–2.

15 Gifford L. Pain, the tissues and the nervous system: a conceptual model. Physiotherapy 1998;84:27–36.

16 Miller P. Pattern Recognition is a Clinical Reasoning Process in Musculoskeletal Physiotherapy (Masters Thesis). Newcastle: The University of Newcastle, Australia 2009.

17 Rivett D. Manual therapy cults (editorial). Manual Therapy 1999;4:125–6.

Chapter 2
Mobilisation with Movement: the art and science of its application

Bill Vicenzino, Wayne Hing, Toby Hall and Darren Rivett

In this chapter we set out to define and operationally describe Mobilisation with Movement (MWM) technique in terms of its parameters and how these may be manipulated in order to achieve clinically beneficial outcomes.

MWM is essentially the application of a specific vector of force to a joint (mobilisation or the first 'M' in MWM), which is sustained while the client performs a previously impaired physical task. The key to successful use of MWM is the skilful and efficient application of this mobilisation force so as to painlessly achieve immediate and long lasting relief of pain.[1] We propose that the mobilisation element of MWM can be adequately described through the parameters of amount, direction and volume of applied force, as well as the location and mode of application of the force. The knowledgeable, judicious and skilful manipulation of these parameters provides the practitioner with the capability whereby to optimise the opportunity for success with MWM.

Notwithstanding the importance of understanding these mobilisation parameters, it is critical to realise that the key feature of a MWM application is the movement or the second 'M' in MWM. We have called this the Client Specific Impairment Measure (CSIM). Specifically, the key to understanding how to apply MWM successfully is in understanding the role of the CSIM in guiding the practitioner on a range of treatment selection issues; for example, in determining the optimum force parameters. Before detailing the mobilisation force parameters of MWM, this chapter will first define in detail the movement element of MWM and along with other chapters demonstrate that it is arguably the most critical element.

This chapter is set out in two parts: the first part is about the CSIM or movement element of MWM whereas the second part is about the mobilisation element of MWM.

PART 1 CSIM: THE MOVEMENT ELEMENT OF MWM

A MWM can only be applied if there is a meaningful clinical measure of the physical task with which the client is having problems. The measure needs to be client-centred and meaningful to the individual client, so consequently we have termed it the Client Specific Impairment Measure (CSIM). To reiterate this point in a slightly different manner, establishing the CSIM is the first criterion that needs to be met. If a CSIM cannot be found then a MWM cannot be used.

The patient's problem

The CSIM is a physical task or functional activity that the practitioner is able to evaluate and that is comparable to the patient's presenting problem, which in many ways is similar to Maitland's[2] comparable sign. That is, the key element of a CSIM is that it needs to reflect the patient's main concern(s). The CSIM assessed in the clinic may be the task itself; for example, placing the hand behind the back to tuck a shirt in for a shoulder problem or walking down a step for a knee problem. That is, a physical activity or task that is easily reproducible in the clinic is likely to be directly incorporated in a MWM, whereas the one that is not readily reproducible in the clinic will need to be approached in a slightly different way. To illustrate this, consider an example of a male patient who indicates that his main problem is throwing a ball. Clearly it is difficult to do a manual therapy technique on a shoulder while the patient is throwing a ball, so in this case the practitioner would conduct a physical examination to find physical signs of impairments that are reproducible in the clinic and for which it is conceivable to apply a MWM. In this example, this may well be shoulder rotation at 90° of elevation in the scapula plane. That is, the more complex or demanding tasks may need to be broken down into some of their critical constituent parts in the clinical context.

In some cases, the CSIM may be a task that is reproducible in the clinic but is not readily amenable to the application of a MWM. For example, a patient may have a severe pain problem with deep squatting or walking down stairs. In this case it may not be desirable to reproduce the deep squat or down stairs walking too many times, so alternatively, the practitioner can break down these tasks into less stressful and presumably with less painful component parts. So in the case of a deep squat perhaps non-weight-bearing knee flexion is limited and less painful than weight-bearing, which could be a starting point for the treatment. If non-weight-bearing knee flexion is only mildly painful, then perhaps 4-point kneeling or partial weight-bearing with a foot up on a step or small stool would be a reasonable and appropriate starting point. In summary, selection of a CSIM, while reflecting the patient's main problem, should also allow a safe MWM to be applied without risk of exacerbating a severe pain problem in fully loaded joints.

To arrive at an appropriate CSIM, the practitioner first identifies, through the interview, a comparable sign or physical task/activity that is problematic (usually painful) to the patient. In doing so, the practitioner should make sure to document the extent to which the physical task interferes with the patient's day-to-day function, as well as the severity and irritability of the condition.[2] Then in the physical examination the practitioner will quantify the CSIM. This quantification will be somewhat variable depending on the presenting problem; that is, it will be different for a painful condition versus a stiffness or weakness problem.

Quantifying the CSIM in painful conditions

In the case of someone presenting with pain as the problem it is essential that the endpoint of the CSIM is the onset of pain (otherwise called a pain threshold endpoint). That is, the physical task, which could be either a movement or muscle contraction, is ceased at the onset of the pain (Table 2.1). It follows that the quantification of the CSIM is the amount of physical activity/task that is possible leading to the onset of pain and not the amount/severity of pain elicited. For example, in the event that the physical problem is a painful movement, the patient would indicate when they first feel pain during the movement and this could be measured with a goniometer, inclinometer, tape measure or some other reference point (e.g. a point on the wall). In the event that a painful muscle contraction is the CSIM, it can be measured with a dynamometer, so that the amount of force generated that leads to the first perception of pain is used to quantify the patient's problem (e.g. grip testing in tennis elbow as illustrated in the case study described in Chapter 13). All these measurements are standard and routine in musculoskeletal healthcare practice.

Using the pain onset as the endpoint of the test (pain threshold) works best in non-irritable presentations and is critical in minimising exacerbation of pain or 'treatment soreness' after the session. It should be used with great care in irritable presentations for which it becomes more important to allow time after performance of the CSIM in order to assess for any latent exacerbation of pain.

CSIM quantification where pain is at end of range or at full strength contraction

The only case in which the foregoing guide may not apply and where pain is the presenting problem is when a patient demonstrates full range of motion (ROM) or

Table 2.1 Defining impairments in terms of endpoint, how measured and target(s) for MWM

Impairment	Endpoint	Measurement or quantity	MWM target(s)
Pain-limited motion[1]	Pain onset	Degrees of motion[2]	Motion (not pain)
Painful arc	Pain onset and offset[3]	Degrees of motion	Arc of motion and motion at onset (not pain)
Pain at full end of range	End of normal range of motion	Pain (NRS or VAS)[4]	Pain (not range of motion)
Limited range of motion with no pain[5]	Range of motion	Degrees of motion	Motion
Force generation less than normal due to pain	Pain onset	Force output	Force generation[6] not pain
Painful contraction without strength deficit	Normal force output	Pain (NRS or VAS)	Pain not force generation
Weakness without pain	Force output	Force output	Force generation

1 The motion could be of joints, muscle or nerve. This applies for all motion functions in this table.
2 In some instances it may not be degrees, but rather a linear distance achieved (e.g. hand behind back using millimetres along the back, bending forward using linear measurement of reach with fingers to the floor).
3 The pain experienced at pain onset should not increase with further movement so as to prevent further movement.
4 VAS (visual analogue scale), NRS (numerical rating scale).
5 This may also include perceptions of stretch and discomfort that the patient does not describe as being painful per se.
6 In order to have a reproducible measure, the force generation is usually isometric, but this only refers to when pain is involved and when pain is the endpoint.

normal muscle strength (usually compared to the other side) at pain onset. In such cases the CSIM can only be measured by the level/severity of pain elicited as measured on a pain visual analogue scale (VAS) or numerical rating scale (NRS) (Table 2.1).

CSIM quantification where pain is not the problem (e.g. weakness, stiffness)

The preceding refers to a patient who has pain on physical activity where pain exacerbation following a provocative treatment session may be a substantial disincentive to continue with the treatment plan. However, those who are seeking help for a limitation in the performance of a task where there is no pain — for example, the person presenting with tight muscles, stiff joint, or muscle weakness — can be managed with reference to discomfort and gains in ROM or muscle force generated. The traction straight leg raise and ankle dorsiflexion MWMs (see Chapter 5, Figure 5.3) are examples of techniques that have been reported to improve ROM where pain is not the main problem.[3, 4]

How to use a CSIM when applying MWM

The critical aspect of a CSIM is that it will guide the MWM application not only immediately during the application of the MWM, but also it will guide modifications of MWM on subsequent applications of a course of treatment. That is, it will be used to judge the effectiveness of the applied MWM within a session and between sessions of a course of treatment. The way in which the CSIM guides the application of a MWM will differ slightly in its implementation when the condition is a predominantly painful condition than when the condition is primarily one of stiffness (or weakness), for example.

This section will outline the use of the CSIM in different generic patient presentations, such as, when a patient presents with a painful condition limiting motion or muscle contraction, or where the patient presents with pain at end of range or full force muscle contraction where it is not the limiting factor, as well as briefly in cases where pain is not present or minimally present, such as in a stiff limited joint.

When the MWM is being used in a painful condition

In terms of the CSIM, the pain-free and immediate effect that is required for an effective MWM is interpreted through a substantial and instantaneous improvement in the quantity being measured at the point of pain onset (Table 2.1). For example, if the ROM was 60° to pain onset out of a possible 160° motion at a joint, then an improvement from 60° to

120° (100%) before pain onset could be viewed as a substantial improvement. Improvements in the order of 50–100% are often cited as targets to be reached in this regard (e.g. McConnell's glide and tilt taping of the patellofemoral joint, which is very much akin to a MWM should improve the patient's pain by 50%[5]), but no hard supportive evidence for MWM exists. Suffice to say that the larger the initial effect, logically the greater the likelihood of success in managing the case with MWM and that pursuing the use of a MWM in a treatment program is a valid course of action. Interestingly, others have shown between session changes are predicted from within session changes.[6, 7] For example, Tuttle[7] showed that for cervical spine manipulation the within session gains in ROM, pain intensity and pain centralisation were highly predictive of between session changes in these measures, of the order of 71–83% predictive. This may be regarded as lending support to the notion of using a CSIM as a guide to clinical decisions on selection of a MWM, or other manual therapy treatment.

It is important to understand the concept of a ceiling effect in determining how much of an improvement is sufficiently substantial. For example, if the ROM deficit between sides is in the order of 10% (or 16° in the case in the previous paragraph) then regaining that small amount of range in a pain-free manner is also a substantial effect. Thus the presenting condition and the associated potential available improvement also impacts on what is deemed to be substantial.

Vicenzino and Wright[8] showed a desired response profile during a MWM application in a case study (Figure 2.1). The patient was a 39-year-old female with chronic tennis elbow who had failed to respond to typical treatment (deep tissue massage, transverse friction massage, electrotherapy). Application of a lateral glide MWM for tennis elbow produced substantial changes in pain-free grip force during its application in the order of 3–4 times baseline measurement (Figure 2.1 (i)). That is, while the practitioner is actually applying the MWM there should be a substantial change from the baseline CSIM measurement. The improvement in the CSIM immediately following the MWM application should also be substantial relative to the pre-treatment measurement of the CSIM, as represented at (ii) in Figure 2.1.

The foregoing has dealt with the CSIM during and immediately after the application of the MWM. There is preliminary evidence that the CSIM may also prove to be useful in predicting the success or otherwise of a course of MWM treatment before it is even applied. There is only one study that we are aware of that addresses the issue of predictors of success with MWM. In this recent study, a preliminary clinical prediction rule (CPR) was developed from a post-hoc analysis of 64 patients with tennis elbow who were treated with an average of five sessions of MWM

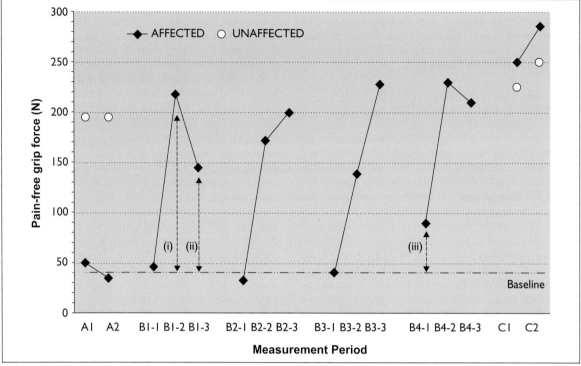

Figure 2.1 Pain-free grip force measurements taken at 8 sessions divided into baseline phase (A) treatment phase (B) and post-treatment phase (C)

The circles represent the unaffected side and the diamonds the affected side. On the affected side, the triplicate measurements in each treatment phase (B1 to B4) represent pre- (-1), during (-2) and post-MWM (-3) measurements. Key points of interest are the grip force during MWM application (i) and post-application (ii), both compared to pre-application for that same session, as well as the pre-application grip force in subsequent sessions (iii) compared to baseline (A and B1-1). In this figure, B4-1 is the first session at which the pre-MWM grip force is substantially higher than the baseline (iii), which we propose is a sign of an adequate volume of MWM being applied by the practitioner and patient, taping and exercise. Figure adapted with permission from Vicenzino & Wright 1995.[8]

and exercise over 3 weeks.[9] One of the univariate predictor variables identified in this analysis was a >25% improvement in pain-free grip force (CSIM) during the application of an elbow lateral glide MWM compared to pre-MWM application. However, this was not retained in the final multivariate CPR model, and it only represented a small effect size (positive likelihood ratio [LR] of 1.5 [95% CI 0.78 to 2.9]), which translates to a small increase in probability of improvement from 79% to 85%.

Interestingly, in the final CPR model, the pre-treatment CSIM (pain-free grip force) was a major determinant of improvement in tennis elbow at 3 weeks. That is, the probability of improvement with this treatment improved to 93% (LR 3.7 [95% CI 1.0 to 13.6]) when two of the following were present in a patient: (a) a high pain-free grip force on the affected side (>112N); (b) a low pain-free grip force on the unaffected side (<336N); and (c) being younger than 49 years.[9] These preliminary findings need to be further explored both clinically and through research. Nevertheless, the results do provide some support for the role of a CSIM

(and possibly the change in CSIM) in an initial MWM application in increasing the confidence with which a practitioner can choose an effective MWM treatment.

An important aspect of MWM is the application of overpressure to the CSIM at the endpoint of the movement, but only if pain-free. This overpressure has been strongly emphasised by Mulligan[1] and is regarded as necessary in order to optimise the effectiveness of the treatment. Either the patient or the therapist can apply overpressure. Certain techniques require the patient to apply the overpressure because the practitioner has both hands otherwise engaged in the MWM. In these circumstances the patient needs to have the process explained to them prior to the application of the MWM and have the capacity to understand and perform the overpressure. Additionally, specific techniques that have an active weight-bearing (e.g. see Chapter 16) or include a gravitational effect (e.g. see Chapter 15), thus effectively an overpressure component, require no manual application of overpressure and are often valuable techniques for a patient to perform as a self-MWM.

In overview, a fundamental rule of MWM for painful conditions is that there needs to be a substantial positive change in the CSIM in terms of an increased ROM or muscle force production to the onset of pain (Table 2.1) at the time of its application and immediately afterwards. The important matter in this regard is the quantity of either the ROM or force production obtained at the first perception of pain on the CSIM.

For the MWM where there is pain at end of range or on full strength contraction

Instead of quantifying the ROM or force generated, in this situation the patient reports their perception of pain using VAS or NRS and the MWM should substantially reduce the pain to no pain or very little pain for it to be of any use in treatment (Table 2.1).

When the MWM is being used in cases where pain is not the problem

The CSIM would be used in much the same way as for when pain is present, but the endpoint of the CSIM is a quantity such as ROM or force generated (Table 2.1).

Summary of Part 1

The CSIM is fundamentally the most critical element of the MWM because it connects the treatment effect to the patient's specific problem. In doing so, it guides the application of the MWM in terms of the practitioner's selection, modification and progression of the various parameters of a technique. In this regard it is vitally important that the practitioner understands the concept of a CSIM and its endpoint for different clinical presentations (e.g. pain-limited function). The following part of this chapter focuses on the applied force or the mobilisation element of MWM.

PART 2: THE MOBILISATION ELEMENT OF MWM

The parameters of the applied force vector, which is the mobilisation element of MWM, will be discussed herein under the separate categories of the direction of force application, the amount of force being applied, the possible interrelationship between direction and amount of force, the locality of the force application, the manner in which the force is applied (e.g. manually, tape, treatment belt) and the overall volume. The overall volume is the sum total of all repetitions of the MWM applied by the practitioner and patient. We propose that manipulation of the mobilisation force parameters, such as the amount, direction and locality of the applied force, impacts directly on the immediacy of effect. Whereas varying the volume is considered to have more to do with

the sustainability of the effect over time. These factors can be considered the input parameters/variables of the mobilisation (or first 'M') part of the MWM (Figure 2.2).

There are two reference points for these parameters (Figure 2.2). One is in reference to the description of the input parameters, such as the amount (N) and direction (degrees) of force. The other reference point is the CSIM and in particular how the parameters impact on the CSIM, which is ascertained through changes in output. The interrelationship between these two reference points is highlighted in a proposed algorithm outlined in Figure 2.3.

Direction of force application

The direction of force application is predicated on the best possible outcome of the CSIM at the time of application and initially afterwards, within that treatment session. The direction of force application refers to the direction of the accessory or passive physiological motion that the practitioner is seeking to exert at the joint. For example, accessory motions may encompass medial, lateral, anterior and posterior translations, traction and rotational joint forces, with the latter constituting physiological motions at some joints. It is uncommon that flexion/extension or abduction/adduction will be used as the mobilisation force. Any of these passively applied forces will be sustained while the patient undergoes a CSIM. It is interesting to note that of all the 25 MWM techniques for peripheral joints specifically described by Mulligan in his book (fourth edition), the lateral glide is mentioned 11 times (44% of all mobilisations described) and appears to be the most favoured direction of choice. Transverse plane glides (56%) are more commonly recommended than glides in the sagittal plane (28%), which seems to be a characteristic feature of MWM that somewhat differentiates it from other manual therapy approaches. While this should only be seen as a record of Mulligan's clinical observations over the course of his practice, it still provides novice practitioners with an expert opinion (from the innovator of the techniques) regarding a starting point to their applications of MWM in individual patients, especially since there appear to be no other scientifically based guidelines for the direction of force application in MWM.

Apart from the recommended direction of force application for a particular MWM described by Mulligan, the practitioner may also employ some other basic guidelines to select the initial mobilisation to use when first applying a MWM, such as the concave–convex rule[10] or simply opposing the direction of the mechanism of injury. In applying any joint glide the practitioner should also be aware of the concept of the 'treatment plane', which is defined as the plane that lies perpendicular to a line drawn

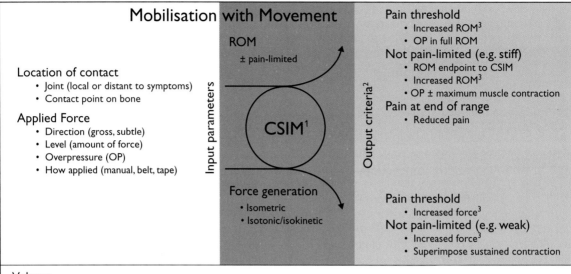

Figure 2.2 Overview of a schematic definition of MWM in which the central feature is the CSIM or the 'movement' element of MWM and its output criteria (right column)
The input parameters of the 'mobilisation' element of MWM are listed in the left column. Pain threshold refers to measuring some quantity of the task other than pain, such as ROM or force generated when the patient first feels the onset of pain. That is, pain is not the variable, but rather the ROM or force generation are the key output criteria. Where pain is not the main limiting feature of the patient's problem then measures of pain, ROM, and force generated become the possible output criteria. From these criteria, decisions can be made to modulate the input parameters (location and force in the left column, and volume in the middle row above footnotes) of the mobilisation (first 'M' in MWM). Implicit in this flow chart is the iterative nature of MWM applications.

from the axis of rotation of the convex member to the centre of the concave member of a joint.[11] An example of the treatment plane is shown in Figure 2.4. It is believed that to be effective, all MWM will be either applied parallel or perpendicular to this treatment plane.

There are two important aspects to the direction of force application: the gross (in foregoing paragraphs) and the subtle. For example, visualise that a practitioner has applied a lateral glide of the tibiofemoral joint in order to improve a pain-limited squat (limited to one-third squat). On first performing the glide the patient is able to go somewhat further but not by any substantial amount (e.g. one-third squat pre-MWM to half squat with the MWM applied). In order to seek a larger effect, the practitioner may wish to modify the glide direction to attain a better outcome, which may be achieved by fine-tuning the inclination of the lateral glide so that it is now slightly posteriorly inclined (~10° posterior to the frontal plane; see Figure 2.4(b) to visualise this, for an example). If this was a successful refinement the squat would then be substantially improved and the patient may be able to fully squat with the application of the MWM. However, if there was no change on initial application of the lateral glide then the practitioner should consider changing the gross direction of the force (e.g. perform a medial or posterior glide, or medial rotation), which would also be the case if the subtle changes in direction were ineffective.

As MWM is a reasonably recent innovation there are limited detailed data in the literature regarding the

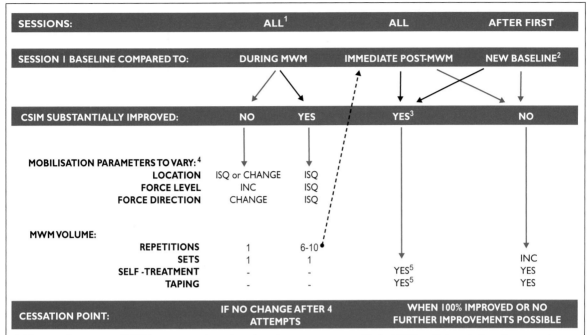

SESSIONS:	ALL[1]		ALL	AFTER FIRST
SESSION I BASELINE COMPARED TO:	**DURING MWM**		**IMMEDIATE POST-MWM**	**NEW BASELINE**[2]
CSIM SUBSTANTIALLY IMPROVED:	NO	YES	YES[3]	NO
MOBILISATION PARAMETERS TO VARY: [4]				
LOCATION	ISQ or CHANGE	ISQ		
FORCE LEVEL	INC	ISQ		
FORCE DIRECTION	CHANGE	ISQ		
MWM VOLUME:				
REPETITIONS	1	6-10		
SETS	1	1		INC
SELF-TREATMENT	-	-	YES[5]	YES
TAPING	-	-	YES[5]	YES
CESSATION POINT:	IF NO CHANGE AFTER 4 ATTEMPTS		WHEN 100% IMPROVED OR NO FURTHER IMPROVEMENTS POSSIBLE	

1. After completing a set of MWM repetitions always do a through range movement with the MWM applied, gradually easing out to the end of range pain-free. Failure to do this commonly results in an exacerbation of pain when the patient first moves after the MWM.

2. If patient does not report 100% recovery (to the extent that is possible for their condition) with the application of only one type of MWM technique (usually applied over several sessions) then consideration needs to be given to new MWM techniques being additionally applied, possibly at other locations also (e.g. spine for peripheral problem, or adjacent joint).

3. Care should be exercised at the first session as it is commonly reported that a rebound effect (worsening in ensuing 24-48 hours) may occur if Volume is too great.

4. In all MWMs with ROM as an endpoint criterion, overpressure is applied. This overpressure may be passive as in pain-limited ROM or it may be a maximal contraction in cases of stiffness or weakness limited ROM.

5. This is not always the case following first sessions, but depends on how successful the MWM was, how well the patient can learn the self-treatment and if tape was possible to apply. After the first session, if the patient is very much better (which occurs in some) then self-treatment and tape may not be required.

Figure 2.3 An overview of a proposed decision matrix that can be incorporated in the clinical reasoning process for the application and progression of MWM in one session and across a number of sessions

For within session decisions on application and progression, the clinical reasoning process largely relies on the response during and immediately post-MWM application compared to that session's pre-application CSIM, whereas for ensuing sessions the pre-application CSIM is compared to the first session's baseline (pre-application) CSIM. Whether or not the CSIM is substantially improved or not will dictate whether changes will be made to the parameters of the MWM and the exact nature of those changes if required. Parameters such as location, level and direction of force are modulated to effect changes during application, whereas volume parameters are usually manipulated to maintain or improve on the post-MWM CSIM, either within or between sessions. As a general guide, a successful MWM session appears to usually involve 1 to 3 sets of 10 repetitions but the exact volume for any individual can only be determined with certainty by using the post-application CSIM response.

contribution of the direction of the force application to improving the CSIM. In a study of 25 patients with tennis elbow, Abbot et al[12] showed that 19 patients responded with greater pain-free grip force when the lateral glide MWM was applied in a pure lateral (n = 9) or slightly (~5°) posterior of lateral direction (n = 10), as opposed to slightly anterior or caudal of lateral (n = 6). In a single case study of a 79-year

old female with a 7-month history of base of thumb pain following a fall, Hsieh et al[13] reported that only the MWM that used a supination glide of the proximal phalanx effected a pain-free full range of flexion of the first metacarpophalangeal joint, whereas MWMs with either a medial or lateral glide component did not improve flexion (see Chapter 14). Teys et al[14] assessed the effect of a shoulder MWM in 24 patients with pain-limited shoulder elevation and reported that the MWM with a posterior glide of the humerus produced a significantly greater improvement in shoulder elevation (~10%) than a sham anterior glide MWM of the humerus. Interestingly, there is some evidence for shoulder manipulations (not MWM) that suggests that the direction of the manipulation of the humeral head significantly impacts on the gains in ROM and pain reduction after treatment.[15]

The gross direction of force application during a MWM and the subtle variations thereof, which have been long advocated by Mulligan, appear to be critical in the successful application of a MWM. Practitioners should consider varying this parameter in improving outcomes.

Amount of force application

The initial change in CSIM is determined to some extent by the amount of force that is applied during the MWM. There is preliminary evidence that there may well be a threshold of force application that governs the outcome in the CSIM. McLean et al[16] evaluated the effect of four incremental force level applications on pain-free grip force in six tennis elbow patients (Figure 2.5). They used a flexible force mat to measure the force applied by the practitioner during the manual application of a lateral glide MWM of the elbow. The practitioner estimated three force levels (a third, half and two-thirds of his maximum force application) and applied these and the maximum force application in a random sequence. The data showed that there was a substantially greater pain-free grip force production

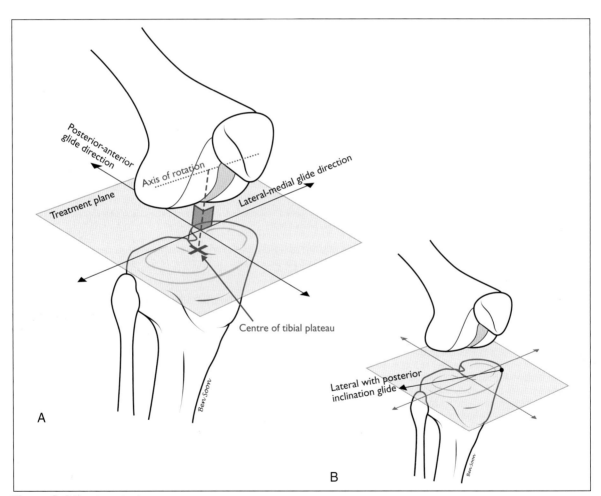

Figure 2.4 Treatment plane
(a) The treatment plane defined with reference to an example at the tibiofemoral joint. The treatment plane is perpendicular to a line drawn from the centre of rotation of the femoral condyles (convex member) to the centre of the tibial plateau (concave member). Glides and rotations that occur in this plane are thought to be the most mechanically effective.
(b) Demonstrates fine-tuning of a lateral glide with a slight posterior inclination with the filled in circle representing the contact point and the arrow the direction. Note how the contact point and application will be modified when fine-tuning the direction.

at the higher two levels of force (approximately 30% greater) than at the lower level (37 N). Interestingly, there was very little difference between maximum (mean force 113 N) and two-thirds maximum (75 N) force application on pain-free grip force production. To our knowledge this is the only study to have evaluated the impact of varying the amount of force application on MWM effects. Even though it is a small preliminary study it does alert the practitioner to be aware of the need to ensure that adequate force is being applied with MWM, such that if the effect on the CSIM is not substantial with MWM application, the practitioner should consider if they have applied sufficient force. This may occur where the patient is relatively large or has very stiff connective tissues and the practitioner is relatively small (small hands) or lacks sufficient strength, in which case the use of treatment belts may assist the practitioner in delivering a therapeutically effective force level (e.g. see Figures 1.2b, 5.3, 13.4 and 17.2). Alternatively, if the effect on the CSIM is substantial then the practitioner could consider if less force would still achieve this effect. Feasibly less force reduces the risk of any side-effect of the treatment affecting the soft tissues. Along these lines, it is prudent to always commence a MWM with a lower level of force, especially soon after injury or in cases of high pain intensity. That is, the least force required to achieve the desired effect on the CSIM should be the aim. (See the following section for a conceptual framework on this.)

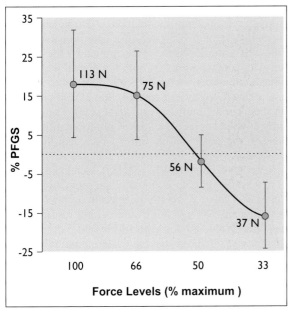

Figure 2.5 A higher-order Bèzier curve approximating the relationship between applied manual force of a MWM and the percentage change in pain-free grip strength (% PFGS). Adapted from McLean et al.[16]

Relationship between direction of force and amount of force applied

In setting up a MWM technique, practitioners should satisfy themselves that they sense that accessory joint play has occurred from the application of the accessory joint glide prior to the patient trying the CSIM. This is an immediate feedback that a practitioner seeks at the moment of the application of a joint mobilisation and provides the earliest affirmation that a joint mobilisation technique will have a chance of being effective. The following is a conceptual framework (Figure 2.6) that will help illustrate how a practitioner may optimise effecting accessory joint play during the application of a MWM.

In the previous sections of this chapter we described separately the direction and the amount of applied force as being important in optimising the effect of a MWM technique. However, the amount of force applied is likely not independent of the orientation/direction of the glide. The successful manual therapy practitioner will need to appreciate the interdependent relationship between direction and amount of force applied in a MWM technique. Above we previously described the treatment plane geometrically, but its practical clinical utility for practitioners is in conceiving the treatment plane as that plane in which the applied MWM glide effects most joint motion with least applied force. A schematic representation of this can be seen in Figure 2.6 in which force is hypothesised to exponentially increase as the practitioner applies the force increasingly out of the treatment plane. An additional dimension can be seen by the integration of the force threshold curve reported by McLean et al[16] (Figure 2.5), such that for any orientation/direction of the glide there is likely a different outcome in CSIM that is dependent on the amount of applied force.

Location of applied force
The location of applied force for MWM is not unlike that for other manual therapy applications in that there is a notion that the therapeutic effects are optimal when the force is applied at the most appropriate location. Similarly, good general joint handling skills are required in the application of MWM to optimise the effects; for example, using manual contact points near the joint line. Some of the other aspects that need to be considered in order to appropriately apply a MWM are:
• localisation/identification of the joint to be mobilised, for example, should the neck or shoulder be treated for proximal arm pain, or should an individual bone, such as the scaphoid, be targeted as opposed to several carpal bones at the wrist being targeted as a functional wrist articulation
• deciding which bone is to be stabilised and which is to be moved
• the direction of the applied glide as this will dictate the contact points

- the amount of tenderness at the contact point may necessitate a slightly different contact point be used, although a foam pad can also sometimes be useful in reducing contact point tenderness
- how fine or gross should the contact point be.

As for many approaches in musculoskeletal healthcare, the practitioner clinically reasons the resolution of these aspects following an examination of the patient prior to first delivering a MWM treatment and

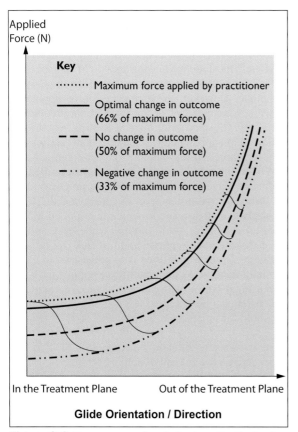

Figure 2.6 Four curves showing a hypothetical relationship between the amount of force in Newtons applied by the practitioner, and the accessory glide orientation of the mobilisation (from within the treatment plane to out of the treatment plane)

Applied force increases exponentially the further out of the treatment plane the practitioner directs the technique, such that practitioners should trial ('tweak') the glide orientation/direction to find the one for which least force is required. Additionally, for any given application of a MWM, the applied force–outcome relationship (see Figure 2.5) also varies in a characteristic way, hence the superimposition of 6 force-outcome higher-order Bèzier-like curves, which show that for any given treatment application the practitioner should be aware that there is likely a range of force levels with differential outcomes on the CSIM (from negative to optimal outcome). That is, practitioners will find that there is an accessory glide direction that will deliver an optimum outcome without overloading the joint or being ineffectual.

then on the basis of ongoing clinical re-examination and reasoning (e.g. see Jones et al[17] and Chapters 8–19). As a general rule in orthopaedics the joints above and below the one at which the patient is reporting problems should be considered in examination and as a possible location for treatment to be applied. In manipulative therapy, it is common practice to also consider the spine as the possible origin of peripherally located symptoms. For example, in managing someone with tennis elbow with MWM, the practitioner needs to consider not only the elbow, but also the neck as a potential site from which pain has been referred and at which a MWM may need to be applied to achieve complete resolution of the patient's problem. Once a joint and general direction of mobilisation is chosen, the MWM is applied once and then on the basis of the response in CSIM (as per the algorithm in Figure 2.3). If there is not a substantial improvement in the CSIM then further refinement of the location may need to occur in order to continue performing the MWM or in order to optimise it further. Alteration of the location of contact may also need to occur on the basis of a change in mobilisation direction (see Figure 2.4b), with the extent to which it will change varying, depending on if it is a gross or fine change in direction.

Most of the foregoing is based on clinical reasoning and a biologically plausible but indirect rationale. Notwithstanding this, there are some preliminary reports that support the notion that localisation of a manual technique is important in terms of its induced effects. One such report studied the effect of a lateral glide MWM for tennis elbow,[18] which is similar to that reported in Chapter 13. The lateral glide MWM was compared to a sham intervention in 24 patients. The sham intervention consisted of a firm pressure to the elbow that mimicked the force applied by the MWM, but with contact points on both the medial and lateral ulna, radius and humerus, which is different to the specific contact points in a lateral glide MWM (i.e. ulna on medial side, humerus on lateral side). The specifically applied lateral glide MWM produced effects that were in the order of five times larger than the sham treatment.

In terms of spinal MWM (SNAG), locating the exact or at least the most appropriate spinal segment to apply the MWM force is usually deemed to be important if not essential. We are not aware of any research that has directly studied this aspect of MWM, but there are several investigations that have looked into other postero–anterior (PA) mobilisation techniques.[19–21] Chiradejnant et al[19] evaluated the specificity of applying accessory glide mobilisations (central and unilateral PA, transverse) to the upper and lower lumbar spine of 140 patients with low back pain by two manipulative therapists. While these investigators reported that the effect on patient outcomes was no better for the therapist-selected spinal level than if randomly selected, they did find that there was a greater analgesic effect gained from the application of the mobilisations to the lower lumbar spinal levels (L_4–L_5). This appears to support the view that the area of pain and its qualities/characteristics, which are obtained through patient interview rather than by manual examination, play an important role in selecting the region of the spine that should be targeted by the MWM. In applying this clinically, after the interview, from which the practitioner has ascertained a region of the spine that is likely the best to target (i.e. narrowed down the range of possibilities to 2 or 3 motion segments), it appears reasonable that an iterative approach as outlined in Figure 2.3 is employed to determine the most effective MWM to apply (location being one of the variables that can be manipulated in this regard). That is, the MWM technique itself can be used to fine-tune the localisation of the segment to which the force is most effectively applied.

HOW MUCH MWM IS REQUIRED?

The amount of MWM that is applied may be conceptualised as a volume, which is defined as the sum total of all MWM applications that a patient experiences. The volume of MWM consists of the MWM that is performed by the practitioner as well as that which the patient does in self-treatment. This is reasonably easy to quantify by multiplying the number of repetitions per set by the number of sets of a specific MWM completed over a period of time. The application of tape is also considered another way of extending the amount/volume of MWM experienced by the patient, but it is relatively less quantifiable and in most cases is only worn for a day or two per application.

In contrast to the studies of the initial effects of level and direction of force application on the CSIM, preliminary as they may be, there is no study yet of the initial effect of manipulating volume in a MWM.[22] In order to get a sense of the relationship between the amount or volume of a MWM delivered and its initial effect, we conducted an analysis of all relevant papers,[4, 14, 18, 23–28] by selecting from the results of the comprehensive search strategy in Chapter 3 only those papers that reported: (1) a study of initial effects; (2) sufficient data to calculate a percent change score; and (3) enough information to allow a volume (number of total repetitions) of the MWM to be determined. The data from this analysis is collated in Figure 2.7. What Figure 2.7 highlights is that there appears to be no relationship between volume and the initial effect of a MWM ($R^2 = 0.063$) when we collapse data from tennis elbow[18, 25–27, 29], ankle[4, 23, 24, 28] and shoulder[14] studies as well as include both force and ROM data (and represent point estimates of effect as a percent change from baseline). The highest degree of association was observed when we examined only the force data for tennis elbow ($R^2 = 0.12$), but this was still very small.

We interpret this as supporting the contention that the volume of the applied MWM is not relevant to its initial effect.

From our clinical experience and the collation of the above data we hypothesise that the volume of the MWM treatment pertains more to the sustainability of the effect (i.e. over two or more sessions) rather than the initial effect, which appears to be better modulated through manipulation of magnitude, direction and location of force application parameters. That is, the manipulation of the volume parameter should be seen more in light of a mode of progressing MWM treatments in order to sustain an effect rather than exacting a larger magnitude of effect (Figure 2.3).

We propose that the manner in which the practitioner manipulates volume (repetition and sets) is determined by taking into account primarily the change in CSIM from pre- to post-application of the MWM (Figure 2.3). For example, the case described in Figure 2.1 shows that initially after application of the lateral glide MWM there was a substantial change (improvement to 150N) compared to the pre-MWM pain-free grip force of 50N (unaffected side ~200N), which we suggest is an indication to the practitioner that sufficient MWM volume was administered at that session (Figure 2.3). However, let us assume that a set of 6–10 repetitions had made a substantial improvement in the CSIM during the application of the MWM, but that this was not maintained immediately after the application of the MWM; for example, lets say it was 75N after MWM application. In this situation it would

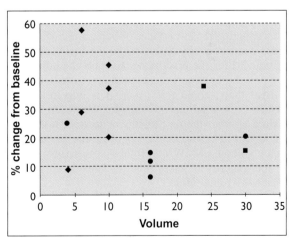

Figure 2.7 Initial effect (y-axis) by volume (x-axis; total number of repetitions performed) plot for MWM for tennis elbow (diamond; pain-free grip force) [18, 25–27, 29], ankle (circle; ankle range of motion) [4, 23, 24, 28] and shoulder disorders (square; shoulder range of motion) [14], highlighting a lack of association between the amount of MWM applied in a session and the immediate effect size

appear reasonable to apply more MWM or, in other words, increase volume by repeating the MWM for another two or three sets in order to seek to sustain the effect. A recent review highlighted that there has been no systematic evaluation of the most appropriate volume of MWM, but that 86% of papers published on case studies and clinical trials of MWM roughly followed Mulligan's initial recommendation of three sets of 10 repetitions, with some studies using one set and others four.[22] The implementation of a MWM self-treatment program along with the addition of a MWM taping technique should also be considered in this regard.

There is one caveat on increasing the volume in the manner described — that it is not uncommon for patients to experience a rebound effect within the 24–48 hours after their first session, especially in those with a severe or irritable disorder, but also in those who have a remarkably substantial improvement in that first session. This is an often repeated cautionary message.[1] An example is seen at measurement period B2-1 in Figure 2.8 [8] which shows a rebound to pre-treatment baseline values in the pain visual analogue scale (VAS) during the 48 hours after the first application of MWM. At the second session (B2) the patient expressed her unhappiness at continuing with treatment if this was to be a common outcome following treatment and required quite a deal of reassurance to continue with this treatment. In this case it was fortunate that the patient did actually return to express such a sentiment; she could have easily not bothered. Withdrawing from the treatment would have been counterproductive in this instance as the patient subsequently demonstrated an excellent response to the MWM program of treatment, underpinning the importance of being somewhat cautious and not overly ambitious in the first session. It is prudent for the practitioner to warn the patient of the possibility of an exacerbation and to reassure the patient that, should this occur, it is only transient. Whilst it is important to consider the possibility of a flare up after the first treatment session, it is more important to ensure that the patient receives an adequate volume of MWM at follow-up sessions, which in the majority of cases requires considerably more than 6–10 repetitions.

While change in the CSIM after the treatment application can be used as a guide to determining the required volume of MWM, comparison of the baseline CSIM with that over ensuing sessions can also be used to monitor the sustainability of the effects gained from the MWM, in addition to the effect of any self-treatments and taping that has been instituted. We propose that it is reasonable to determine that an adequate volume of MWM has been reached when the baseline CSIM for a given treatment session changes substantially from the baseline of the first session. For example, this can be seen in Figure 2.1 (iii) in which there was a sizeable elevation (~50–100%) in pain-free grip force from the baseline measure of the first to that of the fourth session. Notable in this case study is the lack of change in the baseline CSIM in the second and third sessions. Guided by this response the practitioner gradually increased the volume of the MWM treatment by adding in MWM self-treatment and elbow taping (see Chapter 13 for techniques). Essentially, if the baseline CSIM at subsequent sessions is not substantially improved, then the volume of the MWM should be progressed by increasing the repetitions and sets performed, but remember this only applies if the MWM produces substantial changes during and immediately after a MWM application. Additional consideration should be given to adding patient MWM self-treatment and taping. Typically 4–6 sessions are required to gradually ramp up the volume of MWM, but this will vary from patient to patient. Failure to improve the baseline CSIM over such a treatment period could be taken to indicate that the MWM should not be continued.

In comparing the ensuing sessions' baseline to the first baseline CSIM, it is important to keep in mind other factors that are not within the MWM treatment program. For example, overall physical activity levels or any unintentional events (such as an unexpected increase in pain-provoking tasks), as well as patient compliance with and adherence to effective self-treatment. These would need to be considered on an individual case-by-case basis and they may also impinge upon the decision to continue with MWM treatment or to modify it by addressing the various other parameters, as well as modulating volume.

SELF-TREATMENT ISSUES

Another element of MWM application that is required for the majority of patients (i.e. those who are not completely recovered after a session or two with the practitioner, see Figure 2.3) is self-treatment in order to ensure complete ongoing resolution of their condition. As outlined above, the volume of MWM experienced by the patient is likely to be a large driver of the sustainability of the MWM effects and, as such, repetition of the MWM will often require the patient to self-treat, which will necessitate their cooperation. The patient needs to cooperate in several ways, the most fundamental being an ability to effectively apply the MWM and then to diligently repeat the application at a volume that has been determined in collaboration with the practitioner.

The patient's ability to effectively apply the self-treatment MWM can be assessed in the same way as the practitioner has been directed herein and in the previous chapter; that is, by using the CSIM to quantify

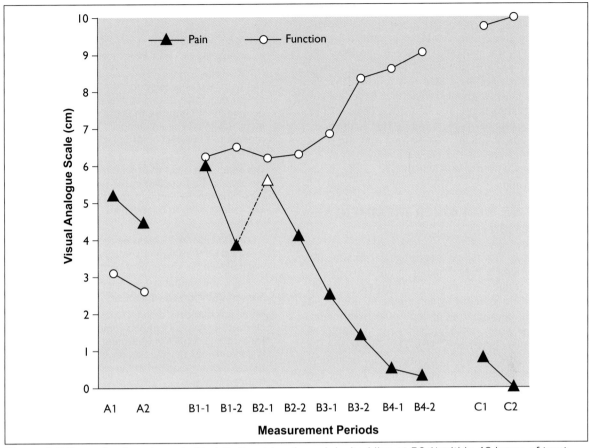

Figure 2.8 Example of a rebound effect (hollow triangle and dashed line at B2-1) within 48 hours of treatment

Visual analogue scale (VAS) for pain (triangle, where 10 is worst pain and 0 is no pain) and function (circle, where 10 is normal function and 0 is 'arm in sling') for a single case of tennis elbow. B represents a 2-week period in which 4 treatment sessions were delivered (number immediately after B is the treatment session number) with the last number in the B phase representing either pre-MWM (-1) or post-MWM (-2). A and C are no treatment (representing baseline) and post-treatment phases, respectively. Figure adapted with permission from Vicenzino & Wright 1995.[8]

the effect of the self-MWM. While it may not be feasible or realistic for the patient to reproduce the same magnitude of the effect that the practitioner is able to bring about, it is futile to have a patient repeating a self-administered MWM that does not effectively change the CSIM in any meaningful way.

Strapping tape that is applied in a manner that seeks to replicate the manually applied MWM (i.e. applied in a similar direction to the mobilisation) is another strategy that is frequently employed to extend the therapeutic effect of the practitioner delivered MWM. Taping relies on the patient being able to tolerate the adhesive without allergic reaction as much as it relies on its skilful application, which in most instances is best accomplished by a practitioner and not the patient. Similar to the self-administered MWM, the tape should have some demonstrable effect on the CSIM if it is to be used as part of the treatment plan.

Compliance and adherence to the self-treatment set by the practitioner is essential in ensuring the success of MWM. This is not unique to MWM but there are some unique features of MWM that can be used to facilitate high levels of compliance and adherence. One of the unique features is that the MWM has a built-in feedback mechanism (i.e. performance on the CSIM) through which the patient and practitioner can judge the compliance of the patient in performing an effective self-application of the specific MWM. The immediacy of feedback on performance of the MWM with respect to the CSIM and the substantial size of the effect are both very strong drivers of 'buy in' by the patient and are critical to seeding a positive attitude in complying with the self-MWM approach. Adherence to a self-MWM protocol can be encouraged by structuring the clinical encounter in such a way that the patient becomes implicitly aware of the importance of the self-treatment. For example, at follow-up sessions after the self-MWM has been given to the patient, the very first thing that should be examined by the practitioner is the patient's ability to perform the self-MWM. Typically this would involve the patient performing the baseline CSIM test followed by the self-MWM. The practitioner would then have two key bits of information that will establish the basis for that treatment session: one being a comparison to the baseline measurement for the first session and the other being an indication of the patient's ability to effectively repeat the self-MWM which was taught in the previous session.

INTEGRATION WITH OTHER TREATMENTS AND FUNCTION

As is the case with many other physical treatments, once the patient is experiencing improved capacity to move, be it due to relief of pain, increase in ROM, improvement in strength or combinations thereof, it is frequently beneficial to include other treatments, often in the form of exercises (e.g. strengthening, endurance, functional, etc). This integration of MWM with other forms of treatment can be undertaken in much the same manner as described for the application of a MWM, by an iterative approach of assessment/re-assessment and intervention to guide the latter.

SUMMARY

In this chapter we operationally defined MWM in terms of a set of parameters and provided the reader with some guidelines on how these parameters may be manipulated in order to optimise treatment effects. We emphasised that the practitioner will usually be able to ascertain if, when, what type and how much of a MWM should be used if they exercise their clinical reasoning skills and apply some basic rules as elucidated upon herein, some of which have some supporting evidence, albeit low level. In the following chapter we present a comprehensive review of the literature pertaining to the clinical efficacy of MWM.

the CSIM endpoint is the onset of pain (pain threshold). That is, the CSIM will measure either ROM of a joint or amount of force output of a muscle to the onset of pain – not pain on a rating scale.

- The parameters of the applied manual force, such as location, force level and direction of force, can be modified to improve the outcome as quantified by the CSIM and should be used in an iterative manner in the selection of the most effective MWM.
- The volume or amount of a MWM applied, inclusive of that applied by the practitioner in the clinic and that self-administered by the patient, will usually need to be modified (often increased) in order to:
  - sustain beyond the treatment session the effects on the CSIM of a successful MWM gained within a treatment session
  - gain a substantial improvement in the pre-treatment CSIM at subsequent sessions.
- While it is currently difficult to provide evidence-based data on the volume required for a successful MWM treatment program, it is generally recognised that several sets of 10 repetitions are required in the clinic to gain long lasting effects.
- If on attempting to apply a MWM it is unsuccessful, no more than four attempts at trying to make the MWM work should be entertained. An unsuccessful MWM in this case being defined as a lack of substantial improvement in the CSIM at the time of application. This definition assumes that the MWM is not making the condition worse; if it was the MWM would be immediately ceased.

References

1 Mulligan B. Manual Therapy — 'NAGS', 'SNAGS', 'MWMS' etc. (5th edn). Wellington: Plane View Services 1999.
2 Maitland G, Hengeveld E, Banks K, English K. Maitland's Vertebral Manipulation (7th edn). Sydney: Butterworths-Heinemann 2007.
3 Hall T, Beherlein C, Hansson U, Teck Lim H, Odermark M, Sainsbury D. Mulligan Traction SLR: A pilot study to investigate effects on range of motion in patients with low back pain. Journal of Manual and Manipulative Therapy. 2006 Jul 22;14(2):95–100.
4 Vicenzino B, Martin D, Prangley I. The initial effect of two Mulligan mobilisation with movement treatment techniques on ankle dorsiflexion. In: Goodman C (ed.) 2001: A Sports Medicine Odyssey: Challenges, Controversies & Change, Australian Conference of Science and Medicine in Sport, 2001; Perth: Australia: Sports Medicine Australia; 2001. Online. Available: http://fulltext.ausport.gov.au/fulltext/2001/acsms/default.asp (accessed 21 April 2010).

KEY POINTS

- The Client Specific Impairment Measure (CSIM) is a key and central feature of the MWM.
- Clear identification and specification of the CSIM (ROM, pain onset or level, muscle strength etc) is required as a basis for determining the most effective MWM technique.
- It is critical to the success of the MWM that in patients with pain-limited function (e.g. ROM, contraction of a muscle or muscle group) that

5 Crossley K, Cowan SM, Bennell KL, McConnell J. Patellar taping: is clinical success supported by scientific evidence? Manual Therapy. 2000;5(3):142–50.

6 Hahne AJ, Keating JL, Wilson SC. Do within-session changes in pain intensity and range of motion predict between-session changes in patients with low back pain? Australian Journal of Physiotherapy. 2004 Jan 1; 50(1):17–23.

7 Tuttle N. Do changes within a manual therapy treatment session predict between-session changes for patients? Australian Journal of Physiotherapy. 2005 Jan 1.

8 Vicenzino B, Wright A. Effects of a novel manipulative physiotherapy technique on tennis elbow: a single case study. Manual Therapy. 1995;1(1):30–5.

9 Vicenzino B, Smith D, Cleland J, Bisset L. Development of a clinical prediction rule to identify initial responders to mobilisation with movement and exercise for lateral epicondylalgia. Manual Therapy. 2008 Sep 30;10.1016/j.math.2008.08.004.

10 Kaltenborn F. Manual Mobilisation of the Extremity Joints, Basic Examination and Treatment Techniques. Norway: Olaf Norlis Bokhandel 1989.

11 Prentice W. Joint Mobilization and Traction Techniques in Rehabilitation. In: Prentice W, Voight M, (eds.) *Techniques in musculoskeletal rehabilitation*. New York: McCraw-Hill 2001:235–58.

12 Abbott JH, Patla CE, Jensen RH. The initial effects of an elbow mobilization with movement technique on grip strength in subjects with lateral epicondylalgia. Manual Therapy. 2001;6(3):163–9.

13 Hsieh CY, Vicenzino B, Yang CH, Hu MH, Yang C. Mulligan's mobilization with movement for the thumb: a single case report using magnetic resonance imaging to evaluate the positional fault hypothesis. Manual Therapy. 2002 Feb;7(1):44–9.

14 Teys P, Bisset L, Vicenzino B. The initial effects of a Mulligan's mobilization with movement technique on range of movement and pressure pain threshold in pain-limited shoulders. Manual therapy. 2008 Oct 25.

15 Johnson AJ, Godges JJ, Zimmerman G, Ounanian LL. The effect of anterior versus posterior glide joint mobilization on external rotation range of motion in patients with shoulder adhesive capsulitis. The Journal of Orthopaedic and Sports Physical Therapy. 2007 Mar 1;37(3):88–99.

16 McLean S, Naish R, Reed L, Urry S, Vicenzino B. A pilot study of the manual force levels required to produce manipulation induced hypoalgesia. Clinical Biomechanics. 2002 May;17(4):304–8.

17 Jones M, Rivett D, (eds.) Clinical Reasoning for Manual Therapists (2nd edn). Edinburgh; New York: Butterworth-Heinemann 2004.

18 Vicenzino B, Paungmali A, Buratowski S, Wright A. Specific manipulative therapy treatment for chronic lateral epicondylalgia produces uniquely characteristic hypoalgesia. Manual Therapy. 2001 Nov;6(4):205–12.

19 Chiradejnant A, Maher CG, Latimer J, Stepkovitch N. Efficacy of 'therapist-selected' versus 'randomly selected' mobilisation techniques for the treatment of low back pain: a randomised controlled trial. Australian Journal of Physiotherapy. 2003 Dec 31;49(4):233–41.

20 Chiradejnant A, Maher C, Latimer J, Stepkovitch N. Does the choice of spinal level treated during postero-anterior (PA) mobilisation affect treatment …. Physiotherapy Theory and Practice. 2002;18:165–74.

21 Tuttle N, Barrett R, Laakso L. Relation between changes in posteroanterior stiffness and active range of movement of the cervical spine following manual therapy treatment. Spine. 2008 Sep 1;33(19):E673–9.

22 Hing W, Bigelow R, Bremner T. Mulligan's Mobilisation with Movement: A review of the tenets and prescription of MWMs. New Zealand Journal of Physiotherapy. 2008;36(3): 144–64.

23 Collins N, Teys P, Vicenzino B. The initial effects of a Mulligan's mobilization with movement technique on dorsiflexion and pain in subacute ankle sprains. Manual Therapy. 2004 May;9(2):77–82.

24 O'Brien T, Vicenzino B. A study of the effects of Mulligan's mobilization with movement treatment of lateral ankle pain using a case study design. Manual Therapy. 1998;3(2):78–84.

25 Paungmali A, O'Leary S, Souvlis T, Vicenzino B. Hypoalgesia and sympathoexcitatory effects of mobilisation with movement for lateral epicondylalgia. Physical Therapy. 2003;83(4):374–83.

26 Paungmali A, O'Leary S, Souvlis T, Vicenzino B. Naloxone fails to antagonise initial hypoalgesic effect of a manual therapy treatment for lateral epicondylalgia. Journal of Manipulative and Physiological Therapeutics. 2004;27(3):180–5.

27 Paungmali A, Vicenzino B, Smith M. Hypoalgesia induced by elbow manipulation in chronic lateral epicondylalgia does not exhibit tolerance. Journal of Pain. 2003;4(8):448–54.

28 Vicenzino B, Branjerdporn M, Teys P, Jordan K. Initial changes in posterior talar glide and dorsiflexion of the ankle after mobilization with movement in individuals with recurrent ankle sprain. The Journal of Orthopaedic and Sports Physical Therapy. 2006 Jul 1;36(7):464–71.

29 Abbott J, Patla C, Jensen R. Grip strength changes immediately following elbow mobilisation with movement in subjects with lateral epicondylalgia. In: Singer K (ed.) *Proceedings of the 7th Scientific Conference of the IFOMT in conjunction with the MPAA*. Perth, Australia: University of Western Australia 2000:8–10.

SECTION TWO

Efficacy

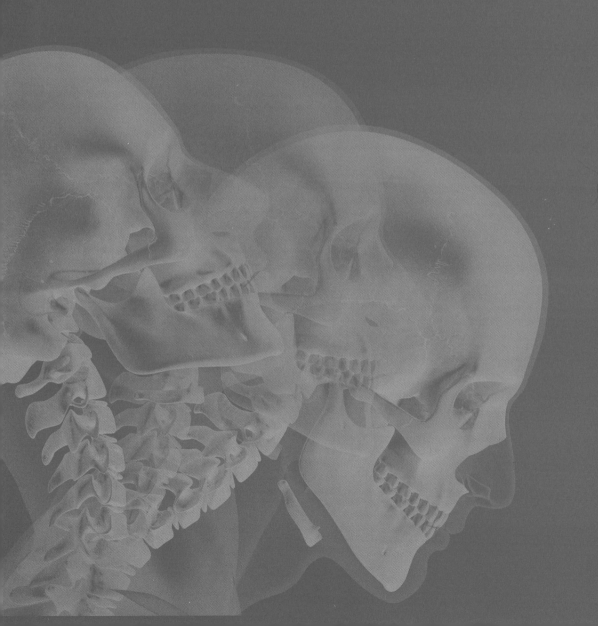

Chapter 3
A systematic review of the efficacy of MWM

Leanne Bisset, Wayne Hing and Bill Vicenzino

INTRODUCTION

The ability of Mobilisation with Movement (MWM) techniques in generating hypoalgesic effects, increasing joint range of motion (ROM), enhancing muscle function, as well as more specifically, treating particular pathologies or post-trauma treatment has been reported in a number of studies of varying quality.[1–6] Studies applying MWM techniques to the shoulder, elbow and ankle have shown them to be effective in reducing pain and increasing joint ROM immediately during and after their application, though the main focus has been to the upper limb joints.[1, 6, 7] Despite a number of studies reporting the clinical effects of MWM, we are not aware of any systematic reviews that have summarised the evidence for this technique's clinical efficacy.

In order for practitioners to make informed decisions about whether a treatment for a particular condition is truly effective, all the available evidence must be evaluated and summarised. There is variety in the quality of evidence presented in the literature and it is therefore important to be informed as to the level of evidence achieved by a particular study or review.[8] A randomised controlled trial (RCT) represents a high level of evidence, as does a meta-analysis or a systematic review, but it is not to say that lower levels of evidence, such as an observational study or a case report, are not also important and included in systematic reviews where insufficient RCTs have been published.[9–11] For example, nascent physical therapies are often initially described through case reports and case studies, prior to undergoing preliminary evaluation through case series or controlled trials of initial effects before any RCT is undertaken. However, for a therapist to be confident that a particular treatment approach, such as MWM, will be effective in the management of their individual patient, the highest levels of evidence are required. Equally, if the evidence for a particular treatment depends only on a few observational studies, it should not be seen as having been proven to be effective. The level of evidence supplied by a particular study or review can be rated using the Oxford Centre for Evidence-based Medicine Levels of Evidence (see Table 3.1; Phillips et al[12]).

The aim of this chapter is to synthesise the evidence for the efficacy of MWM techniques. It achieves this through a systematic review of the literature about the effects of MWM techniques on clinically relevant outcomes for musculoskeletal conditions. There is a focus on defining and providing information on the levels of evidence, quality issues and how this is reflected in the literature on MWM techniques. This chapter does not deal with potential mechanism(s) of action of MWM effects, nor of the effects of MWM, which are dealt with in Chapters 4–7, but rather this chapter deals with the clinical efficacy of MWM.

METHODS

Search strategy

One reviewer searched the full set of the following databases to 21 October 2009, without language restrictions, using the recommended Cochrane Library search strategy: MEDLINE, CINAHL, Web of Science, SPORTdiscus, and Physiotherapy Evidence Database (PEDro).[13] The Cochrane Controlled Trial Register was searched for RCTs on MWM, and references from retrieved articles and systematic reviews were also screened. The refined key terms included Mobilisation with Movement* OR mobilization with movement* OR MWM*; manual therapy AND (mobilisation* OR mobilization*); mulligan; mulligan mobilisation* OR mulligan mobilization*. In addition, cross referencing was undertaken through communication with experts in the field.

Selection

For this systematic review we included all studies that met the following conditions: participants with a diagnosis of a musculoskeletal condition, as confirmed by a clinical diagnosis and/or other investigations (e.g. radiographic), and who were treated with a MWM technique. Studies that included other treatments in addition to MWM were also included as the multi-modal approach is standard in contemporary physiotherapy. A MWM technique was defined as any passive joint mobilisation that was applied and sustained during a passive or active movement of

Table 3.1 Levels of evidence, adapted[12]	
Level	**Therapy/prevention, aetiology/harm**
1a	SR (with homogeneity*) of RCTs
1b	Individual RCT (with narrow Confidence Interval)
1c	All or none§
2a	SR (with homogeneity*) of cohort studies
2b	Individual cohort study (including low quality RCT; e.g., <80% follow-up)
2c	'Outcomes' Research; Ecological studies
3a	SR (with homogeneity*) of case-control studies
3b	Individual case-control study
4	Case-series (and poor quality cohort and case-control studies§§)
5	Expert opinion without explicit critical appraisal, or based on physiology, bench research or 'first principles'

RCTs = randomised controlled trials; SR = systematic review.

* homogeneity = a systematic review that is free of worrisome heterogeneity in the directions and degrees of results between individual studies. Studies displaying worrisome heterogeneity should be tagged with a '-' at the end of their designated level.

§ Met when <u>all</u> patients died before the Rx became available, but some now survive on it; or when some patients died before the Rx became available, but <u>none</u> now die on it.

§§ Poor quality <u>cohort</u> study = one that failed to clearly define comparison groups and/or failed to measure exposures and outcomes in the same (preferably blinded), objective way in both exposed and non-exposed individuals and/or failed to identify or appropriately control known confounders and/or failed to carry out a sufficiently long and complete follow-up of patients. Poor quality <u>case-control</u> study = one that failed to clearly define comparison groups and/or failed to measure exposures and outcomes in the same (preferably blinded), objective way in both cases and controls and/or failed to identify or appropriately control known confounders.

Quality assessment

All articles included in this review were ranked according to the Oxford Centre for Evidence-based Medicine Levels of Evidence.[12] As non-randomised trials were also included, the Quality Index[14] was used to evaluate the quality of the studies. The Quality Index is a checklist that can assess the methodological quality not only of randomised controlled trials but also non-randomised studies (Appendix 3.1). This checklist has previously been shown to provide a profile of an individual paper, alerting reviewers to its particular methodological strengths and weaknesses. On average, the Quality Index has been shown to have high internal consistency (Kuder-Richardson 20: 0.89), test-retest (r 0.88) and inter-rater (r 0.75) reliability.[14] The Quality Index consists of five categories including reporting (/10), external validity (/3), internal validity (bias) (/7), internal validity (confounding or selection bias) (/6) and power (/1), totalling 27 criteria. Two experienced raters (LB and NC) rated all papers independently and blind to each other. Both raters were also blind to the name of the authors, institution and journal, as these identifying features were removed prior to rating.[15] Disagreement on any criterion was reassessed by both reviewers and any disagreement that was unresolved by general consensus was taken to a third reviewer (BV), who was independent to the initial deliberations, and a final consensus was reached.

Each criterion was accompanied by a strict descriptive list and was rated either 'yes', 'no' or 'unable to determine' to minimise ambiguity. Each criterion was then given a score: yes = 1 point, no = 0 point, unable to determine = 0 point; except for criterion 5, which scored a maximum of 2 points (Appendix 3.1). A total score for the methodological quality of each study was calculated by summing up the number of positive criteria (maximum score of 28). The last item in this tool, regarding the power of a study, was modified due to its complexity.[16] While all studies were included in this review, data pooling for further meta-analyses were limited to studies rating 50% or more ($\geq$14/28) in order to ensure adequate methodological quality and reliable interpretation of results. It has been previously shown that the inclusion of poorer quality studies in a meta-analysis may alter the estimate of benefit and therefore may alter the interpretation of the effect of an intervention.[17]

Inter-rater reliability

Inter-rater reliability was evaluated by reporting the percentage of initial agreement and the Kappa statistics, both for overall agreement as well as for each criterion.[18]

Data management and statistical analysis

Key data such as participant characteristics, description of the treatments given, outcome measures used and results were extracted from all articles. Summary

the joint or contraction of muscles. By definition, the studies also required the use of one clinically relevant outcome measure, such as pain, grip strength or range of movement, however studies with no data were still included in the review process. Non-randomised trials were also included as there are very few RCTs published on this emergent therapy.

Abstracts of papers identified by the search strategy were screened for inclusion by one reviewer (LB). If there was any indecision, the full text was retrieved and reviewed by three reviewers (LB, WH, BV). A full copy of all identified articles was then retrieved.

data, where available, was extracted and if the studies were clinically homogeneous, then a meta-analysis was performed using RevMan 5.0[19] to provide an overall effect estimate for each comparison. If the study compared at least two groups, the between group Standardised Mean Difference (SMD) with 95% confidence intervals (CI) (SMD; 95% CI) and Relative Risk (RR; 95% CI) were calculated on a random effects model. A positive SMD represents an effect in favour of the intervention, with values greater than 0.8 considered a large clinical effect, 0.5 a moderate effect and 0.2 a weak effect.[20, 21] To rate clinical significance for the RR, we followed Smidt et al[22] and set it at 0.7 as favouring the placebo/control group and 1.5 as favouring the intervention. Where possible, the mean change scores and standard deviations of the change scores were used to calculate the SMD. If this was not possible, and provided the baseline scores were not significantly different, the SMD and 95% CI were calculated from the post-intervention mean and standard deviation scores. All data entry and conversion was performed by one investigator (LB) and then checked by another (BV). Confidence interval that contained 0 represented a null effect.

If valid data was lacking or the studies were too clinically or statistically heterogeneous, then the meta-analysis was not performed and only an analysis of the quality of the studies was performed. Various levels of evidence to the effectiveness of MWM were assigned using the Oxford Centre for Evidence-based Medicine Levels of Evidence [12] (Table 3.1).

Where studies failed to include a comparison group, the effect size (post-intervention mean – pre-intervention mean/standard deviation mean) for the individual group was calculated.

RESULTS

The systematic review process of identifying, refining and final selection of studies into this review is illustrated in Figure 3.1. A total of 38 papers were rated using the Quality Index.

Inter-rater reliability

Out of a total of 1026 criteria rated, there were 57 (5.6%) initial disagreements between raters with a Kappa statistic of 0.894. The median (lower to upper quartile) for inter-rater agreement for each criterion was 0.903 (0.729 to 0.9695) (Table 3.2). After a consensus meeting between the two reviewers (LB and NC), seven (<1%) decisions could not be resolved and the third reviewer (BV) was called upon to make the final decision.

Methodological quality

Methodological quality, as rated by the Downs and Black Quality Index,[14] ranged from 2 to 24 out of a maximum of 27 rateable criteria, and a maximum of 28 points (criterion number 5 awarded a maximum of 2 points).

Following rating by reviewers, 17 studies (Table 3.3) scored above the *a-priori* minimum quality score of 50% (i.e. 14 out of 28 points) to be included in further meta-analyses, where possible. The most common features of the studies that rated less than 50% were the lack of a control group, lack of randomisation and lack of blinding. All of the poorer quality studies were single case studies, except for five studies: Manchanda and Grover[23] and Naik et al[24] were RCTs, Kochar and Dogra[25] was a quasi-randomised trial and Abbott[7] and Merlin et al[26] used a single group pre- post-test design (Table 3.3 — quality rating results).

As illustrated in Table 3.4, cross-over RCTs in which participants acted as their own control achieved the highest mean score for methodological quality (average score = 19.9/28), closely followed by full RCTs and then single group pre- post-test design. The quasi-randomised study,[25] single case studies and case reports rated below 14/28 on the quality rating scale, except for Creighton et al.[27] Even though the study by Creighton et al[27] used a non-experimental design and did not specifically label the intervention as a MWM, it scored 50% (14/28) and met the inclusion criteria of an applied joint glide in conjunction with a movement or exercise, and was therefore included in this review.

The sub-category of reporting was the only one that averaged greater than 50%, with significant weaknesses across all studies in reporting on the external validity sub-scale (Table 3.4). The majority of studies also reported poorly on the internal validity (confounding) sub-scale, with the mean score of 1.9 (SD 1.6) out of a possible 6 points across all studies.

Figure 3.2 illustrates the relationship between methodological quality and estimated effect size of the MWM intervention. It is evident that studies of lesser quality reported larger effects than studies of higher quality. Importantly, 15/21 studies that rated below 50% on the Quality Index did not report sufficient data to allow estimation of an effect size.

Outcome measures

Pain scores were reported in the majority of studies using either a continuous visual analogue scale (VAS) or an ordinal points system (Table 3.5). Joint ROM was reported in several studies (ROM; 18 studies; 47%) as was pain-free grip strength (PFGS; 8 studies; 21%). Table 3.5 lists the outcome measures used across the included studies. Thirty-two studies reported at least one short-term outcome assessment ($\leq$ 6 weeks), whilst only two studies [28, 29] included a long-term follow-up ($\geq$ 6 months) of the primary outcome measures. Fourteen studies only looked at the immediate post-intervention effects of the primary outcome measure, with nine studies not reporting any outcome data.

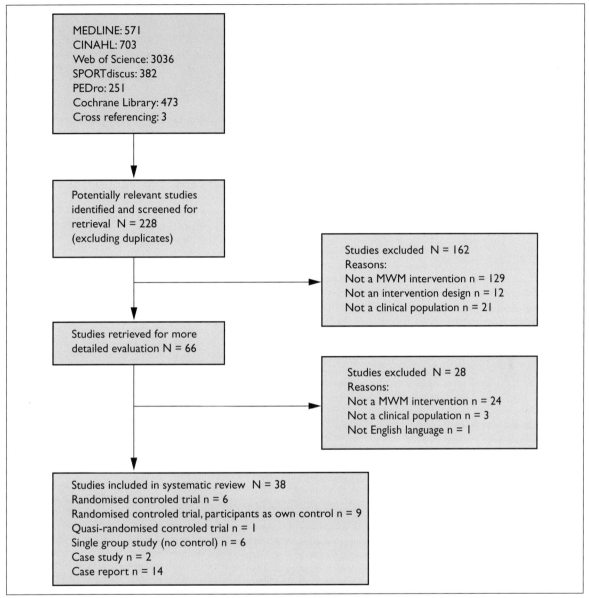

Figure 3.1 Number of hits for each database, obtained using a sensitive search strategy and numbers remaining after application of exclusion filters

Characteristics of studies

The study characteristics are reported in Table 3.6. There were a number of body regions investigated across the studies, with six studies assessing MWM techniques on shoulder conditions (two non-specific, two impingement, one frozen shoulder), 12 studies assessed lateral epicondylalgia (LE) populations, four studies assessed wrist and hand disorders (two de Quervain tenosynovitis, one thumb pain, one Colles' fracture), seven assessed spinal populations (two cervicogenic headache, one cervicogenic dizziness, one acute thoracic pain, three low back pain), one study assessed

lateral hip pain, one study assessed patellofemoral pain syndrome and seven studies assessed ankle pain. Overall, only 15 studies compared a MWM intervention with another intervention; the remaining studies did not include a comparison group. The study designs ranged from RCTs to single case reports (Tables 3.4 and 3.6).

MWM for lateral epicondylalgia

Twelve studies assessed the effects of a MWM lateral glide to the elbow in patients with a clinical diagnosis of LE. Of these, six studies satisfied the criteria of 50%

Table 3.2 Evaluation criteria and inter-rater reliability, with number of studies that did or did not meet each criterion

Criteria	Number of articles		Inter-rater reliability
	Adequate	Inadequate*	(Kappa)
1 Is the hypothesis/aim/objective of the study clearly described?	31	7	0.891
2 Are the main outcomes to be measured clearly described in the Introduction or Methods section?	27	11	1.000
3 Are the characteristics of the subjects included in the study clearly described?	28	10	0.914
4 Are the interventions of interest clearly described?	33	5	0.247
5 Are the distributions of principal confounders in each group of subjects to be compared clearly described?	31†	7	0.903
6 Are the main findings of the study clearly described?	29	9	0.716
7 Does the study provide estimates of the random variability in the data for the main outcomes?	21	17	0.812
8 Have all the important adverse events that may be a consequence of the intervention been reported?	9	29	0.569
9 Have the characteristics of patients lost to follow-up been described?	26	12	0.742
10 Have actual probability values been reported (e.g. 0.035 instead of <0.05) for the main outcomes except where the probability value is less than 0.001?	18	20	0.818
11 Were the subjects asked to participate in the study representative of the entire population from which they were recruited?	0	38	1.000
12 Were the subjects who were prepared to participate representative of the entire population from which they were recruited?	0	38	1.000
13 Were the staff, places, and facilities where the patients were treated representative of the treatment the majority of patients received?	9	29	0.582
14 Was an attempt made to blind study subjects to the intervention they have received?	3	35	0.529
15 Was an attempt made to blind those measuring the outcomes of the intervention?	13	25	0.937
16 If any of the results of the study were based on 'data dredging', was this made clear?	22	16	0.807
17 In trials and cohort studies, do the analyses adjust for different lengths of follow-up of patients, or in case-control studies, is the time period between the intervention and outcome the same for cases and controls?	20	18	0.939
18 Were the statistical tests used to assess the main outcomes appropriate?	23	15	1.000
19 Was compliance with the interventions reliable?	9	29	0.779
20 Were the main outcome measures used accurate (valid and reliable)?	22	16	1.000
21 Were patients in different intervention groups (trials and cohort studies) or were cases and controls (case-control studies) recruited from the same population?	16	22	0.937
22 Were study subjects in different intervention groups (trials and cohort studies) or were cases and controls (case-control studies) recruited over the same period of time?	5	33	0.716
23 Were study subjects randomised to intervention groups?	16	22	1.000

(Continued)

Table 3.2 Evaluation criteria and inter-rater reliability, with number of studies that met or didn't meet each criterion—cont'd

Criteria	Number of articles		Inter-rater reliability
	Adequate	Inadequate*	(Kappa)
24 Was the randomised intervention assignment concealed from both patients and healthcare staff until recruitment was complete and irrevocable?	8	30	0.904
25 Was there adequate adjustment for confounding in the analyses from which the main findings were drawn?	2	36	0.637
26 Were losses of patients to follow-up taken into account?	25	13	0.914
27 Did the study have sufficient power to detect a clinically important effect, where the probability value for a difference being due to chance is less than 5%?	8	30	1.000

* Includes articles where raters were unable to determine whether or not criterion was met.
† includes studies that only partially fulfilled this criterion (i.e. scored either 1 or 2 points for this criterion).

or more on the quality rating scale to be included in further analyses. It was possible to pool data from two studies,[4, 30] which showed a positive immediate effect of MWM on measures of PFGS (SMD 1.28; 95% CI 0.84 to 1.73; Figure 3.3) and pressure pain threshold (SMD 0.49; 95% CI 0.08 to 0.90; Figure 3.3). One limitation of this research is that it involved only a single treatment session and there was no long-term follow-up.

Two RCTs[23, 28] compared a co-intervention of MWM lateral glide to the elbow and exercise, with comparator groups. Bisset et al[28] compared the MWM intervention with corticosteroid injections and a wait-and-see approach, whereas Manchanda and Grover[23] compared the MWM intervention to a co-intervention of wrist manipulation, ultrasound and exercise as well as an ultrasound/exercise group. There were several methodological differences between the two RCTs that meant no meta-analyses were possible. For Bisset et al,[28] which scored highly on the Quality Index, the primary endpoints were 6- and 52-weeks follow-up. The authors reported a significant difference between MWM and wait-and-see groups in the measure of global improvement at 6 weeks; 41/63 (65%) participants reported success with MWM compared with 16/60 (27%) with wait-and-see (MWM versus wait-and-see RR 2.44; 95% CI 1.55 to 3.85). There was no significant difference between the MWM and corticosteroid injection group, with 51/65 (78%) reporting success with corticosteroid injections (MWM versus injections RR 0.83; 95% CI 0.66 to 1.03). At 52-weeks follow-up, the MWM group was significantly better on all outcomes compared with the corticosteroid injection group, but no different to the wait-and-see group, as most participants had either greatly improved or completely recovered (MWM 59/63; wait-and-see 56/62; injection 44/65)

(Table 3.7). Manchanda and Grover,[23]who scored below 50% on the Quality Index, had a maximum follow-up of 15 days (i.e. end of treatment) and found no difference between the MWM and the wrist manipulation intervention for measures of pain and function. However, both the MWM and wrist manipulation interventions were superior to the ultrasound intervention. There were several methodological flaws in the reporting of this study, and as such, the conclusions drawn by the authors must be considered with caution.

Kochar and Dogra,[25] in a quasi-randomised study, compared a co-intervention of MWM lateral glide to the elbow, ultrasound and exercise to a co-intervention of ultrasound and exercise. In addition, they included a non-randomised control group. Outcomes were assessed at 3 weeks and 12 weeks. The authors reported that most participants in the MWM group made a complete recovery, but did not specify the follow-up time period for this observation. They also reported five recurrences in the ultrasound group, but there was no mention of how a recurrence was defined. Overall, the MWM group appeared to be significantly improved at 12 weeks compared with both the US and control groups. Minimal data was supplied, thus making any further analyses impossible.

Paungmali et al[31] investigated the effects of naloxone, saline and a no-substance control intervention on PFGS, pressure pain threshold (PPT), thermal pain threshold and an upper limb neural provocation test (ULTT2b), immediately after the application of a MWM lateral glide to the elbow. The authors reported no significant difference between naloxone, saline and control conditions, which implicated a non-opioid-mediated pain modulation mechanism of action for MWM in participants with LE. There was insufficient data reported to enable further analyses.

Table 3.3 Quality rating results using a modified Quality Rating Scale[14]

Criteria First author	1	2	3	4	5	6	7	8	9	10	11	12	13
Konstantinou[48]	1	1	1	1	2	1	1	0	1	1	0	0	1
Bisset[28]	1	1	1	0	2	1	1	1	1	0	0	0	0
Paungmali[4]	1	1	1	1	2	1	1	1	1	1	0	0	0
Reid 2008[50]	1	1	1	1	1	1	1	1	1	1	0	0	0
Vicenzino[5]	1	1	1	1	2	1	1	1	1	1	0	0	0
Vicenzino[30]	1	1	1	1	2	1	1	1	1	1	0	0	0
Paungmali[31]	1	1	0	1	2	1	1	1	1	1	0	0	0
Hall[29]	1	1	1	1	2	1	1	0	1	1	0	0	0
Paungmali[34]	1	1	1	1	2	1	1	1	1	1	0	0	0
Reid[41]	1	1	1	1	1	1	1	0	1	1	0	0	0
Teys[6]	1	1	1	1	1	1	1	1	1	1	0	0	0
Collins[1]	1	1	1	1	1	1	1	1	1	1	0	0	0
Yang[37]	1	1	1	0	2	1	1	0	0	0	0	0	0
Kachingwe[38]	1	1	1	1	2	1	1	0	1	1	0	0	0
Hall[46]	1	1	1	1	2	1	1	0	0	1	0	0	0
Abbott[32]	1	1	1	1	2	1	1	0	1	0	0	0	0
Creighton[27]	1	1	1	1	1	1	1	0	1	1	0	0	0
Abbott[7]	1	1	1	1	1	1	1	0	1	1	0	0	0
Manchanda[23]	1	1	0	1	1	1	1	0	0	1	0	0	1
Kochar[25]	1	1	1	1	1	1	1	0	0	0	0	0	1
DeSantis[2]	1	1	1	1	2	1	0	0	1	0	0	0	1
McLean[33]	1	1	0	1	0	0	1	0	0	1	0	0	0
Vicenzino[35]	1	1	0	1	1	1	0	0	1	0	0	0	0
O'Brien[43]	1	1	0	1	1	0	0	0	1	0	0	0	0
Naik[24]	1	0	1	0	0	1	0	0	0	1	0	0	1
Hsieh[53]	1	1	0	1	1	1	0	0	1	0	0	0	1
Backstrom[51]	1	1	1	1	1	1	0	0	1	0	0	0	0
Richardson[49]	1	0	1	1	2	1	0	0	0	0	0	1	0
Stephens[36]	0	0	1	1	2	1	0	0	1	0	0	0	0
Penso[44]	1	1	1	1	0	1	0	0	0	0	0	0	1
Horton[47]	0	0	1	1	1	0	0	0	1	0	0	0	0
Exelby[3]	0	0	1	1	1	0	0	0	1	0	0	0	0
Gebhardt[39]	1	0	0	0	0	1	0	0	1	0	0	0	0
Carpenter[55]	1	0	1	0	2	0	0	0	0	0	0	0	0
Folk[52]	0	0	1	1	1	0	0	0	0	0	0	0	0
Hetherington[42]	0	0	0	1	0	0	0	0	0	0	0	0	1
Merlin[26]	0	0	0	1	0	0	0	0	0	0	0	0	0
Mulligan[40]	0	0	0	1	0	0	0	0	1	0	0	0	0
total	30	26	27	32	46	28	20	8	25	17	0	0	9
%	81	70	73	86	62	76	55	22	68	46	0	0	24

(Continued)

Table 3.3 Quality rating results using a modified Quality Rating Scale—cont'd

14	15	16	17	18	19	20	21	22	23	24	25	26	27	total	%
1	1	1	1	1	1	1	1	1	1	1	0	1	1	24	86
0	1	1	1	1	1	1	1	1	1	1	1	1	1	22	79
0	1	1	1	1	1	1	1	0	1	1	0	1	1	22	79
0	1	1	1	1	1	1	1	0	1	1	0	1	1	21	75
0	1	1	1	1	1	1	1	0	1	0	0	1	0	20	71
0	1	1	1	1	0	1	1	0	1	1	0	1	0	20	71
1	1	1	1	1	1	1	0	0	1	1	0	1	0	20	71
1	1	1	1	1	0	1	0	0	1	1	0	1	1	20	71
0	0	1	1	1	1	1	1	0	0	0	0	1	1	19	68
0	1	1	1	1	1	1	1	0	1	0	0	1	1	19	68
0	1	1	1	1	0	1	1	0	1	0	0	1	0	18	64
0	1	1	1	1	0	1	1	0	1	0	0	1	0	18	64
0	1	1	1	1	0	1	1	0	1	1	1	1	1	18	64
0	1	1	0	1	0	1	1	0	1	0	0	1	0	17	61
0	0	1	1	1	1	1	1	1	0	0	0	0	0	16	57
0	0	1	1	1	0	1	0	0	0	0	0	1	0	14	50
0	0	1	0	1	0	1	1	0	0	0	0	1	0	14	50
0	0	0	1	1	0	1	0	0	0	0	0	1	0	13	46
0	0	1	1	1	0	0	0	0	1	0	0	0	0	12	43
0	0	1	0	1	0	0	1	0	0	0	0	0	0	11	39
0	0	0	0	0	0	1	0	0	0	0	0	1	0	11	39
0	0	1	1	1	0	1	0	0	1	0	0	0	0	10	36
0	0	0	1	1	0	1	0	0	0	0	0	1	0	10	36
0	0	1	0	1	0	1	0	0	0	0	0	1	0	9	32
0	0	0	0	0	0	0	1	1	1	0	0	0	0	8	29
0	0	0	0	0	0	0	0	0	0	0	0	1	0	8	29
0	0	0	0	0	0	0	0	0	0	0	0	1	0	8	29
0	0	0	0	0	0	0	0	0	0	0	0	0	0	7	25
0	0	0	0	0	0	0	0	0	0	0	0	1	0	7	25
0	0	0	0	0	0	0	0	0	0	0	0	0	0	6	21
0	0	0	0	0	0	0	0	0	0	0	0	1	0	5	18
0	0	0	0	0	0	0	0	0	0	0	0	0	0	4	14
0	0	0	0	0	0	0	0	0	0	0	0	1	0	4	14
0	0	0	0	0	0	0	0	0	0	0	0	0	0	4	14
0	0	0	0	0	0	0	0	0	0	0	0	0	0	3	11
0	0	0	0	0	0	0	0	1	0	0	0	0	0	3	11
0	0	1	1	0	0	0	0	0	0	0	0	0	0	3	11
0	0	0	0	0	0	0	0	0	0	0	0	0	0	2	7
3	12	21	19	22	8	21	15	5	15	7	2	24	7		
8	32	57	51	59	22	57	41	14	41	19	5	65	19		

Table 3.4 Study designs, scores and methodological data variation

Study design N = 38	Authors	Reporting (/11)	External validity (/3)	Bias (/7)	Con-founding (/6)	Power (/1)	Total (/28)	Quality score mean (SD)
RCT (6)	Bisset[28]	9	0	6	6	1	22	16.7 (5.6)
	Reid[50]	10	0	6	4	1	21	
	Hall[29]	10	0	6	3	1	20	
	Kachingwe[38]	10	0	4	3	0	17	
	Manchanda & Grover[23]	7	1	3	0	0	12	
	Naik7[24]	4	1	0	0	0	8	
RCT with participants as own control (9)	Konstantinou[48]	10	1	7	5	1	24	19.9 (2.0)
	Paungmali[4]	11	0	6	4	1	22	
	Paungmali[31]	10	0	7	3	0	20	
	Vicenzino[30]	11	0	5	4	0	20	
	Vicenzino[5]	11	0	6	3	0	20	
	Reid[41]	9	0	6	3	1	19	
	Collins[1]	10	0	5	3	0	18	
	Teys[6]	10	0	5	3	0	18	
	Yang[37]	7	0	5	5	1	18	
Quasi-randomised trial (1)	Kochar & Dogra[25]	7	1	2	1	0	11	11
Single group pre- post-test design (6)	Paungmali[4]	11	0	5	2	1	19	12.5 (5.5)
	Hall[46]	9	0	5	2	0	16	
	Abbott 2001a[7]	9	0	4	1	0	14	
	Abbott 2001b[32]	9	0	3	1	0	13	
	McLean[33]	5	0	4	1	0	10	
	Merlin[26]	1	0	2	0	0	3	
Case study (2)	Vicenzino & Wright[35]	6	0	3	1	0	10	9.5 (0.7)
	O'Brien & Vicenzino[43]	5	0	3	1	0	9	
Case report (14)	Creighton[54]	9	0	3	2	0	14	6.0 (3.5)
	DeSantis & Hasson[2]	8	1	1	1	0	11	
	Backstrom[51]	7	0	0	1	0	8	
	Hsieh[53]	6	1	0	1	0	8	
	Stephens[36]	6	0	0	1	0	7	
	Richardson[49]	6	1	0	0	0	7	
	Penso[44]	5	1	0	0	0	6	
	Horton[47]	4	0	0	1	0	5	
	Exelby[45]	4	0	0	0	0	4	
	Gebhardt[39]	3	0	0	1	0	4	
	Folk[52]	3	0	0	0	0	3	

(Continued)

Table 3.4 Study designs, scores and methodological data variation—cont'd

Study design N = 38	Authors	Reporting (/11)	External validity (/3)	Bias (/7)	Con-founding (/6)	Power (/1)	Total (/28)	Quality score mean (SD)
	Hetherington[42]	1	1	0	1	0	3	
	Mulligan[40]	2	0	0	0	0	2	
	Carpenter[55]	2	0	0	0	0	2	
Mean (SD)		7.1 (3.0)	0.2 (0.4)	2.9 (2.5)	1.9 (1.6)	0.2 (0.4)	12.1 (6.7)	
Range		1–11	0–1	0–7	0–6	0–1	2–24	

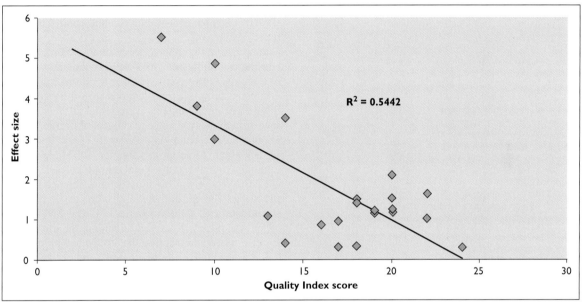

Figure 3.2 Effect size versus Quality Index score for pain-free grip strength and range of motion outcomes, where available

Four studies[7, 32–34] reported pre- to post-test data for a single group intervention, all involving a MWM lateral glide to the elbow. Abbott et al[32] reported an immediate improvement in PFGS and maximum grip strength on the affected side after the application of a single session of MWM lateral glides to the elbow (effect size, Table 3.8). Paungmali et al[34] also assessed the effects of MWM lateral glides to the elbow on outcomes of PFGS, as well as PPT in participants with unilateral LE. However, this intervention differed from Abbott et al[32] in that the participants received six treatment sessions in total. The authors reported a significant improvement in PFGS over the course of the treatments (45.29%; P = 0.05), but not in PPT (P = 0.59), concluding that the hypoalgesic effect of the MWM technique did not reduce, or become tolerant to, repeated applications of the technique. This suggested that opioid peptides do not play a significant role in the hypoalgesic properties of the MWM technique in participants with LE. Abbott[7] also investigated the immediate effects of a MWM lateral glide to the affected elbow on outcomes of shoulder internal and external rotation ROM. He found significant improvement in both internal and external rotation ROM for both the affected and unaffected sides. Finally, McLean et al[33] investigated the required force for optimal changes in PFGS during a MWM lateral glide to the affected elbow, and demonstrated that best results are gained when a MWM is applied at either 66% or 100% of maximum force.

One single case study[35] and one single case report[36] both reported positive effects in terms of pain and grip strength, in an individual with LE. Raw data was estimated from figures within the Vicenzino and Wright[35] study to allow calculation of an effect size (Table 3.8).

Table 3.5 Outcome measures in 38 studies of MWM treatments

Outcome measures	Number of studies
PAIN SCALES TOTAL:	16
Numerical rating scale (NRS) 0–10	5
Visual analogue scale (VAS) 0–100 mm	7
Unspecified	4
PAIN/SYMPTOM & FUNCTION RATING SCALES TOTAL:	14
Patient assessment of subjective improvement	6
Functional VAS 0–100 mm	2
Severity of dizziness VAS 0–100 mm	1
Assessor's rating of severity VAS 0–100 mm	1
Shoulder function questionnaires:	1
• Flexi-level Scale of Shoulder Function (FLEX-SF) Pain-Free Index	1
• Shoulder Pain and Disability Index (SPADI)	2
• Disability of Arm, Shoulder and Hand scale (DASH)	1
Pain-free function questionnaire (elbow)	2
Functional pain scale for tennis elbow	1
Kaikkonen ankle function questionnaire	1
Quality of Life Short Form 36 (SF-36)	1
Headache severity index	2
Dizziness handicap inventory	1
Lower Extremity Functional Score (LEFS)	1
Western Ontario and McMaster University Index (WOMAC)	1
Harris Hip Function Scale	1
Thumb Motion Scale and Functional Assessment Tool (origin unknown)	1
PHYSICAL EVALUATION TOTAL:	30
Pain-free grip strength	8
Maximum grip strength	3
Pressure pain threshold	8
Range of motion	18
Manual muscle test (0–5)	2
Muscle length	2
Weights test	2
Posterior talus glide	1
Sympathetic nervous system indicators	1
Thermal pain threshold	3
Upper limb tension test 2b	1
Standing balance	2

Note: several papers used more than one outcome measure in each category.

Insufficient data was available from two studies to enable calculation of effect size.[25, 36]

In summary, there is level 1b evidence that MWM in combination with an exercise program is superior to a wait-and-see approach in the short term and superior to corticosteroid injections in the long term. As a single treatment, there is level 2a evidence that a MWM treatment is superior to placebo and control treatments for measures of PFGS, immediately after the intervention has been applied.

MWM for shoulder pain

Six studies assessed the effects of a MWM technique to the shoulder in patients with shoulder pain. Of these, three studies satisfied the criteria of 50% or more on the quality rating scale to be included in further analyses.[6, 37, 38] Due to heterogeneity in participant populations, outcome measures and follow-up time periods, it was not possible to pool data from any studies.

Teys et al[6] investigated the immediate effects of a MWM technique on ROM and PPT in participants with shoulder pain that limited elevation ROM. They found that the MWM intervention resulted in significantly greater improvement in ROM (P<0.02) and PPT (P<0.05) compared with placebo and control interventions (Table 3.7).

Yang et al[37] compared three interventions (MWM, end-range mobilisation, mid-range mobilisation) across two groups with frozen shoulder syndrome, with each group receiving all interventions in a different order. Significant improvements were found at 12 weeks follow-up in the MWM and end-range mobilisation groups in outcomes of disability assessment (Flexi-level Scale of Shoulder Function), shoulder ROM (elevation, internal/external rotation) and scapulohumeral rhythm (P<0.01). There was no significant difference between the MWM and end-range mobilisation group except in scapulohumeral rhythm (Table 3.7). The MWM technique was poorly described, including the direction of the arm movements during the MWM technique.

Kachingwe et al[38] compared 6 weeks of MWM glides to the shoulder with three other groups who received either passive glenohumeral joint mobilisations, exercises or a control intervention, in 33 patients with a diagnosis of primary shoulder impingement. The timing of follow-up measures was unclear, but the authors reported that all groups showed significant improvements in pain, ROM and function over time, however, there was no significant difference between groups at follow-up. It should be noted that the group numbers were small (between seven and nine participants per group) and no sample size calculations were performed, so it is likely that a Type II error occurred and results should be interpreted with caution.

Studies by DeSantis and Hasson[2], Gebhardt et al[39] and Mulligan[40] were all case reports that gave raw data outcomes across a variety of shoulder conditions, including 'subacromial impingement', 'painful dysfunctional shoulder' and 'shoulder impingement'. All three papers reported positive findings using the MWM technique either as a sole intervention[40] or in combination with other techniques such as ice, exercise, education, other joint mobilisations and pain-relieving modalities[2, 39]. There was insufficient data from these three studies to calculate pre- to post-intervention effect size for MWM.

Table 3.6 Characteristics of all studies

Author	Participants	Intervention	Outcome measures	Results	Comments
Abbott[7]	25 participants with LE. 17 men, 8 women. Mean age: 46 years (range 29–60 years).	MWM lateral glide of proximal medial forearm with the distal humerus stabilised, whilst participant performed previously painful movement (fist, gripping, wrist extension, 3rd finger extension), to both affected and unaffected arms. Frequency: 1 session.	PFGS. MGS.	PFGS and MGS were significantly increased post-intervention for the affected limb only. PFGS was found to be more responsive to change compared with MGS.	Single group pre-test/ post-test of initial effects, order of treating and testing the affected and unaffected arms were randomised. Excluded any person who responded negatively to MWM at initial assessment.
Abbott[32]	23 participants with LE. 18 men, 5 women, age not reported. Duration of condition mean 16 months (range 1 month to 8 years).	MWM lateral glide of proximal medial forearm with the distal humerus stabilised, whilst participant performed previously painful movement (fist, gripping, wrist extension, 3rd finger extension), to both affected and unaffected arms. Frequency: 1 session.	Passive ROM of shoulder internal and external rotation using a gravity dependent goniometer.	Shoulder external rotation range on the affected side was significantly less compared with unaffected side pre-intervention, with no significant difference between affected and unaffected shoulder internal rotation pre-intervention. Both IR and ER on affected side significantly increased post-intervention, with some suggestion of increased ROM on the unaffected side also.	Single group pre-test/ post-test of initial effects, order of treatment and testing of affected and unaffected arms were randomised. Excluded any person who responded negatively to MWM at initial assessment.
Back-strom[51]	61-year-old female with de Quervain's tenosynovitis of the right wrist.	Manipulation of capitate on first session only, MWM, elastic splint with horseshoe type insert (introduced on session 6), eccentric and concentric strengthening, active ROM, tendon gliding, transverse friction, anti-inflammatories and HEP (ROM, strengthening, tendon gliding, frictions, self-MWM) MWM: radial glide of proximal row of carpal bones. Three sets of 10 repetitions for each movement (wrist flexion, extension, ulna and radial deviation, and thumb radial or palmar abduction), applied at all sessions. Weight-bearing technique — participant weight bears through the hand and the same radial glide was performed as participant progressively weight-bearing through the right upper limb. Ulna glide of trapezium and trapezoid for thumb radial abduction. Self-MWM — weight-bearing through upper limb. Participant applied ulnar glide on forearm (therefore radial glide of carpal bones), shifted body weight (wrist flexion/extension) with thumb abducted.	Pain: VAS. Observation. ROM (goniometer). Wrist flexion, extension, radial and ulnar deviation. Thumb palmer and radial abduction. Strength — isometric and MMT. Accessory motion testing. Palpation. Finklestein test.	Rapid reduction in pain level, 25% after first session, and 50% after third session. After 12 sessions (2 month treatment period) all impairments resolved except 0.5 cm of swelling at the right wrist. There were no painful limitations for activities of daily living. At 12 month follow-up there was still no evidence of wrist/thumb pain or functional deficits whatsoever.	Single case study.

(Continued)

Table 3.6 Characteristics of all studies—cont'd

Author	Participants	Intervention	Outcome measures	Results	Comments
Bisset[28]	198 participants with LE. 128 men, 70 women. Mean age: 48 (SD 7.8) years. Median duration of condition 22 weeks (range 12–42 weeks).	Group 1: 8 sessions of physiotherapy. Group 2: corticosteroid injection. Group 3: wait-and-see. Physiotherapy: 8 sessions for 30 min over 6 weeks. Included MWM, isometric/concentric/eccentric exercises and taping. MWM lateral glide of proximal medial forearm with the distal humerus stabilised, whilst participant performed previously painful movement (fist, gripping, wrist extension, 3rd finger extension). Corticosteroid injection: 1 injection, and a 2nd one if necessary after 2 weeks. Wait-and-see: advice, education on modification of activity, encourage non-provocative activity, use of analgesic drugs, heat, cold and braces as required.	3, 6, 12, 26 and 52 weeks (primary endpoints 6 and 52 weeks). Global improvement. Pain-free grip force. Assessor's rating of severity. Pain VAS. Elbow disability (pain-free function questionnaire). Success.	Corticosteroid injection showed significantly better effects at 6 weeks but with high recurrence rates thereafter (47/65 suffered a recurrence in their elbow pain) and significantly poorer outcomes in the long-term compared with the physiotherapy group. Physiotherapy was superior to wait-and-see at 6 weeks but there was no difference at 52 weeks with both reporting a successful outcome. Physiotherapy was superior to injections after 6 weeks.	RCT, blinded assessor, concealed allocation, intention to treat analysis.
Carpenter[55]	53-year-old woman with 3 month history left lateral hip pain.	Three treatment sessions over 4 weeks, consisting of anterior passive mobilisations followed by MWM for hip flexion, therapeutic exercise.	NPRS: 0-10. Lower Extremity Functional Score (LEFS) Western Ontario and McMaster University Index (WOMAC) Harris Hip Function Scale Global Rating of Change	NPRS: 1/10. LEFS: 62/80. WOMAC: 44/96. Harris Hip Function Scale: 88/100. Global Rating of Change: 'a great deal better'.	Single case study.
Collins[1]	16 participants. 8 men, 8 women. Mean age: 28 (14 participants analysed) sub-acute Grade II lateral ligament ankle sprain. Mean duration of condition 40 (SD 24) days.	Group 1: MWM. Group 2: placebo. Group 3: control. MWM: at talocrural joint. Participant weight-bearing in stance position with affected leg forward. Belt around therapist's pelvis and distal tibia and fibula. Therapist leaned back to create postero-anterior glide, with talus and forefoot stabilised by therapist's hand and other hand over proximal tibia and fibula to maintain leg alignment. Placebo: a/a with belt over calcaneum and minimal force, with stabilising hand over metatarsals. Control: participant in stance position for 5 minutes with no manual contact of therapist.	Before and after treatment weight-bearing DF ROM. PPT. TPT.	DF ROM: significantly increased in only the MWM group. PPT and TPT: no significant results, except an increase in PPT in the placebo group post-intervention.	Within subject, repeated measures randomised cross-over trial of initial effects, with participants acting as their own control.

(Continued)

Table 3.6 Characteristics of all studies—cont'd

Author	Participants	Intervention	Outcome measures	Results	Comments
Creighton[54]	Six participants with clinical diagnosis of unilateral anterior knee pain (patellofemoral pain syndrome). Age range 35–74 years.	Stretching rectus femoris in side lie with sustained anterior translation of proximal tibia for 2 minutes; versus open kinetic chain assisted knee extension with anterior translation glide of proximal tibia, for 20 minutes with 30 seconds rest every 5 minutes. Results of 6 treatments reported.	NPRS 0–10. Passive knee flexion ROM in prone (goniometer).	Both techniques significantly reduced NPRS: open chain exercise reduced pain to 0.92 (range 0–1.6; p = 0.016). Rectus femoris stretch reduced pain to 0 (p = 0.016); knee ROM also significantly increased (p = 0.000).	Case series, unclear if all subjects received both interventions. Within subject pre-post-intervention over six treatment sessions.
DeSantis & Hasson[2]	27-year-old male with left shoulder supraspinatus tendinopathy.	Physiotherapy 3 times a week for 30 minutes for total 12 sessions. Warm-up: 5 min warm-up on cycle ergometer prior to each session. Phase 1: focused on decreasing pain (education on rest, cryotherapy, restoring ROM with MWM). MWM: AP glide with abduction movement (guiding movement of the scapular and humerus with both hands). Phase 2: focused on strengthening rotator cuff, scapular stabilising muscles, improving function, education regarding posture. Each session ended with 10 min of cryotherapy.	NPRS and abduction ROM at every session. Active abduction ROM measured with a goniometer, manual muscle test, impingement tests (Neer, Hawkins-Kennedy, empty can, apprehension), functional status (Shoulder Pain and Disability Index), SF-36 (global self-report questionnaire).	During each MWM session, NPRS score was reduced by 2–3 points. Rx sessions 4–6 of MWM improved pain-free ROM by 30–45°; by the last session = 175° (overall increase = 80°) (clinically sig). MWM stopped on seventh session as participant no longer reported pain during active abduction, had achieved near-full active ROM and had very little pain on overhead activities. At discharge the patient had improved function, improvement (>10%) on disability scales with no positive impingement tests.	Single case study.
Exelby[45]	46-year-old female with 3 day history right-sided low back pain.	Cephalad SNAG L4 in 4-point knee, 5 repetitions, followed by cephalad SNAG L5 with anterior pelvic tilt, tape across erector spinae at L4. 4-point rocking and anterior pelvic tilt were prescribed as home exercises.	None reported.	None reported.	Single case report.
Folk[52]	39-year-old female, 4.5 weeks after strain to 1st MCP, with diagnosis of de Quervain's of the left hand.	Received occupational therapy (7 sessions in 6 weeks), then referred for trigger thumb release surgery, then back to occupational therapy, which then referred to physiotherapy. Prior treatment included 2 corticosteroid injections, splint and gutter use, active ROM exercises, surgical release of trigger thumb. Physiotherapy treatment: MWM at 1st metacarpophalangeal joint with sustained pain-free internal axial rotation, with overpressure at the end.	Follow-up at 2 months and 1 year post treatment. Pain (metacarpophalangeal extension). Swelling. ROM (metacarpophalangeal extension). MMT. Grip strength. Upper limb tension tests. Cervical spine assessment. de Quervain's tests (Finkelstein, pincer strength, palpation).	Occupational therapy treatment had not improved patient's symptoms overall over past 10 months. Patient had persistent loss of motion, tenderness, trigger symptoms and loss of daily function. Patient's preoperative symptoms had not improved after the operation. Once referred to physiotherapy, and performed MWM treatment, 1 session of MWM treatment abolished pain with metacarpophalangeal extension and the patient cancelled second physiotherapy appointment, as all activities were now symptom-free. At follow-up (2 months and 1 year) the patient confirmed she had remained symptom-free post the MWM treatment.	Single case report.

(Continued)

Table 3.6 Characteristics of all studies—cont'd

Author	Participants	Intervention	Outcome measures	Results	Comments
Geb-hardt[39]	48-year-old male with several week history of right shoulder pain of insidious onset; decreased shoulder ROM, hypomobile glenohumeral and acromioclavicular joints, rotator cuff and scapula muscle weakness.	MWM of the shoulder girdle.	Disability of arm, shoulder and hand scale (DASH). Global rating of change scale (GROC).	Initial DASH 14.2, post-intervention DASH 3.7. GROC 'a great deal better'.	Single case report, unknown number of sessions, unclear exactly what technique was used, number of repetitions, ROM outcomes not reported.
Hall[46]	19 participants (11 women, 8 men, mean age 37 SD 12 years), with current episode of LBP and limited SLR, mean duration 2 years 9 months, mean pain over previous week 4.6 (SD 2.4) cm on 10cm VAS.	MWM single treatment session. Traction SLR with passive SLR to onset discomfort for 3 repetitions.	Pre- post-intervention. SLR range.	SLR increased by 11° (22%) after intervention, mechanosensitivity did not influence outcome.	Single group pre-test/ post-test of initial effects within a single session.
Hall[29]	32 participants with clinical diagnosis of cervicogenic headaches and restricted ROM of at least 10° on the flexion-rotation test; 19 women; mean age 36 (SD 3) years, mean history of headaches 6 (SD 3.5) years.	Single treatment session of C1-C2 self-SNAG using a cervical self-SNAG strap or placebo (3-second sustained forward glide on C1 using the strap, but no movement of the head); 3 familiarisation trials followed by 2 repetitions of treatment.	Cervical flexion-rotation test (only measured immediately post-intervention of a single session). A headache questionnaire, pain severity (10 cm VAS), and questionnaire to assess participant compliance with exercise program were measured at 4 weeks and 12 months follow-up.	Flexion-rotation test improved in both groups post-intervention, although significantly greater in the self-SNAG group: mean difference 15° (SD 9°) versus 5° (SD 5°) for placebo. Headache questionnaire had a mean improvement at 4 weeks for the self-SNAG group of 22/100 (95% CI 16 to 27) and 0 (95% CI -7 to 6) for placebo. At 12 months, the self-SNAG group showed mean improvement of 28/100 (95% CI 22 to 35) and 6 (95% CI 1 to 12) for placebo.	Randomised controlled trial, patient blinded, assessor blinded, single intervention session with primary outcome measure follow-up at 4 weeks and 12 months.
Hether-ington[42]	Patients post ankle sprain with limited and painful ROM.	Majority of patients were treated only with MWMs and taping. No electro-physical therapies were used. MWM: lateral malleolus of fibula glided posteriorly with active inversion (with and without a belt). Taping: two strips of 25mm tape approximately 15cm in length. Posterior glide applied and then tape applied over the lateral malleolus and travelled around the lower leg (taping changed after 24 hrs).	Before, during and after treatment. Pain on inversion. ROM. One-leg standing test (balance — eyes closed). Swelling. Gait patterns.	Re-evaluation of pain-free movement after the MWMs resulted in a marked increase in pain-free ROM. One-leg standing test (eyes closed) post MWMs and taping revealed increased balance equal to that of the uninjured side. Gait patterns also substantially improved.	Case report.

(Continued)

Table 3.6 Characteristics of all studies—cont'd

Author	Participants	Intervention	Outcome measures	Results	Comments
Horton[47]	20-year-old male university student, acute left side thoracic pain.	Central SNAG to T8 with postural correction, x4 repetitions, taping to T8-9 thoracic segment for 1 treatment session, followed by passive joint mobilisations for 1 treatment session.	No outcome measures reported.	Patient reported 94% improvement on second treatment.	Single case study, no outcome measures reported.
Hsieh[53]	79-year-old female with right thumb pain.	MWM was applied to the proximal phalanx. MRI was taken before, during MWM, then after a course of MWM treatment. Participant performed self-MWMs: flexing the thumb while sustaining a supination glide of the proximal phalanx of the thumb using the other hand's index finger and thumb.	MRI: pre treatment, during 1st treatment, after treatment. Week 1: pain, ROM, distraction/compression, passive ROM. Week 2 — a/a. Week 3 — a/a, grip strength. MRI. Pain: VAS. AROM: goniometer (flexion of interphalangeal and metacarpophalangeal joints). Passive ROM: thumb radial abduction. Grip strength: hand dynamometer. Compression/distraction of the metacarpophalangeal joint.	During MWM, positional fault was corrected (under MRI). End of week 1 — still had pain, limited ROM, pain on distraction, pain with passive ROM. End of week 2 — pain, limited ROM, pain with distraction. End of week 3 — no pain, normal ROM, normal grip strength, pain-free distraction. MRI demonstrated patient still had a positional fault.	Single case report.
Kachingwe[38]	33 participants with shoulder impingement. 17 men, 16 women. Mean age: 46.4 years.	Group 1: supervised exercises 1 x weekly for 6 weeks. Group 2: supervised exercises plus glenohumeral joint passive accessory mobilisations 3 sets of 30 seconds, 1 x weekly for 6 weeks. Group 3: supervised exercises plus glenohumeral joint MWM posterior glide with active shoulder flexion 3 sets of 10 repetitions, 1 x weekly for 6 weeks. Group 4: control group, received advice and home exercise program during the initial examination session.	Worst pain VAS over 24 hours. Pain VAS with Neer Impingement test. Pain VAS with Hawkins-Kennedy test. Pain-free active shoulder flexion and scaption ROM (goniometer). Shoulder Pain And Disability Index (SPADI).	All groups had significantly less pain on Worst Pain, Neer and Hawkins-Kennedy tests, and significantly greater ROM and SPADI, but no significant difference between groups for any of the measures. Percentage change also showed no significant difference between groups.	Randomised controlled pilot study, with power calculations done post hoc. Timing of follow-up measures is unclear.

(Continued)

41

Table 3.6 Characteristics of all studies—cont'd

Author	Participants	Intervention	Outcome measures	Results	Comments
Kochar & Dogra[25]	66 participants with LE. 36 men, 30 women. Mean age: 41 years.	Group 1: combination of US and MWM on 10 sessions (different treatment on alternate days) completed in 3 weeks and an exercise program (9 weeks). Group 2: US only on 10 sessions completed in 3 weeks and an exercise program (9 weeks). Group 3 (control): no treatment. US: 3 MHz, 1.5 W/cm2, pulsed 1.5, 5 min. MWM: elbow extended, forearm pronated, 10 repetitions, no pain, glide sustained while participant lifted weight that previously produced pain, for 3 sets, 10 sessions. Progressed MWM by increasing weights by 0.5kg. Exercise: stretching, isometric/concentric/eccentric.	Week 1, 2 and 3. Follow-up at 4 months. Pain — VAS scale. Ability to lift 0-3kg weights with no pain, 24 hrs after treatment. Grip strength. Weights test.	Subjective: treatment group 1 — pain decreased by 5.9cm (p<0.01), and in treatment group 2 by 1.67 cm (p<0.01). Treatment group 1 was superior to the control and group 2 in the assessment score at 12 weeks. Objective: treatment group 1 was able to lift heavier weights than group 2 and control group (p<0.01) from the 2nd week onwards. Grip strength in group 1 improved from 22.7 kg — 31.6 kg in the 3 weeks, and was significantly different from the control. No significant differences were found in group 2. Overall control group showed no statistically significant changes in any parameter. Most patients in the intervention groups showed complete recovery. Five recurrences in the US group.	Three groups, two of which were randomised and a non-randomised control group. Follow-up was only for the two randomised groups.
Konstantinou 2007[48]	26 participants with LBP (pain on lumbar flexion and limited flexion ROM). 15 men, 11 women. Mean age: 38.3 (SD 11.7) years. Duration of symptoms 26.8 (SD 47.9) months.	Flexion MWM central or unilaterally 1 to 3 spinal levels, 2-3 sets x 4-6 repetitions on each level. Placebo: participant lying comfortably on couch for same length of time as MWM intervention (approximately 3 minutes).	Primary outcomes: true and total lumbar spine flexion ROM. Secondary outcomes: pain during lumbar flexion (10 cm VAS) and total lumbar spine extension ROM. ROM measured with two inclinometers, one at spinal level T12 and the second at S2.	Using clinical improvement score of ≥ 7° in ROM and ≥ 2 cm on VAS, 11 and 14 participants after the MWM improved on true lumbar flexion and total lumbar flexion respectively, compared with 6 and 5 participants after the placebo intervention; 11 versus 6 (MWM vs placebo) improved on pain VAS. MWM significantly greater improvement than placebo intervention for true and total flexion, but not total extension or pain VAS.	Single group pre-post-test design, received two interventions in a randomised order, within a single session, assessor blinded to the order of interventions.
Manchanda & Grover[23]	30 participants with LE. 15 men, 15 women. Mean age: Group 1: 39.3 (8.73) years; Group 2: 37 (6.7) years; Group 3: 41.1 (6.95) years.	Group 1: Mulligan MWM 3 sets of 10 repetitions, plused US for 5 minutes, graduated therapeutic exercise program. Group 2: Wrist manipulation 3 sets of 10 repetitions, plused US for 5 minutes, graduated therapeutic exercise program. Group 3: pulsed US for 5 minutes, graduated therapeutic exercise program. Each group received 15 treatment sessions, each lasting approximately 30 minutes.	Pain VAS for worst pain in last 24 hours. Weights test: able to lift the weight of their own arm, then 1 kg, 2 kg or 3 kg etc. as required without pain. Functional pain scale for tennis elbow. Follow-ups at day 1, 5, 10 and 15.	All 3 groups improved over time in pain VAS, weights test and function scores. No significant difference between groups for pain VAS or functional pain scale. MWM (group 1) was significantly better than plused US (group 3) at days 10 and 15 on the weights test (P< 0.05).	Randomised controlled trial, no blinding of participants, therapists or outcome assessors, no concealed allocation, no intention to treat analyses. Participants received 15 treatment sessions in 15 days.

(Continued)

Table 3.6 Characteristics of all studies—cont'd

Author	Participants	Intervention	Outcome measures	Results	Comments
McLean[33]	Six participants with LE. 2 men, 4 women. Mean age: 49 years (range 39–58 years).	MWM force levels were determined at assessment for 33%, 50%, 66% and maximum. All participants received applications of the 4 force levels in a random order. MWM: directed towards the medial aspect of the ulna. Duration of each treatment technique was no more than 10 seconds. Three applications with contraction for baseline measure. Two applications of the 4 force levels, with 2 min rest intervals.	Before and after treatment PFGS. Muscle force: measured with a flexible pressure sensing mat between hand and elbow.	Mean raw force data ranged from 36.8N–113N. Mean standardised force data was 1.2N/cm and 3.8N/cm. The two lower standardised force level scores (1.2 and 1.9N/cm) caused a drop in PFGS, whereas the higher two (2 and 3.8N/cm) caused an increase in PFGS. A-priori contrasts showed no significant change in PFGS between the two lower force levels, but was significantly greater for the third (66%) force level. Overall, level of force applied during a MWM determines the hypoalgesic effects. Grip strength changes observed = 15–18%.	Single group, repeated measures over two sessions (one assessment, one testing), pre- post-test design.
Merlin[26]	Eight participants with recent history of sprain to the ankle lateral ligament complex.	MWM posterior/cephalad directed glide to the lateral malleolus with active ankle plantar flexion/inversion, 3 sets of 10 repetitions.	Before and after treatment ROM, pain VAS and single leg standing balance with eyes closed. Position of fibula measured using MRI, tip of fibula to sole of foot.	Significant improvement in ROM and standing balance, but no significant difference in pain was reported.	Single group, pre-post-test design of a single treatment session. Unable to utilise data due to a lack of clarity of the units of measurement and variability reported.
Mulligan[40]	30-year-old female with 2 year history of shoulder pain and limited ROM, 45-year-old female with 1 year history of shoulder pain and limited ROM, 24-year-old male with 3 day history of shoulder pain and limited ROM, 35-year-old male with shoulder pain of unknown duration.	Each patient received a varying number of treatments (range 1–4 sessions).	No outcome measures reported.	No outcome data reported.	Four individual case reports, two patients had one session, one patient had two sessions and one patient had four sessions.

(Continued)

Table 3.6	Characteristics of all studies—cont'd				
Author	Participants	Intervention	Outcome measures	Results	Comments
Naik[24]	30 participants with radiological diagnosis of Colles' fracture who have undergone external fixation and removed after 2 months. No demographics of participants given.	Group 1: moist heat 15 minutes, Maitland mobilisations (Grade 1 and 2) for 1st week, then Grade 3 and 4 for 2nd week.. Group 2: moist heat 15 minutes, 'Mulligan manipulations'.	Wrist ROM (flexion/ extension, radial/ulnar deviation, supination/ pronation). Thumb Motion Scale and Functional Assessment Tool.	MWM (Group 2) reported greater pain relief (p = 0.029) compared with the Maitland mobilisations (Group 1). The results for ROM are unclear, but it appears there was no significant difference between pre- and post-intervention for any ROM except active wrist flexion, which showed a significant increase after the Maitland mobilisation (p = 0.02). There was no significant difference for either group for the Functional Assessment Tool.	Randomised trial. It is unclear what is meant by 'external fixation' in the inclusion criteria for these participants. Colles' fractures rarely require external fixation, so it is likely the authors mean closed reduction with plaster or fibreglass fixation. Number of treatments unclear, no blinding of participant, therapist or assessor, no concealed allocation, no intention to treat analyses. It is unclear how pain was measured, and the reported data for all outcomes are ambiguous.
O'Brien & Vicenzino[43]	Two male participants with recent (2–3 days) lateral ankle sprains. Aged 17 and 18 years.	To determine the effectiveness of MWM applied at the ankle for acute lateral ankle pain. MWM treatment: posterior glide of distal fibula while participant inverted the ankle. Passive overpressure was applied. Repeated 4 times. Treatment 1: 6 sessions over 2 weeks. Treatment 2: 3 sessions over 1 week. No Treatment 1: 3 sessions over 1 week. No Treatment 2: 5 measurement sessions over 1 week. Strapping tape was applied to maintain the posterior glide after every treatment session.	Before, during (pain, inversion ROM) and after each treatment. Pain: VAS. ROM: inversion using a modified pedal goniometer. DF ROM measured in weight-bearing knee to wall. Functional performance (Kaikkonen scale). Function VAS.	ROM: (inversion) improved during MWM and to a lesser extent post treatment. DF improved post MWM treatment. Pain: improved during MWM and to a lesser extent post treatment. Function: increased with treatment. Functional performance: strong positive correlation between MWM treatment and function. Strong correlations between functional performance and function, pain and function, functional performance and pain, functional performance and DF, DF and function. Moderate correlations with pain and function, inversion and DF, functional performance and inversion, inversion and function.	Two single case studies with BABC AND ABAC designs. A = non-intervention period. B = intervention period. C = post-treatment session of home exercises.

(Continued)

Table 3.6 Characteristics of all studies—cont'd

Author	Participants	Intervention	Outcome measures	Results	Comments
Paung-mali[4]	24 participants with LE. 17 men, 7 women. Mean age: 49 (SD 7.2) years, mean duration of condition 8.9 (SD 8.4) months, all right hand dominant, 20 participants were right side affected.	Each participant completed the 3 randomised treatment groups (treatment, placebo, control), at same time of day. 48 hrs in between each session. Treatment group: lateral glide MWM to the ulna and radius with pain-free dynamometer gripping. Participant supine, with shoulder internally rotated, elbow extended, forearm pronation. 10 repetitions, for 6 seconds, 15 second rest period. Placebo: PT applied a firm manual contact with both hands over the elbow joint whilst the participant gripped the dynamometer pain-free. Control: involved the pain gripping action only (no manual force applied).	Before, during and after treatment. PFGS. PPT. TPT. Sympathetic nervous system indicators: • cutaneous blood flux • skin conductance • skin temperature • blood pressure • heart rate.	PFGS significantly improved in the MWM group during and after treatment, but not during or following the placebo and control groups. PPT significantly improved in the MWM group after treatment, but not following the placebo and control groups. There was no change in TPT for the MWM or placebo group, but it decreased (i.e. got worse) after the control intervention. The sympathetic nervous system changes with the MWM intervention, but no changes for placebo or control interventions.	Within subject, repeated measures randomised cross-over trial, with participants acting as their own control, immediate pre- post-intervention measures.
Paung-mali[34]	24 participants with LE. 19 men, 5 women. Mean age: 50 years.	All participants received lateral glide MWM. Applied on 6 occasions, approximately 48 hours apart. MWM: patient supine with shoulder in internal rotation, elbow extended and supinated. Therapist stabilised the humerus and applied lateral glide at forearm. Technique performed was pain-free with participants maintaining a grip for approximately 6 seconds and repeated 10 times with 15 seconds rest intervals.	Before and after every treatment. PFGS. PPT.	MWM technique produced a mean Maximal Possible Effect of 38.84% (SEM 7.05) in PFGS during the treatment and 45.29% (SEM 8.12) immediately after the treatment application, and 17.51% (SEM6.95) in PPT across all experimental sessions. There were no significant differences between sessions indicating that tolerance did not develop in the hypoalgesic effect of MWM.	Single group, repeated measures over six sessions.
Paung-mali[31]	18 participants with LE. 14 men, 4 women. Mean age 49 (SD 2.4) years, 94% right side dominant, 78% right side affected.	Intravenous administration of naloxone (0.8 mg in 2mL of 2% lidocain), placebo of 2 mL normal saline administered as per the naloxone procedure and a no-substance control condition. Each was administered on separate occasions over 3 days. Each participant received MWM to the affected elbow: participant supine with shoulder in internal rotation, elbow extended and supinated. Therapist stabilised the humerus and applied lateral glide at forearm. Technique performed was pain-free with participants maintaining a grip for 6 repetitions with 15 second rest intervals.	PFGS. PPT. TPT. Upper limb neural provocation test 2b (ULTT2b).	MWM technique produced a mean improvement of 29% (SEM 5.6) in PFGS, 18% (SEM 4.3) in PPT, 1.6% (SEM 0.4) in ULTT2b and 0.2% (SEM 0.7) in TPT across all experimental conditions. There was no significant difference between naloxone, saline and control interventions. Naloxone did not antagonise the initial hypoalgesic effect, suggesting that the MWM technique induces a non-opioid form of analgesia.	Within subject, repeated measures randomised cross-over trial, with participants acting as their own control, immediate pre- post-intervention measures.

(Continued)

Table 3.6 Characteristics of all studies—cont'd

Author	Participants	Intervention	Outcome measures	Results	Comments
Penso[44]	25-year-old female runner, chronic left medial ankle pain during 7–10 km 2 × weekly run. Pain VAS 8/10 with running and stretching calf. Recurrent ankle sprains for 17 years.	MWM — anteroposterior glide of distal tibia with stabilisation of posterior foot, with active ankle dorsiflexion in weight-bearing. 2 × 10 repetitions for 2 treatment sessions. Follow-up after each treatment, and at 1 month and 4 months.	Active and passive pain-free ankle ROM dorsiflexion, plantarflexion, inversion, eversion. Muscle length of gastrocnemius and soleus.	Able to run pain-free after 2 sessions. Dorsiflexion ROM improved from 21° (active and passive) at baseline to 36° (active)/37° (passive) after 2nd treatment and 35° (active)/36° (passive) at 4 months follow-up. Gastrocnemius muscle length improved from 3.25 cm (distance heel to lower step) to 2.5 cm after the second treatment, which was maintained at 4 months follow-up and equal to the unaffected side.	Single case report of 2 treatment sessions. No mention of how ROM outcome measures were taken. Pain and function not measured.
Reid[41]	23 participants. 8 men, 15 women. Unilateral sub-acute ankle sprain sustained within the past 2 years (not within the past 8 weeks), limited ankle dorsiflexion in weight-bearing. Mean age: 25 (SD 9) years, (range 13–47 years).	MWM — weight-bearing ankle dorsiflexion with glide applied (via a padded belt) to the posterior lower leg, the inferior margin of the belt level with the inferior margin of the medial malleolus. Therapist applied a counterforce to fix the talus and calcaneus with her hands, allowing an anterior draw of the tibia via the belt. Force applied to 200 (SD 20) mm Hg measured by a biofeedback pressure device. Sham — participant prone lie, splint applied to the dorsal foot/ankle and therapist performed passive knee flexion/extension with no ankle movement. A single session of 2 sets of 10 repetitions with a 2 minute rest in between sets was applied for each condition, 7 days apart.	Weight-bearing ankle dorsiflexion ROM.	Change in dorsiflexion with MWM technique (0.63, SD 0.89 cm) was greater than change with sham technique (0.18, SD 0.35 cm) p = 0.02. Mean difference in dorsiflexion ROM between the 2 interventions 0.45 cm (95% CI 0.08–0.82).	23 participants, crossover within subjects design, randomised order of intervention, immediate pre- post-test assessments.
Reid[50]	34 participants. 13 men, 21 women. Clinical diagnosis of cervicogenic dizziness. Mean age: 63.5 (SD 13.4) years.	SNAG at C1 or C2 with active cervical movement in the direction that predominantly caused dizziness, 6 repetitions, progressing to 10 repetitions. Sham — detuned laser, 6 applications of 20 s to various sites on upper cervical spine. Both groups received interventions 4–6 times over 4 weeks.	Severity of dizziness (VAS). Dizziness Handicap Inventory (DHI). Frequency of dizziness (6-point rating scale). Pain VAS. Global perceived effect (GPE, 6-point Likert scale). Standing balance (eyes open and closed; sway index). Cervical ROM.	SNAG group significantly less severity of dizziness, lower scores on DHI, and less pain severity than sham group post-treatment and at 6 weeks, but no difference at 12 weeks follow-up. GPE was significantly higher in SNAG group compared to sham at all time points. No significant difference between groups at any time point for frequency of dizziness or cervical ROM.	Randomised controlled trial. The authors reported that participants were blind to treatment or placebo groups, but it is difficult to know if participants would credibly think that the MWM was a placebo, any more so than the laser. Follow-up was post-treatment, 6 weeks and 12 weeks.

(Continued)

Table 3.6 Characteristics of all studies—cont'd

Author	Participants	Intervention	Outcome measures	Results	Comments
Richard-son[49]	29-year-old woman with left-sided sub-occipital headaches of cervicogenic origin of 6 months' duration.	Treatment 3 times per week for 4 weeks, total 11 treatment sessions. SNAGs and reverse SNAGs between occiput and C2, 10 second holds for 6–10 repetitions, massage, ischaemic tissue release, education, therapeutic exercises, moist heat, electrical stimulation.	Pain VAS. Cervical lateral flexion and rotation ROM. Headache Rating System Score.	At discharge: Headache Rating Score: 3/15 Pain VAS: 0/10 Cervical lateral flexion active ROM: 48° left and right Cervical rotation active ROM: 83° right, 84° left.	Single case report, total 11 treatments, no statistical analyses.
Ste-phens[36]	43-year-old woman with left sided 1 year history of LE, past history of bilateral carpal tunnel syndrome requiring surgery, instability of the right carpometacarpal joint resulting in thumb pain and managed with a wrist and thumb splint.	MWM: (a) lateral mobilisation of the forearm at the elbow during active wrist extension, forearm supination and gripping; (b) dorsal glide of the hand applied at the wrist during radial deviation; and (c) metacarpal of the thumb was mobilised palmarly at the carpometacarpal joint during thumb opposition. US: 20% cycle 3 MHz, 1.0 to 1.2 W/cm2 to the lateral elbow for 5 minutes. Transverse friction massage, taping, exercises, gripping with dynamometer, ice massage of trigger points, trigger point massage, stretching of wrist extensors. Home: ice 3 x daily for 20 minutes each. Home exercise program, self mobilisations were performed against a doorway to provide pain relief, advice to avoid aggravating activities. Treatment: 3 x weekly for 4 weeks, then 1 x weekly for 4 weeks, then 1 x fortnightly for 6 weeks.	Pain: NPRS. Active ROM: shoulder, elbow and thumb. Strength: shoulder, elbow, wrist and grip.	No outcome data presented at end of treatment, except for grip strength which improved from 40 with pain to 95 lbs pain-free.	Single case study. Total of 23 treatments, no statistical analyses, poor reporting of data.
Teys[6]	24 participants with shoulder pain. 11 men, 13 women. Mean age: 46 (SD 46.1) years. Unable to elevate arm beyond 100° in plane of the scapula due to shoulder pain.	Group 1: MWM treatment. Group 2: placebo. Group 3: control. MWM: posterolateral glide with patient seated. Therapist placed hands over posterior scapula and the thenar eminence of other hand over anterior aspect of head of humerus. Posterolateral glide applied to humeral head. Participant actively elevated arm in plane of the scapula, 3 x 10 repetitions. Placebo: as above, but hands of therapist were anteriorly on the clavicle and sternum, and posteriorly on humeral head, an anterior glide with minimal force was applied to humerus and participant asked to elevate arm in plane of the scapula to only half available range, 3 x 10 repetitions. Control: no manual contact of therapist for approximately the same time period as the other two interventions. Single session of each intervention given with a minimum 24 hours in between sessions.	Before and after treatment, on 3 sessions. Active pain-free shoulder ROM in the plane of the scapula (goniometer) and PPT.	ROM: mean increase of 16° (p = 0.000) for MWM, 4° (p = 0.06) for placebo and no change (p = 0.84) for control intervention. The MWM had a significantly greater improvement than the placebo (10°) and control (11°). PPT: mean increase of 63 kPa (p = 0.000) for MWM, 26 kPa (p = 0.05) for placebo and 20 kPa (p = 0.07) for control intervention. MWM had a significantly greater improvement than the placebo (45 kPa) and control (46 kPa) interventions.	Within subject, repeated measures randomised cross-over trial, with participants acting as their own control, immediate pre- post-intervention measures.

(Continued)

47

Table 3.6 Characteristics of all studies—cont'd

Author	Participants	Intervention	Outcome measures	Results	Comments
Vicenzino[30]	24 participants with LE. 14 men, 10 women. Mean age: 46 (SD 1.68) years, (range 34–66 years). Duration of condition 8.3 (SD 1.71, range 2–36) months. 83% right arm dominant, 74% right side affected.	MWM: lateral glide of the elbow. One hand gliding the proximal forearm, and other stabilising the distal humerus, while the participant performed pain-free gripping, six repetitions with 15 second rest between repetitions. Placebo: firm manual contact over elbow joint with no glide. Control: no manual contact by the therapist for approximately the same time period as the other two interventions. Each participant received a single session of each intervention on three separate days at least 48 hours apart.	PFGS. PPT.	PFGS on the affected side significantly improved for the MWM intervention (46% change, p<0.000), but not for the placebo (10% change) or control (3% change). There was a significant improvement in PPT for affected side for MWM (10% change) compared with placebo (4% change) and control (0% change).	Within subject, repeated measures randomised cross-over trial, with participants acting as their own control, immediate pre-post-intervention measures.
Vicenzino[5]	16 participants with history of unilateral recurrent lateral ankle sprain (no acute ankle sprain within the past 6 months). 8 males, 8 females. Mean age: 19.8 (SD 2.3) years.	Group 1: weight-bearing MWM. Group 2: non-weight-bearing MWM. Group 3: control. All participants experienced 1 of the 3 conditions in a randomised sequence on 3 separate days (at least 48 hours apart). Weight-bearing MWM: in standing with therapist manually stabilising the foot on the plinth, using belt to apply force and participant moving into DF. Non-weight-bearing MWM: applied with the participant in supine lying, tibia resting on plinth and ankle on the edge. Control: no manual contact or movement. The participant stood for a similar period of time similar to the treatment time for the other two groups.	Before and after treatment, over three sessions. Posterior talar glide. Weight-bearing ankle DF (tape measure).	Posterior talar glide significantly improved for both weight-bearing (55%; SEM 40) and non-weight-bearing (50%; SEM 32) MWM techniques compared to the control group (17%; SEM 22, p<0.001). Weight-bearing dorsiflexion range of movement also improved significantly for weight-bearing (26%; SEM 24) and non-weight-bearing (26%; SEM 29) MWM techniques compared to control (9%; SEM 10, p<0.017).	Within subject, repeated measures randomised cross-over trial, with participants acting as their own control.
Vicenzino & Wright[35]	39-year-old female with right side LE.	Six treatment sessions over 5 weeks. Included 2 weeks assessment, 2 weeks intervention (4 sessions), and 6 weeks home exercise program. Treatment: MWM — lateral glide applied at the proximal part of the forearm whilst stabilising the lateral aspect of the distal humerus (participant in supine, shoulder internal rotation, elbow extended, forearm pronated). Participant was taught self mobilisation and taping (taping was used to replicate the lateral force applied at the elbow by the MWM).	VAS. PPT. Grip strength. Function VAS. Pain-free function questionnaire.	PFGS increased during treatment phases. All 6 items on the pain-free function questionnaire, which caused pain before, had improved following treatment. Improvement in grip strength was correlated with improvements in function and decrease in pain. At 6 weeks: no pain, full function, a strong correlation was illustrated that as function increased, pain decreased (r = -0.92, p<0.0001).	Single case study.

(Continued)

Table 3.6 Characteristics of all studies—cont'd

Author	Participants	Intervention	Outcome measures	Results	Comments
Yang[37]	28 participants with frozen shoulder syndrome. Group 1: 13 women, mean age 53.3 (SD 6.5) years, duration of symptoms 18 (SD 8) weeks, dominant arm affected 8. Group 2: 11 women, mean age 58 (SD 10.1) years, duration of symptoms 22 (SD 10) weeks, dominant arm affected 7.	Multiple intervention design. Group 1: A-B-A-C. Group 2: A-C-A-B. A = mid-range mobilisation. B = end-range mobilisation. C = MWM. 3 weeks for each phase of the interventions, twice weekly for 30 minutes per session. Mid-range mobilisation: participant supine, 10–15 repetitions of passive mobilisation at 40° shoulder abduction. End-range mobilisation: therapist held close to the glenohumeral joint with humerus in maximal range in different directions, for 10–15 repetitions of intensive mobilisation. MWM: participant sitting, belt placed around the head of humerus, counterpressure applied to the scapula by therapist's hand and glide applied through the belt, along with slow active shoulder movements to the end of pain-free range; 3 x 10 repetitions.	Flexi-level Scale of Shoulder Function (FLEX-SF) 3D motion analysis (FASTRAK). Elevation in the plane of the scapula. Hand-to-neck (shoulder external rotation). Hand-to-scapula (shoulder internal rotation). Scapula tipping. Scapulohumeral rhythm.	FLEX-SF, arm elevation, scapulohumeral rhythm, shoulder internal and external rotation significantly improved (p<0.01) for both end-range mobilisation and MWM over time. There was no significant difference between the end-range mobilisation and MWM groups for any measure except scapulohumeral rhythm, where MWM had greater improvement than end-range mobilisation at 6 and 12 weeks follow-up.	Randomised cross-over design, two groups each receiving both treatments in the opposite order A-B-A-C and A-C-A-B, where A = mid-range mobilisation, B = end-range mobilisation and C = MWM. The direction of the MWM glide and direction of arm movements were not specified.

a/a = as above; DF = dorsiflexion; ER = external rotation; HEP = home exercise program; IR = internal rotation; LE = lateral epicondylalgia; LBP = low back pain; MGS = maximum grip strength; MMT = manual muscle testing; MRI = magnetic resonance imaging; MWM = mobilisation with movement; NPRS = numerical pain rating scale; PFGS = pain-free grip strength; PPT = pressure pain threshold; RCT = randomised controlled trial; ROM = range of motion; SD = standard deviation; SLR = straight leg raise; SNAG = sustained natural apophyseal glide; TPT = temperature pain threshold; US = ultrasound; VAS = visual analogue scale.

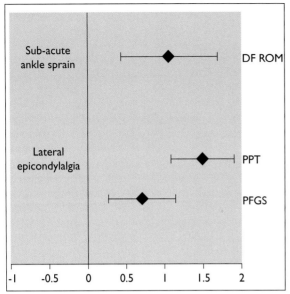

Figure 3.3 Pooled results for outcome measures of pain-free grip strength (PFGS), pressure pain threshold (PPT) and range of motion (ROM) for MWM treatment for participants with lateral epicondylalgia[4, 30] and sub-acute ankle inversion sprain,[1, 41] immediately post-intervention

In summary, due to the heterogeneity of the study populations and timing of outcome measures, we were unable to pool data across studies of shoulder MWM. Based on the inconsistent findings of three studies of adequate methodological quality, there is insufficient evidence to either support or refute the use of MWM in patients with shoulder conditions.

MWM for ankle conditions
Three studies of adequate methodological quality (rated 18, 18 and 20 respectively),[1, 5, 41] looked at the immediate effects of a talocrural joint MWM on ankle dorsiflexion ROM in participants with a history of ankle sprains. It was possible to pool data from Reid et al[41] and Collins et al[1], as these two studies included participants with a clinical diagnosis of sub-acute lateral ankle inversion sprain. The pooled data showed a positive immediate effect of talocrural MWM on measures of ankle dorsiflexion ROM (SMD 1.18; 95% CI 0.55 to 1.81) in this population (Figure 3.3).

Vicenzino et al[5] utilised a population of recurrent ankle sprains, and were therefore unable to be included in the pooled analyses due to population heterogeneity, however, the authors reported similar results, with both a weight-bearing and non-weight-bearing MWM technique demonstrating significant improvements in weight-bearing ankle dorsiflexion ROM (26% for both) and posterior talar glide (55% and 50% respectively), compared with a control condition.

The findings of these studies of adequate methodological quality are supported by the findings of four lesser quality studies,[26, 42–44] three of which reported beneficial effects of a MWM postero–cephalad glide to the lateral malleolus in individuals with a history of inversion ankle sprain.[26, 42, 43] One single case report found beneficial effects of a MWM antero–posterior glide to the distal tibia in reducing medial ankle pain associated with recurrent ankle sprains in a 25-year old female recreational runner.[44] There was insufficient data from these latter studies[26, 42, 44] to allow calculation of an effect size.

In summary, there is level 2a evidence that a MWM intervention is superior to a placebo and control intervention for assessment of immediate effects using outcomes of ankle dorsiflexion ROM, in patients with sub-acute lateral ankle inversion sprain. There is level 2b evidence that a MWM intervention is superior to a control intervention for assessment of immediate effects using outcomes of ankle dorsiflexion ROM, in patients with recurrent ankle sprains.

MWM for spinal conditions
Six studies assessed the effects of MWM on a range of spinal conditions,[29, 45–49] with three of these studies deemed of adequate methodological quality.[29, 46, 48]

Hall et al[29] in a double-blind RCT, compared a home program of self-MWM (also termed 'sustained natural apophyseal glides' or SNAGs) using a cervical self-SNAG strap (Manual Concepts, Booragoon, Australia), with a placebo intervention on participants with a clinical diagnosis of cervicogenic headaches. ROM was measured immediately following a single intervention session, and headache severity was measured at 4 and 52 weeks follow-up using a headache questionnaire. The MWM group demonstrated significantly greater improvement in cervical rotation ROM than the placebo group immediately following the intervention, with an increase of 15° (SD 9°) in the MWM group compared with 5° (SD 5°) in the placebo group (P<0.001; Table 3.7). Similarly, headache severity was significantly reduced at 4 and 52 weeks in the MWM grap compared with the placebo group (Table 3.7). The authors also reported that exercise compliance was greater in the MWM group than in the placebo group at 4 weeks follow-up.

Reid et al,[50] in an assessor-blinded RCT, compared a 4-week treatment program of SNAGs to C1 or C2 with active cervical ROM to a sham laser intervention. The SNAG intervention was superior to the sham laser intervention at post-treatment and 6 week follow-up, on measures of dizziness severity (P = 0.03), Dizziness Handicap Inventory (P = 0.02, 0.05), and in pain severity (P = 0.001, 0.048). The SNAG intervention was superior to the sham intervention at all follow-up time points (post-treatment, 6 and 12 weeks; P<0.001) for global perceived effect. In addition, it appears that standing balance with cervical spine extension improved

Table 3.7 MWM interventions

Intervention First author	Score	Sample size (N)	INT (n)	Week	Other SMD/RR (95% CI)	ROM/PFGS SMD (95% CI)	PPT SMD (95% CI)
Cervicogenic headache							
C1-C2 SNAG versus placebo					Headache severity index	Cervical flexion-rotation ROM	
Hall[29]	19	32	1	0		1.34 (0.56 to 2.12)	
				4	1.58 (0.77 to 2.38)		
				52	2.09 (1.21 to 2.97)		
Cervicogenic dizziness							
C1-C2 SNAG versus sham laser					Global perceived effect		
Reid[50]	21	33	4-6	0	1.63 (0.83 to 2.43)		
				6	1.54 (0.75 to 2.33)		
				12	1.78 (0.96 to 2.60)		
Lateral epicondylalgia							
MWM versus placebo						Pain-free grip force (strength)	
Vicenzino[30]	20	24	1	0		1.23 (0.61 to 1.85)	0.63 (0.04 to 1.21)
Paungmali[4]	21	24	1	0		1.34 (0.70 to 1.97)	0.36 (-0.21 to 0.93)
MWM + exercise versus corticosteroid injection					Success RR		
Bisset[28]	21	128	8	6	0.83 (0.66 to 1.03)	-0.74 (-1.1 to -0.38)	
				52	1.38 (1.16 to 1.66)	0.31 (-0.03 to 0.66)	
MWM + exercise versus wait-and-see (control)							
Bisset[28]	21	123	8	6	2.44 (1.55 to 3.85)	1.01 (0.63 to 1.38)	
		125		52	1.04 (0.93 to 1.15)	0.22 (-0.14 to 0.57)	
MWM versus control							
Vicenzino[30]	20	24	1	0		1.51 (0.86 to 2.16)	0.24 (-0.32 to 0.81)
Paungmali[4]	21	24	1	0		1.63 (0.97 to 2.29)	0.67 (0.09 to 1.25)
Manchanda[23]	12	20	15	2	Pain VAS 0.58 (-0.31 to -1.48) Functional Pain Scale 0.69 (-0.22 to 1.59)	Weights test (strength) 1.41 (0.40 to 2.41)	
MWM versus wrist manipulation							
Manchanda[23]	12	20	15	2	Pain VAS 0 (-0.88 to 0.88) Functional Pain Scale 0.3 (-0.58 to 1.18)	Weights test (strength) 0.8 (-0.11 to 1.72)	

(Continued)

Table 3.7 MWM interventions—cont'd

Intervention First author	Score	Sample size (N)	INT (n)	Week	Other SMD/RR (95% CI)	ROM/PFGS SMD (95% CI)	PPT SMD (95% CI)
Shoulder							
Pain-limited shoulder ROM							
MWM versus placebo							
Teys[6]	18	24	1	0		Shoulder elevation 0.99 (0.38 to 1.59)	0.82 (0.23 to 1.41)
MWM versus control							
Teys[6]	18	24	1	0		Shoulder elevation 1.50 (0.85 to 2.15)	0.87 (0.28 to 1.47)
Frozen shoulder							
MWM versus end-range mobilisation							
Yang[37]	17	22		6		Shoulder elevation -0.22 (-1.02 to 0.59) Shoulder internal rotation 0.74 (-0.11 to 1.59) Shoulder external rotation -0.11 (-0.93 to 0.71) Scapulohumeral rhythm 1.40 (0.47 to 2.33)	
				12		Shoulder elevation 0.11 (-0.71 to 0.93) Shoulder internal rotation -0.73 (-1.58 to 0.12) Shoulder external rotation -0.14 (-0.96 to 0.68) Scapulohumeral rhythm 0.95 (0.08 to 1.82)	
Shoulder impingement							
MWM versus passive mobilisation							
Kachingwe[38]	18		6	6	Pain VAS 0.3 (-0.63 to 1.23) SPADI 0.04 (-0.88 to 0.97)	Flexion 0.70 (-0.26 to 1.66) Scaption 0.93 (-0.06 to 1.91)	
MWM versus exercise							
Kachingwe[38]	18		6	6	PVAS 0.41 (-0.56 to 1.37) SPADI 0.20 (-0.75 to 1.16)	Flexion 0.49 (-0.48 to 1.46) Scaption 0.85 (-0.16 to 1.86)	
MWM versus control							
Kachingwe[38]	18		6	6	PVAS 0.47 (-0.54 to 1.48) SPADI -0.49 (1.49 to 0.52)	Flexion 0.15 (-0.84 to 1.14) Scaption 0.90 (-0.15 to 1.95)	

(Continued)

Table 3.7 MWM interventions—cont'd

Intervention First author	Score	Sample size (N)	INT (n)	Week	Other SMD/RR (95% CI)	ROM/PFGS SMD (95% CI)	PPT SMD (95% CI)
Lumbar spine							
MWM versus placebo							
Konstantinou[48]	23	26	1	0	Pain VAS during lumbar flexion 0.04 (-5.0 to 5.9)	True lumbar flexion 0.25 (-0.29 to 0.80) Total lumbopelvic flexion 0.31 (-0.23 to 0.86) Total lumbopelvic extension 0.25 (-0.3 to 0.8)	
Ankle							
Non-weight-bearing MWM versus control – Recurrent ankle sprain							
Vicenzino[5]	20	16	1	0		Posterior talar glide 1.17 (0.41 to 1.93) Weight-bearing ankle dorsiflexion 0.76 (0.04 to 1.49)	
Weight-bearing MWM versus control – Recurrent ankle sprain							
Vicenzino[5]	20	16	1	0		Posterior talar glide 1.15 (0.39 to 1.90) Weight-bearing ankle dorsiflexion 0.90 (0.17 to 1.63)	
Weight-bearing MWM versus placebo –Sub-acute ankle sprain							
Collins[1]	18	14	1	0	Thermal pain threshold — ATFL -0.53 (-1.29 to 0.23)	Weight-bearing ankle dorsiflexion 0.16 (-0.58 to 0.9)	Pressure pain threshold - ATFL -0.16 (-0.90 to 0.59)
Reid[41, 50]	18	23	1	0		Weight-bearing ankle dorsiflexion 1.18 (0.55 to 1.81)	
Weight-bearing MWM versus control – Sub-acute ankle sprain							
Collins[1]	18	14	1	0	Thermal pain threshold - ATFL -0.47 (-1.22 to 0.28)	Weight-bearing ankle dorsiflexion 0.31 (-0.44 to 1.05)	Pressure pain threshold - ATFL- 0.22 (-0.97 to 0.52)

Summary of validity score, sample size, and effect size (95% confidence interval) for pain, maximum grip strength (MGS), pain-free grip strength (PFGS) and pressure pain threshold (PPT) for study time intervals on included interventions (first author cited). Effect size measured as standardised mean difference (SMD) for continuous outcome measures and relative risk (RR) for dichotomous outcome measures. Score = quality rating score, INT = number of treatment sessions, Week = timing of outcome measures from baseline. CI containing 0 indicate null effect.

ATFL = anterior talofibular ligament; MWM = mobilisation with movement; ROM = range of motion; SLR = straight leg raise; SNAG = sustained natural apophyseal glide; VAS = visual analogue scale.

Table 3.8 Effect size for single group interventions and case studies

Intervention First author	Score	Sample size (N)	INT (n)	Week	PFGS effect size	ROM effect size	Other effect size
Lateral epicondylalgia							
MWM at 33% maximum glide force McLean[33]	10	6	1	0	2.02		
MWM at 50% maximum glide force McLean[33]					3.18		
MWM at 66% maximum glide force McLean[33]					4.85		
MWM at 100% maximum glide force McLean[33]					4.19		
Lateral ulna glide MWM McLean[33]							
Abbott[7]	14	25	1	0	0.40		MGS 0.12
Abbott[32]	13	23	1	0		Affected shoulder internal rotation ROM 1.07 Affected shoulder external rotation ROM 0.36	
Vicenzino[35]	10	1	4	2	2.98		PVAS 2.07 FVAS 5.47
Paungmali[34]	18	24	6	2	1.14		PPT 0.51
Paungmali[31]	20	18	1	0	0.70		PPT 0.58 ULTT2b 0.57 TPT 0.04
Low back pain							
Traction SLR							
Hall[46]	16	19	1	0		True SLR 0.86 Pelvic rotation with SLR 0.46	
Acute thoracic spine pain							
SNAG							
Creighton[54]						ROM quadriceps length 3.5	PVAS (stretch) 3.6 PVAS (isometric contraction) 2.6
Cervicogenic headache							
SNAG and reverse SNAG							
Richardson[49]	7	1	11	4			Headache Rating Scale 4.6 PVAS 5.5
Ankle							
MWM posterior talus glide							
O'Brien[43]	9	2	6	4.7		Ankle dorsiflexion ROM 2.8 Ankle inversion ROM 3.8	PVAS 4.7 Kaikkonen scale 41.0 FVAS 18.4

INT = number of treatment sessions, MGS = maximum grip strength, ROM = range of motion, PVAS = pain visual analogue scale, FVAS = function, visual analogue scale, PPT = pressure pain threshold, ULTT2b = upper limb tension test 2b (radial nerve bias), TPT = thermal pain threshold, SLR = straight leg raise, SNAG = sustained natural apophyseal glides.

significantly in the SNAG intervention group at 12 week follow-up (P = 0.05), and worse in the sham intervention group for quiet standing balance at 12 week follow-up (P = 0.01). There was no significant difference between groups for cervical ROM at any time point.

Konstantinou et al[48] compared a MWM lumbar flexion technique with a placebo intervention. The authors reported an immediate positive effect of the MWM technique on measures of lumbar flexion ROM (49.2° SD 16.4) over a placebo intervention (45.3° SD 14.1). There was no significant difference in pain scores between the two groups (Table 3.7). The SMDs calculated from the post-intervention means and SDs did not reach significance (Table 3.7).

Hall et al[46], using a single group pre- post-test design, assessed the effects of a single session of straight leg raise (SLR) with traction MWM on SLR ROM in a cohort with a current episode of low back pain and pain-limited SLR ROM. In this population, the authors reported a significant improvement of 11° (95% CI 9 to 13) in SLR ROM following the MWM technique. However, there was no placebo or control group with which to compare these results.

Exelby[45], Horton[47] and Richardson[49] presented single case reports on the effectiveness of central and unilateral spine SNAGs. Exelby[45] and Horton[47] each had a single patient with a clinical diagnosis of an acute locked facet joint (lumbar spine and thoracic spine respectively), whereas Richardson[49] reported on a single patient with a 6-month history of cervicogenic headaches. Central and unilateral SNAGs and reverse SNAGs were performed in conjunction with a variety of other modalities (e.g. tape, heat, electrical stimulation, soft tissue releases). All three reports found the interventions successfully reduced pain in these patients, however effect size was only calculated for Richardson[49] (Table 3.8), as the other two studies did not supply data to allow further analyses.

In summary, three RCTs and four non-randomised studies all found in favour of a beneficial effect in the use of MWMs in the management of a range of spinal conditions. Heterogeneity in study populations and lack of adequate methodological quality, limits any possible conclusions, except that there is level 1b evidence that cervical spine MWM appears to be beneficial for short- and long-term outcomes in participants with cervicogenic headache (self-SNAG) and in dizziness, though the latter was not followed up in the long term.

MWM for wrist and hand
One RCT and three case reports presented outcomes for MWM techniques for individuals with de Quervain's tenosynovitis,[51] traumatic thumb injury,[52] chronic thumb pain[53] and post-surgical management of Colles' fracture.[24] None of the studies were of adequate methodological quality and none provided sufficient data to allow calculation of effect size for the MWM

intervention. However, all three studies reported a reduction in pain and improvement in function with the application of MWM techniques.

There is insufficient evidence to draw a conclusion from one RCT and three case reports of poor methodological quality (level 4 evidence), regarding the efficacy of MWM in the management of wrist and hand conditions.

MWM for patellofemoral pain syndrome
Only one study of adequate methodological quality reported on a case series of patients who underwent a MWM for treatment of patellofemoral pain syndrome.[54] While the authors did not explicitly label the intervention as a MWM, it nevertheless met the definition of a passive joint mobilisation that was applied and sustained during a passive or active movement of the joint or contraction of muscles. The MWM applied in this study involved an anterior tibial translation with either passive knee flexion in hip extension (i.e. rectus femoris stretch) or assisted knee extension (open kinetic chain assisted quadriceps exercise). The authors reported that the addition of the MWM successfully reduced the level of pain experienced during the exercise or stretch. Raw data from six participants was reported, therefore an effect size was calculated for pain severity and ROM measures (Table 3.8).

There is insufficient evidence to draw a conclusion for the effectiveness of MWM in the management of patients with patellofemoral pain syndrome, from one case series (level 4 evidence).

MWM for lateral hip pain
One single case report[55] utilised a combination of MWM, passive accessory mobilisations and therapeutic exercise on a patient with a 3-month history of lateral hip pain. The author reported successful outcomes in terms of pain and global rating of change scores after three treatment sessions, however, insufficient data was supplied to allow calculation of an effect size. No conclusions can be drawn as to the efficacy of MWM in patients with lateral hip pain, based on a single case report.

Discussion
In this systematic review, the methodological quality of 38 studies was assessed, and the quality was found acceptable in 17 studies. Where possible, data from these studies were extracted and reported as effect sizes (SMD; 95% CI) for continuous data and relative risk (95% CI) for categorical data. Where there was no comparison group, effect size for the difference in pre- and post-intervention measures was calculated. Conclusions drawn in this systematic review are dependent on our a priori decision rules. These include the clinical relevancy of results, the quality assessment schema used (modified Downs and Black Quality

Rating Scale, Appendix 3.1) and that all papers were accepted for inclusion into this systematic review, regardless of quality. In addition, if a rating criterion was not relevant to the study design (e.g. single case report), then a '0' for 'unable to determine' or 'no' was given. For example, all single case reports received 0 points for criterion #17, regarding the similarity of time period between the intervention and outcome assessment between groups. Only those studies that rated 50% or higher were included in further meta-analyses.

Of the 27 criteria rated, 13 were conspicuously absent in more than 50% of papers (Tables 3.2 and 3.4). Only six of the 38 of the rated studies were true RCTs, and another nine studies used a within-participant cross-over randomised design. The remaining 23 studies lacked randomisation of all participants. Two of the RCTs[28, 29] were the only studies to provide long-term follow-up data. Fifteen out of 20 studies that rated below 50% on the Quality Index scale did not report sufficient data to allow estimation of a treatment effect size. Of those that did, we found the reported treatment effects were larger than studies of higher methodological quality (Figure 3.2). This supports previous findings, where poorer quality studies have been linked with larger effect sizes.[56] It is thought that poorer quality studies overestimate the treatment effect, which underpins the need for better quality studies to allow clinicians to establish a true impression of the effectiveness (or otherwise) of a treatment. Furthermore, the small number of participants in individual studies, that is, low power (criterion 27), also contributes to the difficulty encountered in comparing studies and interpreting results. Non-randomised studies rank lower in the hierarchy of evidence, because they are inherently susceptible to bias. Furthermore, in the absence of a control group, the relationship between interventions and outcomes cannot be definitely established. Despite their limitations, non-randomised studies for novel interventions are frequently undertaken and published. It has been suggested that a systematic review of novel interventions should include non-randomised studies when RCTs are not available, as the findings of non-randomised studies may confirm the findings of RCTs.[9, 10] If non-randomised studies are included in a review, potential biases should be taken into account, including biases in study design and publication bias.[11]

The sub-scale of Reporting in the Quality Index scale was the only sub-scale that averaged greater than 50% compliance, with significant weaknesses across all studies in reporting on the External Validity sub-scale (Tables 3.2 and 3.4). This may be a function of the rating system itself, as the criteria concerning external validity (#11–13) have previously been shown to lack both inter- and intra-rater reliability.[14] Alternatively, a poor score on the External Validity sub-scale may suggest that generalisation of the results to a greater population is limited.

Sixteen out of 38 rated studies in this review were single case or case series studies. On average, the single case and case series studies rated below 50% on the sub-scales for External Validity and Internal Validity (Table 3.4). A low score for the Internal Validity sub-scales is suggestive of bias in the selection of study participants and in the measurement of effect. Single case studies are good at describing the time course of a treatment on an example (N = 1) of a condition. However, it is difficult to generalise the findings of a single case study to the greater population for that particular condition. Results from single case studies that show a positive effect for a MWM intervention should therefore be interpreted with caution. The more patients enrolled in a study, the more likely that the results can be generalised to the total patient population. Studies with larger participant populations will report the variability of responses across the population, not only those who respond positively to a particular intervention. RCTs are important because they can provide reliable evidence of treatment effects and rank highly on the hierarchy of evidence (Table 3.1). The degree to which a practitioner may utilise the findings from a RCT can also be ascertained in part from the inclusion criteria for study participants, which is usually based on a diagnosis. This allows the reader to determine if the patient they see in the clinic is similar in characteristics to the participant population enrolled in a particular study.

The lack of long-term follow-up studies for MWMs limits any firm inferences to clinical practice. Notwithstanding this, we found evidence of positive small to large effects (see the earlier section, 'Data management and statistical analysis') for MWM in all musculoskeletal conditions. The most common significant results found were increase in strength, reduction in pain levels, increase in pressure pain threshold and overall function improvements when compared with placebo or control.

SUMMARY

To summarise the findings of this systematic review, there is level 2a to 1b evidence that MWM is effective in the management of patients with tennis elbow. Twelve studies assessed the immediate, short- and long-term effects using a range of outcome measures on patients with a clinical diagnosis of tennis elbow. We were able to calculate the effect size from 10 studies that all demonstrated a positive benefit of MWM in the short term,[4, 7, 23, 28, 30–35] with additional positive benefits in the long term when compared with corticosteroid injections.[28] Furthermore, Bisset et al[28] reported a Number Needed to Treat index of 3 at 3 months, 2 at 6 months and 4 at 12 months follow-up, when comparing a physiotherapy intervention of MWM and exercise with corticosteroid injections. This translates, for example, to one more successful outcome at 12 months if four patients received physiotherapy rather than corticosteroid injections, which is considered a clinically relevant difference in long-term effects.

For shoulder pain, there is conflicting evidence of the effectiveness of MWM in improving outcomes in patients with shoulder conditions. There is level 2a evidence that MWM is superior to placebo and/or control groups in patients with sub-acute lateral ankle inversion sprain and recurrent ankle sprains. For spinal conditions, heterogeneity in study populations and lack of adequate methodological quality limits any possible conclusions, except for level 1b evidence that cervical spine MWM (SNAG) appears to be beneficial in short- and long-term follow-up in patients with cervicogenic headache and dizziness (latter not followed up in long-term). Finally, there is low-level evidence (level 4) that MWM may be effective in patients with wrist/hand injuries or patellofemoral pain syndrome.

Further studies are required that employ more rigorous methodology, greater participant numbers and a longer follow-up timeframe, before conclusions can be drawn as to the efficacy of MWM in the majority of musculoskeletal conditions. Overall, in all studies regardless of methodological quality, it appears that MWM provides some positive benefits in patients with a range of musculoskeletal conditions.

KEY POINTS

- We identified 38 papers that studied participants with a musculoskeletal condition who were treated with a MWM technique; six were true randomised controlled trials and a further nine, while randomised, included a cross-over feature. Of the 23 other trials, 16 reported single cases.

- The majority of the randomised trials focused on initial and short-term effects.

- Pooled data from a number of trials show the immediate effects of MWM for lateral epicondylalgia on pain-free grip strength and pressure pain threshold to be superior to control or placebo. There is one high quality RCT that shows MWM in combination with exercise is superior to control at 6 weeks and superior to corticosteroid injections in the long-term.

- Pooling of immediate effect studies indicate that MWM at the ankle improves dorsiflexion beyond that of control comparators in patients with recurrent ankle sprains.

- Cervical MWM (SNAG) has been shown to be efficacious in managing cervicogenic head symptoms (headache, dizziness) in separate RCTs.

- Given the dearth of high-quality studies, there is insufficient published evidence to support or refute the use of MWM in the shoulder, wrist/hand, spine (with the exception of cervicogenic headache/symptoms [dizziness]), hip, knee and ankle (except for short-term effects).

- There is a need for further RCTs of MWM, and a need for longer-term follow-up of outcomes.

Acknowledgments: Natalic collins, Renee Bigalow, Toni Bremner.

References

1 Collins N, Teys P, Vicenzino B. The initial effects of a Mulligan's mobilization with movement technique on dorsiflexion and pain in sub-acute ankle sprains. Manual Therapy. 2004 May;9(2):77–82.

2 DeSantis L, Hasson SM. Use of mobilization with movement in the treatment of a patient with subacromial impingement: a case report. Journal of Manual and Manipulative Therapy. 2006;14(2):77–87.

3 Exelby L. Peripheral mobilisations with movement. Manual Therapy. 1996 Jun;1(3):118–26.

4 Paungmali A, O'Leary S, Souvlis T, Vicenzino B. Hypoalgesic and sympathoexcitatory effects of mobilization with movement for lateral epicondylalgia. Physical Therapy. 2003 Apr;83(4):374–83.

5 Vicenzino B, Branjerdporn M, Teys P, Jordan K. Initial changes in posterior talar glide and dorsiflexion of the ankle after mobilization with movement in individuals with recurrent ankle sprain. Journal of Orthopaedic and Sports Physical Therapy. 2006 Jul;36(7):464–71.

6 Teys P, Bisset L, Vicenzino B. The initial effects of a Mulligan's mobilization with movement technique on range of movement and pressure pain threshold in pain-limited shoulders. Manual Therapy. 2008 Feb;13(1):37–42.

7 Abbott JH. Mobilization with movement applied to the elbow affects shoulder range of movement in subjects with lateral epicondylalgia. Manual Therapy. 2001 Aug;6(3):170–7.

8 Fitzpatrick JM. Evidence-based medicine 'up front'. BJU International. 2006;97(6):1141.

9 Chambers D, Rodgers M, Woolacott N. Not only randomized controlled trials, but also case series should be considered in systematic reviews of rapidly developing technologies. Journal of Clinical Epidemiology. 2009;doi: 10.1016/j.jclinepi.2008.12.010.

10 Linde K, Scholz M, Melchart D, Willich SN. Should systematic reviews include non-randomized and uncontrolled studies? The case of acupuncture for chronic headache. Journal of Clinical Epidemiology. 2002;55(1):77–85.

11 Higgins JPT, Green S (eds). Cochrane Handbook for Systematic Reviews of Interventions 4.2.6. Online. Available: http://www.cochrane.org/resources/handbook/hbook.htm (updated September 2006).

12 Phillips B, Ball C, Sackett D, Badenoch D, Straus S, Haynes B, et al. Oxford Centre for Evidence-based Medicine Levels of Evidence (May 2001). Online. Available: http://www.cebm.net/index.aspx?o = 1025 (accessed 10 June 2008).

13 Clarke M, Oxman AD. Medline highly sensitive search strategies for identifying reports of randomized controlled trials in Medline. Cochrane Reviewers' Handbook 4.1.6 The Cochrane Library. Online. Available: http://www.cochrane.org/resources/handbook/hbook.htm (updated January 2003); appendix 5b (accessed 3 April 2003).

14 Downs SH, Black N. The feasibility of creating a checklist for the assessment of the methodological quality both of randomised and non-randomised studies of health care interventions. Journal of Epidemiology and Community Health. 1998;52:337–84.

15 van Tulder MW, Assendelft WJJ, Koes BW, Bouter LM. Method guidelines for systematic reviews in the Cochrane Collaboration Back Review group for spinal disorders. Spine. 1997;22(20):2323–30.

16 Monteiro POA, Victora CG. Rapid growth in infancy and childhood and obesity in later life — a systematic review. Obesity Reviews. 2005;6:143–54.

17 Moher D, Pham B, Jones A, Cook D, Jadad A, Moher M, et al. Does quality of reports of randomised trials affect estimates of intervention efficacy reported in meta-analysis? Lancet. 1998 Aug 22;352(9128):609–13.

18 Fleiss J, Levin B, Paik M. Statistical methods for rates and proportions (3rd edn). Hoboken, NJ: J Wiley 2003.

19 Review Manager (RevMan) [Computer program]. Version 4.2 for Windows edn. Oxford, England: The Cochrane Collaboration 2003.

20 Cohen J. Statistical power analysis for the behavioral sciences (2nd edn). Hillsdale, NJ: Lawrence Erlbaum 1988.

21 Cohen J. A power primer. Psychological Bulletin. 1992;112(1):155–9.

22 Smidt N, Assendelft WJ, Arola H, Malmivaara A, Greens S, Buchbinder R, et al. Effectiveness of physiotherapy for lateral epicondylitis: a systematic review. Annals of Medicine. 2003;35(1):51–62.

23 Manchanda G, Grover D. Effectiveness of movement with mobilization compared with manipulation of wrist in case of lateral epicondylitis. Indian Journal of Physiotherapy and Occupational Therapy. 2008;2(1).

24 Naik VC, Chitra J, Khatri S. Effectiveness of Maitland versus Mulligan mobilization technique following post surgical management of Colles' fracture — RCT. Indian Journal of Physiotherapy and Occupational Therapy. 2007;1(4).

25 Kochar M, Dogra A. Effectiveness of a specific physiotherapy regimen on patients with tennis elbow: clinical study. Physiotherapy. 2002 Jun;88(6):333–41.

26 Merlin D, McEwan I, Thom J. Mulligan's mobilisation with movement technique for lateral ankle pain and the use of magnetic resonance imaging to evaluate the 'positional fault' hypothesis. Isokinetic: Education Research Department. 2005. Online. Available: http://www.isokinetic.com/index.cfm?page = centro_studi/congressi/congresso_2005 (accessed 22 April 2010).

27 Creighton D, Krauss J, Pascoe S, Patel H, Pierce J. The effects of tibio-femoral joint traction mobilization on patients with limited passive knee flexion: a case series. Journal of Manual and Manipulative Therapy. 2006;14(3):173–4.

28 Bisset L, Beller E, Jull G, Brooks P, Darnell R, Vicenzino B. Mobilisation with movement and exercise, corticosteroid injection, or wait and see for tennis elbow: randomised trial. British Medical Journal. 2006;333(7575):939–41.

29 Hall T, Chan HT, Christensen L, Odenthal B, Wells C, Robinson K. Efficacy of a C1–C2 self-sustained natural apophyseal glide (SNAG) in the managment of cervicogenic headache. Journal of Orthopaedic and Sports Physical Therapy. 2007;37(3):100–7.

30 Vicenzino B, Paungmali A, Buratowski S, Wright A. Specific manipulative therapy treatment for chronic lateral epicondylalgia produces uniquely characteristic hypoalgesia. Manual Therapy. 2001;6(4):205–12.

31 Paungmali A, O'Leary S, Souvlis T, Vicenzino B. Naloxone fails to antagonize initial hypoalgesic effect of a manual therapy treatment for lateral epicondylalgia. Journal of Manipulative and Physiological Therapeutics. 2004 Mar–Apr;27(3):180–5.

32 Abbott JH, Patla CE, Jensen RH. The initial effects of an elbow mobilization with movement technique on grip strength in subjects with lateral epicondylalgia. Manual Therapy. 2001 Aug;6(3):163–9.

33 McLean S, Naish R, Reed L, Urry S, Vicenzino B. A pilot study of the manual force levels required to produce manipulation induced hypoalgesia. Clinical Biomechanics. 2002 May;17(4):304–8.

34 Paungmali A, Vicenzino B, Smith M. Hypoalgesia induced by elbow manipulation in lateral epicondylalgia does not exhibit tolerance. Journal of Pain. 2003 Oct;4(8):448–54.

35 Vicenzino B, Wright A. Effects of a Novel Manipulative Physiotherapy Technique on Tennis Elbow: A Single Case Study. Manual Therapy. 1995;1(1):30–5.

36 Stephens G. Lateral epicondylitis. Journal of Manual and Manipulative Therapy. 1995;3(2):50–8.

37 Yang J, Chang C, Chen S, Wang S, Lin J. Mobilization techniques in subjects with frozen shoulder syndrome: randomized multiple-treatment trial. Physical Therapy. 2007 Oct;87(10):1307–15.

38 Kachingwe AF, Phillips B, Sletten E, Plunkett SW. Comparison of manual therapy techniques with therapeutic exercise in the treatment of shoulder impingement: a randomized controlled pilot clinical trial. Journal of Manual and Manipulative Therapy. 2009;16(4):238–47.

39 Gebhardt TL, Whitman JM, Smith MB. Mobilization with movement as part of a comprehensive physical therapy program for a patient with shoulder impingement: a case report. Journal of Manual and Manipulative Therapy. 2006;14(3):176.

40 Mulligan B. The painful dysfunctional shoulder. A new treatment approach using 'Mobilisation with Movement'. New Zealand Journal of Physiotherapy. 2003 Nov;31(3):140–2.

41 Reid A, Birmingham TB, Alcock G. Efficacy of mobilization with movement for patients with limited dorsiflexion after ankle sprain: a crossover trial. Physiotherapy Canada. 2007 Summer;59(3):166–72.

42 Hetherington B. Lateral ligament strains of the ankle, do they exist? Manual Therapy. 1996;1(5):274–5.

43 O'Brien T, Vicenzino B. A study of the effects of Mulligan's mobilization with movement treatment of lateral ankle pain using a case study design. Manual Therapy. 1998 May;3(2):78–84.

44 Penso M. The effectiveness of mobilisation with movement for chronic medial ankle pain: A case study. South African Journal of Physiotherapy. 2008;64(1): 13–6.

45 Exelby L. The locked lumbar facet joint: Intervention using mobilizations with movement. Manual Therapy. 2001;6 (2):116–21.

46 Hall T, Beyerlein C, Hansson U, T. LH, Odermark M, Sainsbury D. Mulligan traction straight leg raise: a pilot study to investigate effects on range of motion in patients with low back pain. Journal of Manual and Manipulative Therapy. 2006;14(2):95–100.

47 Horton SJ. Acute locked thoracic spine: treatment with a modified SNAG. Manual Therapy. 2002;7(2):103–7.

48 Konstantinou K, Foster N, Rushton A, Baxter D, Wright C, Breen A. Flexion mobilizations with movement techniques: the immediate effects on range of movement and pain in subjects with low back pain. Journal of Manipulative and Physiological Therapeutics. 2007 Mar–Apr;30(3):178–85.

49 Richardson CJ. Treatment of cervicogenic headaches using Mulligan 'SNAGS' and postural reeducation: a case report. Orthopaedic Physical Therapy Practice. 2009;21(1):33–8.

50 Reid SA, Rivett DA, Katekar MG, Callister R. Sustained natural apophyseal glides (SNAGs) are an effective treatment for cervicogenic dizziness. Manual Therapy. 2008 Aug 1;13(4):357–66.

51 Backstrom KM. Mobilization with movement as an adjunct intervention in a patient with complicated de Quervain's tenosynovitis: a case report. Journal of Orthopaedic and Sports Physical Therapy. 2002 Mar;32(3):86–94.

52 Folk B. Traumatic thumb injury management using mobilization with movement. Manual Therapy. 2001 Aug;6(3):178–82.

53 Hsieh CY, Vicenzino B, Yang CH, Hu MH, Yang C. Mulligan's mobilization with movement for the thumb: a single case report using magnetic resonance imaging to evaluate the positional fault hypothesis. Manual Therapy. 2002 Feb;7(1):44–9.

54 Creighton D, Krauss J, Kondratek M, Huijbregts PA, Wilt A. Use of anterior tibial translation in the management of patellofemoral pain syndrome in older patients: A case series. The Journal of Manual and Manipulative Therapy. 2007;15(4):216–24.

55 Carpenter G. The effects of hip mobilization and mobilization with movement in the physical therapy management of a person with lateral hip pain: a case report. Journal of Manual and Manipulative Therapy. 2008;16(3):170.

56 Schultz K, Chalmers I, Hayes R, Altman D. Empirical evidence of bias. Dimensions of methodological quality associated with estimates of treamtent effects in controlled trials. Journal of the American Medical Association. 1995;273:408–12.

APPENDIX 3.1 CHECKLIST FOR MEASURING STUDY QUALITY

Reporting

1 Is the hypothesis/aim/objective of the study clearly described?

response	score	location of response
Yes	1	
No	0	

2 Are the main outcomes to be measured clearly described in the 'introduction' or 'methods' section?

If the main outcomes are first mentioned in the 'results' section, the question should be answered no.

response	score	location of response
Yes	1	
No	0	

3 Are the characteristics of the patients included in the study clearly described?

In cohort studies and trials, inclusion and/or exclusion criteria should be given. In case-control studies, a case- definition and the source for controls should be given.

response	score	location of response
Yes	1	
No	0	

4 Are the interventions of interest clearly described?

Treatments and placebo (where relevant) that are to be compared should be clearly described.

response	score	location of response
Yes	1	
No	0	

5 Are the distributions of principal confounders in each group of subjects to be compared clearly described?

A list of principal confounders is provided.

response	score	location of response
Yes	2	
Partially	1	
No	0	

6 Are the main findings of the study clearly described?

Simple outcome data (including denominators and numerators) should be reported for all major findings so that the reader can check the major analyses and conclusions. (This question does not cover statistical tests which are considered below.)

response	score	location of response
Yes	1	
No	0	

7 Does the study provide estimates of the random variability in the data for the main outcomes?

In non-normally distributed data the inter-quartile range of results should be reported. In normally distributed data the standard error, standard deviation or confidence intervals should be reported. If the distribution of the data is not described, it must be assumed that the estimates used were appropriate and the question should be answered yes.

response	score	location of response
Yes	1	
No	0	

8 Have all important adverse events that may be a consequence of the intervention been reported?

This should be answered yes if the study demonstrates that there was a comprehensive attempt to measure adverse events. (A list of possible adverse events is provided.)

response	score	location of response
Yes	1	
No	0	

9 Have the characteristics of patients lost to follow-up been described?

This should be answered yes where there were no losses to follow-up or where losses to follow-up were so small that findings would be unaffected by their inclusion. This should be answered no where a study does not report the number of patients lost to follow-up.

response	score	location of response
Yes	1	
No	0	

10 Have actual probability values been reported (e.g. 0.035 rather than <0.05) for the main outcomes except where the probability value is less than 0.001?

response	score	location of response
Yes	1	
No	0	

External validity

All the following criteria attempt to address the representativeness of the findings of the study and whether they may be generalised to the population from which the study subjects were derived.

11 Were the subjects asked to participate in the study representative of the entire population from which they were recruited?

The study must identify the source population for patients and describe how the patients were selected. Patients would be representative if they comprised the entire source population, an unselected sample of consecutive patients, or a random sample. Random sampling is only feasible where a list of all members of the relevant population exists. Where a study does not report the proportion of the source population from which the patients are derived, the question should be answered as unable to determine.

response	score	location of response
Yes	1	
No	0	
Unable to determine	0	

12 Were those subjects who were prepared to participate representative of the entire population from which they were recruited?

The proportion of those asked who agreed should be stated. Validation that the sample was representative would include demonstrating that the distribution of the main confounding factors was the same in the study sample and the source population.

response	score	location of response
Yes	1	
No	0	
Unable to determine	0	

13 Were the staff, places, and facilities where the patients were treated representative of the treatment the majority of patients received?

For the question to be answered yes the study should demonstrate that the intervention was representative of that in use in the source population. The question should be answered no if, for example, the intervention was undertaken in a specialist centre unrepresentative of the hospitals most of the source population would attend.

response	score	location of response
Yes	1	
No	0	
Unable to determine	0	

Internal validity — bias

14 Was an attempt made to blind study subjects to the intervention they have received?

For studies where the patients would have no way of knowing which intervention they received, this should be answered yes.

response	score	location of response
Yes	1	
No	0	
Unable to determine	0	

15 Was an attempt made to blind those measuring the main outcomes of the intervention?

response	score	location of response
Yes	1	
No	0	
Unable to determine	0	

16 If any of the results of the study were based on 'data dredging', was this made clear?

Any analyses that had not been planned at the outset of the study should be clearly indicated. If no retrospective unplanned subgroup analyses were reported, then answer yes.

response	score	location of response
Yes	1	
No	0	
Unable to determine	0	

17 In trials and cohort studies, do the analyses adjust for different lengths of follow-up of patients, or in case-control studies, is the time period between the intervention and outcome the same for cases and controls?

Where follow-up was the same for all study patients the answer should be yes. If different lengths of follow-up were adjusted for by, for example, survival analysis the answer should be yes. Studies where differences in follow-up are ignored should be answered no.

response	score	location of response
Yes	1	
No	0	
Unable to determine	0	

18 Were the statistical tests used to assess the main outcomes appropriate?

The statistical techniques used must be appropriate to the data. For example, non-parametric methods should be used for small sample sizes. Where little statistical analysis has been undertaken but where there is no evidence of bias, the question should be answered yes. If the distribution of the data (normal or not) is not described it must be assumed that the estimates used were appropriate and the question should be answered yes.

response	score	location of response
Yes	1	
No	0	
Unable to determine	0	

19 Was compliance with the interventions reliable?

Where there was non-compliance with the allocated treatment or where there was contamination of one group, the question should be answered no. For studies where the effect of any misclassification was likely to bias any association to the null, the question should be answered yes.

response	score	location of response
Yes	1	
No	0	
Unable to determine	0	

20 Were the main outcome measures used accurate (valid and reliable)?

For studies where the outcome measures are clearly described, the question should be answered yes. For studies which refer to other work or that demonstrates

the outcome measures are accurate, the question should be answered as yes.

response	score	location of response
Yes	1	
No	0	
Unable to determine	0	

Internal validity — confounding (selection bias)

21 Were the patients in different intervention groups (trials and cohort studies) or were the cases and controls (case-control studies) recruited from the same population?

For example, patients for all comparison groups should be selected from the same hospital. The question should be answered unable to determine for cohort and case-control studies where there is no information concerning the source of patients included in the study.

response	score	location of response
Yes	1	
No	0	
Unable to determine	0	

22 Were study subjects in different intervention groups (trials and cohort studies) or were cases and controls (case-control studies) recruited over the same period of time?

For a study which does not specify the time period over which patients were recruited, the question should be answered unable to determine.

response	score	location of response
Yes	1	
No	0	
Unable to determine	0	

23 Were study subjects randomised to intervention groups?

Studies which state that subjects were randomised should be answered yes except where method of randomisation would not ensure random allocation. For example alternate allocation would score no because it is predictable.

response	score	location of response
Yes	1	
No	0	

response	score	location of response
Unable to determine	0	

response	score	location of response
Yes	1	
No	0	
Unable to determine	0	

24 Was the randomised intervention assignment concealed from both patients and healthcare staff until recruitment was complete and irrevocable?

All non-randomised studies should be answered no. If assignment was concealed from patients but not from staff, the question should be answered no.

response	score	location of response
Yes	1	
No	0	
Unable to determine	0	

25 Was there adequate adjustment for confounding in the analyses from which the main findings were drawn?

This question should be answered no for trials if: the main conclusions of the study were based on analyses of treatment rather than intention to treat; the distribution of known confounders in the different treatment groups was not described; or the distribution of known confounders differed between the treatment groups but was not taken into account in the analyses. In non-randomised studies if the effect of the main confounders was not investigated or confounding was demonstrated but no adjustment was made in the final analyses then the question should be answered no.

26 Were losses of patients to follow-up taken into account?

If the numbers of patients lost to follow-up are not reported, the question should be answered as unable to determine. If the proportion lost to follow-up was too small to affect the main findings, the question should be answered yes.

response	score	location of response
Yes	1	
No	0	
Unable to determine	0	

Power

27 Did the study have sufficient power to detect an important effect with 5% significance?*

A sample size that would give sufficient power to detect an effect with 5% significance was determined *a priori*.

response	score	location of response
Yes	1	
No	0	

---

* Modified according to Monteiro and Victora.[16]

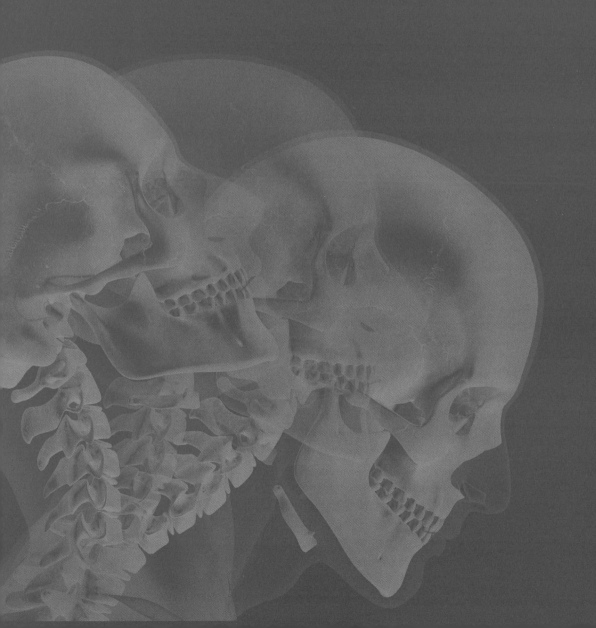

SECTION THREE

Mechanisms and effects

Chapter 4
Mulligan's positional fault hypothesis: definitions, physiology and the evidence

Wayne Hing, Toby Hall, Darren Rivett and Bill Vicenzino

INTRODUCTION

Brian Mulligan first proposed the positional fault hypothesis (PFH) after noticing that many of his patients who presented with peripheral joint dysfunction demonstrated remarkable improvements in pain and range of motion (ROM) following application of a novel manual therapy technique.[1, 2] These improvements were seen after a passive joint mobilisation (usually a sustained accessory glide applied at right angles to the plane of movement) was coupled with the pain-provoking active physiological movement. Importantly, Mulligan found that the direction of glide was critical to the outcome of the technique. This direction specificity led him to speculate that these patients presented with a positional fault at the injured joint and that his treatment technique corrected this fault.[3, 4] The positional fault could be thought of as a bony incongruence that may occur after a sprain, strain or other (micro- or macro-) injury and is responsible for the ongoing symptoms and interference with normal function.

In most healthcare professions, for a variety of reasons, practitioners are compelled to seek explanations for treatments that exert remarkable effects.[5] In the relatively short history of the field of manual therapy, there are many examples of this phenomenon such as the intervertebral disc derangement hypothesis of McKenzie[6] in physiotherapy in relation to repeated active movements, and the vertebral subluxation theory of Palmer[7] in chiropractic in relation to spinal manipulation or adjustment. A schematic representation of the possible evolution of the PFH is shown in Figure 4.1. Apart from providing a simple schematic description of the PFH (in the 'Inferred Clinical Application' box), it overviews the clinical observations and the likely interpretative steps leading up to the proposal of the PFH.

This chapter will provide a perspective on the PFH in regard to: (a) the evidence for the existence of positional faults and their measurement or detection; (b) an explanation of how positional faults may produce pain, impairment and disability; as well as (c) the capacity of Mobilisation with Movement (MWM) to reverse these faults. As such, this chapter addresses a separate matter (of an hypothesised mechanism of action of MWM) to that addressed in the preceding chapter on clinical efficacy.

DO POSITIONAL FAULTS EXIST?

There is both direct research into the PFH as it relates to the MWM concept and also research into joints such as the patellofemoral and glenohumeral that has not directly investigated the MWM concept but which includes studies into the presence of possible minor positional incongruities that highlight key aspects of the PFH. To date, the direct MWM research has focussed on the inferior tibiofibular joint and the proposal that the fibula exhibits an anterior (or posterior) positional fault. This section will evaluate if positional faults have been shown to exist by reviewing relevant literature pertaining to the ankle, patellofemoral and shoulder joints.

Tibiofibular joint

The direct investigation of the PFH in the application of MWM has been heavily focused on the ankle joint, in particular the position of the distal fibula in relation to the tibia following ankle injury. It is likely that the ankle has been the focus of research into the PFH because it is reasonably accessible to measure, commonly injured and therefore frequently presenting to therapists, and particularly because it has strong clinical relevance to MWM through Mulligan's interpretation of his clinical observations when treating chronic ankle pain. Most notably, Mulligan has suggested that in some patients during a plantarflexion-inversion ankle sprain the anterior talofibular ligament (ATFL) remains largely intact and the injury forces are transmitted through to the fibula, causing it to be anteriorly and caudally displaced relative to the tibia.[4] In this position, the ATFL is hypothesised to be slack which may contribute to chronic instability and the recurrence of ankle problems.[8] Hetherington further suggested that this positional fault is maintained after injury due to swelling and adhesions.[9] The ability of the ligament to withstand high forces during inversion injuries is evidenced by avulsion fractures.

Mulligan introduced this hypothesis after discovering that a patient, who was still suffering from pain and

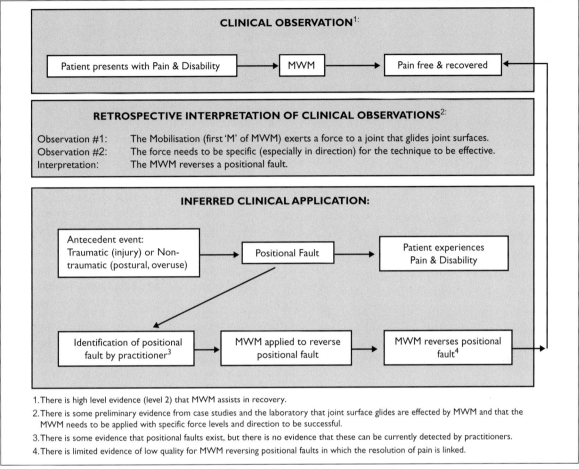

Figure 4.1 A schematic representation of the possible evolution of the PFH

limited ROM 6 weeks after an inversion sprain of the lateral ankle, had an immediate positive response after applying a MWM that involved a posterior glide (with cephalad inclination) to the distal fibula[2] (see Chapter 19 for full description and case example). This evolutionary development of the PFH concept at the ankle demonstrates the process highlighted in Figure 4.1. That is, a practitioner applies a novel manual therapy technique to a chronic unresolved problem with rapid and remarkable results. This then beckons explanation. A simple explanation is that the forces exerted by the practitioner reversed some bony incongruence, which then becomes extrapolated to the presence of the bony incongruence prior to treatment. This bony incongruence could also explain why the patient's symptoms persisted after the usual healing period for ligamentous sprains.

Since the PFH at the ankle was proposed there have been a number of studies that have directly investigated the position of the fibula in relation to the tibia by using fluoroscopy, computed axial tomography (CAT) and magnetic resonance imaging (MRI) in patients with sub-acute ankle sprain and chronic ankle instability. There are discrepancies in the findings of these studies with some reporting an anteriorly positioned fibula, while others report a posteriorly positioned fibula or no positional fault at all in patients with chronic ankle instability. It would appear that these discrepancies are largely due to the method of measurement used. For example, the studies reporting an anteriorly positioned fibula have in the main used fluoroscopy and measured the distance between the anterior edge of the lateral malleolus and the anterior edge of the tibia from a lateral view[10] (Figure 4.2), whereas the studies reporting mixed findings or no positional displacement of the fibula used CAT- and MRI-derived indices of fibular position.

The sagittal plane fluoroscopy studies of Hubbard et al[10, 11] have reported an anteriorly positioned fibula. Hubbard et al reported a mean difference in fibular position between injured ankles and non-injured ankles of 2.9 mm (95% confidence interval [CI]: 1.01 to 4.79) in a group of subjects with sub-acute ankle sprains (n = 11), which also differed to the control

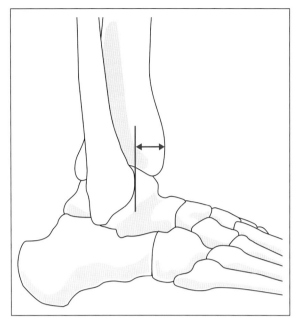

Figure 4.2 Fibular position was measured by the distance in millimeters between the anterior edge of the distal fibula and the anterior edge of the distal tibia

group (mean differences between sides of -0.33 mm [95% CI:-1.15 to 0.5]).[11] There was a strong relationship between swelling and the positional fault (r = 0.8), lending support to Hetherington's proposal.[9] Interestingly, the mean difference was largely driven by two outliers (differences of 11 mm and 5.4 mm, with a data range: 0 to 11), but even with their removal from the analysis there was still a statistically significant, albeit smaller, difference of 1.72 mm (95% CI: 0.73 to 2.71). The 2.9 mm difference is larger than the standard error and the minimal reliable change of the measurement (0.72 mm and 1.996 mm, respectively) and so is most probably real. The findings of Hubbard et al's[11] study on sub-acute ankle injuries closely reflects the changes reported by Hubbard et al in chronic ankle instability. Hubbard et al reported a 2.4 mm (95% CI: 0.72 to 4.08) difference between unstable and unaffected ankles,[10] which was close to the minimal reliable change of 1.996 mm.

While the magnitude of the differences, in the main, exceeds the error of the measurement taken on fluoroscopy, it remains to be seen if this can be reliably detected on clinical assessment (Figure 4.1, footnote 3). Other palpatory tests in manual therapy such as passive physiological intervertebral movements (PPIVMs) have consistently shown poor inter-rater reliability (e.g. see Refshauge and Gass[12]). This does not portend well for the ability of manual therapists to accurately detect positional faults, which similarly involves simultaneous palpation of the relative position of two bony landmarks and a judgment of normalcy. It should be noted however, that palpatory detection of a positional fault is not a requirement for the successful application of MWM.

Studies that used CAT- and MRI-derived indices report results that are less consistent than the fluoroscopy studies of Hubbard and colleagues. The CAT and MRI derived indices reflect relative fibular position in the transverse plane in two ways: (1) the axial malleolar index (AMI) and (2) the intermalleolar index (IMI).[13] The AMI references the lateral malleolus to the talus and as such its validity as a measure of relative positioning of the fibula to tibia is compromised.[14] The IMI references the lateral malleolus to the medial malleolus.[13] Furthermore, the AMI overestimates fibular malposition in chronic ankle instability because in this condition the talus is frequently rotated within the mortise, hence the reason for studies that have used AMI concluding that the fibula is in a posterior position. Lebrun et al[13] have succinctly demonstrated the problems encountered with using AMI by showing that in the same cohort of chronically unstable ankles (n = 21) the AMI would erroneously categorise the injured ankle as having a posteriorly positioned fibula, in stark contrast to the IMI, which showed that there was no difference in fibular position between the normal (n = 60) and chronically unstable ankles.

In contrast to the findings of Lebrun et al[13], an MRI study by Mavi et al[15] reported an anteriorly positioned fibula of on average 2.5 mm (95% CI: 0.22 to 4.78) in 10 males with recurrent ankle sprains when compared to non-injured subjects (n = 43). Females with recurrent ankle sprains (n = 8) did not show a significant difference (1.3 mm, 95% CI: -0.84 to 3.44) when compared to normals (n = 32). Mavi et al[15] measured the distance between the anterior tibia and anterior lateral malleolus, which was relatively similar to that measured on fluoroscopy by Hubbard et al[11] but taken from transverse slices.

Patellofemoral joint

The concept of mal-tracking or lateral displacement of the patella, which is arguably an example of a positional fault, appears to have become widely accepted clinically as a factor in patellofemoral pain syndrome.[16, 17] Many authors ascribe this to Merchant et al[18] who originally described a practical skyline radiographic technique in a group of normal asymptomatic people (n = 200 knees). In their paper, they included a comparison group of 25 knees with proven recurrent dislocations of the patella. The congruence angle, which is the angle between the point of the most posterior edge of the articular ridge of the patella and the bisector of the intercondylar sulcus angle (subtends lines drawn from most anterior part of the medial and lateral condyles to the deepest most point of the intercondylar sulcus), was on average -6°

(99% CI: -8 to -4) in the normal population and 23° in dislocators.[18] Aglietti et al[19] used a similar measure in 150 normal knees with comparison groups of patients with a subluxing patella (n = 37) and chondromalacia patellae (n = 53). Their findings were similar to that of Merchant[18] with normal congruence angle being -8° in the asymptomatic group and 16° in the subluxing group. The chondromalacia patellae group registered a mean congruence angle of -2°, which is marginally greater than Merchant's normal data.[18]

If congruence angle reflects accurately patellar position (or tracking), these data indicate that there is likely a small positional fault present in patellofemoral pain syndrome (presuming chondromalacia patellae is equivalent) that may be difficult to differentiate from the asymptomatic patellofemoral joint.[17] That is, positional faults exist in unstable patellofemoral joints to a much larger extent than in patellofemoral pain syndrome (without instability). Laurin et al[20] used a qualitative method and showed similar findings when comparing 100 chondromalacia patellae knees to 30 recurrent subluxers and 100 normals. In a recent comprehensive literature review, Wilson[17] has indicated that more sophisticated imaging technology (e.g. MRI, CAT scan, ultrasound) and a myriad of other measurement indices (lateral patellar displacement, bisect offset angle, lateral patellofemoral angle, patellar tilt angle, congruence angle, lateral patellar tilt) have not resolved the issue because the focus was still predominantly on comparing instability to normal, but there were also conflicting results when patellofemoral pain was studied.

A number of other issues that stream through the literature on patellar position or tracking are: the reliability and validity of measures; large population variability on all measures; the position of the knee (extended or various angles of flexion); the contraction (relaxed or contracted) status of the quadriceps muscles; whether the limb was weight-bearing or not;[17] and the lack of 3-dimensional biomechanical analyses of the patella for both rotation and translation in all planes (i.e. 6 degrees of freedom[21]). It is salient to the PFH, correction of which has been proposed as a mechanism for MWM, that there exists such a lack of clinical research consensus for a condition like patellofemoral pain syndrome, a condition so widely perceived to relate to a positional fault. The message for practitioners using MWM is that it appears difficult to reliably and validly measure positional faults, even with sophisticated imaging technology.

If the PFH is to be clinically useful for the practitioner (i.e. as well as in the explanation of MWM mechanisms) it is reasonable to expect that the practitioner should be able to reliably and accurately detect positional faults on clinical examination (Figure 4.1) (or at the very least have compelling evidence of such that can be explained to the patient). Unlike the inferior tibiofibular joint, there is a clinical examination protocol for detecting positional faults of the patellofemoral

joint in patients with patellofemoral pain syndrome[22] that should provide insight into the clinical utility of such examination techniques. In brief, the examination techniques involve palpation and visual inspection of the patella relative to the thigh and femoral condyles — with the knee in approximately 20° of flexion — in order to describe the patellar position in the frontal plane (medial–lateral translation and rotation), the transverse plane (lateral pole posterior tilt), and the sagittal plane (inferior pole anterior–posterior tilt).[22]

It appears that most research has focused on the lateral displacement (medial–lateral position in the frontal plane) positional test, which has been described in two ways: that of McConnell[22, 23] and the other from Herrington.[24] The McConnell method has the therapist placing the index fingers of each hand on the medial and lateral epicondyles of the knee and both thumbs nail to nail over the mid point of the patella. The thumbs being approximately equidistant from each epicondyle signifies a normal alignment.[22] In the Herrington method, the therapist marks both epicondyles and the mid-patellar point onto an applied strip of rigid adhesive tape before removing the tape and measuring the distance with a ruler.[24]

A recent systematic review by Smith et al[25] found nine studies (n = 237 patients with 306 knees studied) that on the whole showed good intra-rater reliability, variable inter-rater reliability and moderate criterion validity of the Herrington method[24] (MRI used as the gold standard). A meta-analysis of these studies was not possible because, in common with the diagnostic imaging studies, there was substantial heterogeneity in many critical aspects. For example, there was poor description of the populations studied (height, weight and conditions [instability versus pain]) and the actual measurement tests were not always clearly described.[25] Notwithstanding these issues, Herrington[24] recently reported that a single rater using his measurement technique was able to differentiate those subjects with patellofemoral pain syndrome from normals by a mean difference of 3.7 mm (95% CI: 1.6 to 5.8) in relative lateral displacement, which far exceeded the minimal clinical difference of 0.6 mm in that study. Perhaps in time to come, measurement of positional faults at other joints may evolve to this stage and beyond, whereby the practitioner would have a simple, reliable and valid clinical test that could be used to help direct MWM applications. For example, it would seem reasonable to expect that if 3–4 mm of difference is detectable at the patellofemoral joint then measurement techniques could be developed to detect a 2–3 mm anterior positional fault of the fibula.

Glenohumeral joint

Abnormal geometric relationships between humeral head and the glenoid fossa have been postulated for some conditions of the shoulder.[26] For example, in impingement syndrome of the shoulder it has been suggested that there is excessive elevation of the humeral head within the glenoid as a result of a disturbed balance of forces between the deltoid muscle and rotator cuff.[27] These abnormal bony relationships appear analogous to positional faults and have been measured with various imaging techniques (ultrasound, MRI, X-ray, CAT scans) and recently by combining palpation and photography in a clinical situation.

A previously studied measure of altered position of the glenohumeral joint is the acromiohumeral distance (AHD),[26–28] which is determined as the tangential distance between the humeral head and the edge of the acromion using longitudinal ultrasound imaging (Figure 4.3) and MRI. The AHD as measured with ultrasound, and verified against X-ray, is significantly smaller in shoulders with more severe rotator cuff injuries[28] and shoulder impingement syndrome,[29] in which it was termed the acromio-greater tuberosity (AGT) distance. While Cholewinski et al[29] reported the median difference between impingement syndrome and normal shoulders was 2.7 mm and their minimal meaningful difference being 2.1 mm, the range of data spanned from -3.9 to 8.6 mm, indicating that positional faults exist in only some of these patients. Using MRI, Hebert et al[30] reported a mean difference between affected and unaffected sides of 1.3 mm (95% CI: 0.87 to 1.73) and 1.2 mm (95% CI: 0.53 to 1.87) at 100° flexion and 80° abduction of the shoulder respectively, but that this was not present in neutral. Combining elevation with isometric muscle contraction significantly reduced the AHD in shoulders with impingement syndrome in a study by Graichen et al[31] in cases where there was no difference in AHD in the relaxed state (1.4 mm vs 4.4 mm). Interestingly, Desmeules et al[32] reported AHD in the neutral shoulder position to be 9.9 mm (SD 1.5, n = 13) but 12 mm (SD 1.9, n = 7) in impingement syndrome, which is a larger AHD in the impingement syndrome shoulders by approximately 2.1 mm (95% CI: -3.72 to -0.48). Furthermore, they reported that greater functional improvement following a comprehensive multi-modal rehabilitation program including both passive joint mobilisations and exercises was strongly associated with a reduction in the narrowing of the AHD. It would appear that in some patients with rotator cuff injury or impingement syndrome there exists a positional fault, but that this appears dependent on a number of factors, such as shoulder elevation position, state of muscle contraction, and severity of the condition.

The use of sophisticated and expensive imaging tools to measure the AHD, place it outside of the realm of most practitioners and clinics, thus there is a need for some clinical measurement of the shoulder to detect if positional faults are present or not. Practitioners often use observation and palpation to obtain a sense of the relative position of the humeral head in the glenoid.

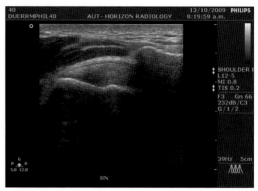

Figure 4.3 Acromiohumeral distance (AHD) on ultrasound imaging

McKenna et al[33] appear to have replicated this by reporting on a combined palpatory–photographic technique for measuring the distance between the anterior margin of the acromion and the anterior border of the humeral head. They investigated the reliability of this clinical measure and determined its validity by comparison to MRI. While the intra-class correlation coefficient for intra-rater repeated measurements was acceptable at greater than 0.85, the minimal reliable change for the palpatory–photographic technique was 6.1 mm, which was larger than the 4.9 mm pathological distance that they had calculated from a meta-analysis of the literature. On this basis, it would appear that further refinements are required before there is a valid method for determining if a glenohumeral joint positional fault exists in a clinical context.

Notwithstanding the efforts as outlined above for tibiofibular, patellofemoral and glenohumeral joints, and in order to improve the practitioner's ability to clinically measure positional faults, should they exist, there is a need for a systematic approach to evaluating the PFH. The issue of large inter-patient variability and heterogeneity, as outlined above, cautions against simply adopting the PFH as the mechanism underlying MWM effects and efficacy.

HOW MAY POSITIONAL FAULTS CAUSE PAIN AND IMPAIRMENT?

The means by which positional faults may cause musculoskeletal pain or loss of range of motion has not been clearly identified to date. Over the recent decade the orthopaedic notion that musculoskeletal pain can be readily (or purely) explained through biomechanical or structural means has evolved to encompass the emerging evidence of the behaviour and properties of biological systems.[34, 35] Dye[35] proposed the 'envelope of function' model, which incorporates the properties of biological systems, to explain the capacity for the musculoskeletal system to adapt to a range of loading conditions homeostatically as a function of some temporal variable (e.g. frequency, timing, duration of loading). That is, the envelope of function defines the range of load that the system can tolerate over a given timeframe before suffering structural macro- or micro-failure due to supra-physiologic overload. The macro- or micro-failure in tissues is then presumed to be the precursor to musculoskeletal pain. There are many factors that would determine the capacity of an individual's tissues to adapt to the load or to succumb to physiological overload and structural failure. For example, there are intrinsic factors including genetics, bony alignment issues (e.g. torsions, varus, valgus), joint mechanics (perhaps including positional faults), previous injury (e.g. ligamentous deficiency), general hypermobility syndrome and nutritional status (protein and micro nutrient); as well as extrinsic factors such as total amount of load being experienced by the tissues and the period of time between the loads. These intrinsic and extrinsic factors may be present in a myriad of possibly interacting and/or interdependent ways in the patient with musculoskeletal pain and injury.

Sahrmann proposes that the biomechanics of motion segments of the human body are similar to the mechanics of other systems in that ideal alignment of moving parts will optimise longevity and problem free function.[36] While acknowledging that biological systems do indeed demonstrate a positive adaptive response to variations from ideal alignment and mechanics, Sahrmann argues that when alignment and movement are not ideal a scenario exists for a breakdown in the system (e.g. degenerative joint changes).[36] The writings of Dye[35] and Sahrmann[36] appear to echo the sentiment of other authorities on the subject and may serve as an explanation of the role of positional faults in musculoskeletal pain and injury.

At any joint (motion segment) the movement of the joint members at any instant during a motion can be described as rotation about the instantaneous axis of rotation.[37] This instantaneous axis of rotation is seldom fixed and during motion follows a path, termed the path of the instantaneous axis of rotation.[38] A positional fault will feasibly result in a deviation from the ideal path of the instantaneous axis of rotation, which may then lead to a change in loading of the supporting joint structures and consequently the experience of pain and associated impairment.[39, 40] Indeed, Comerford and Mottram[41] describe the deviations from the ideal path of the instantaneous axis of rotation in terms of abnormal translatory accessory glides which abnormally load the supporting joint structures, thus causing micro-stress that, with repetition, eventually leads to tissue breakdown and pain.

We believe that this concept of movement deviation leading to abnormal tissue stress and pain may well serve as a contemporary model of the PFH that can be used by practitioners to describe the possible mechanical relationship between a positional fault and the presenting musculoskeletal condition. It must be remembered that further research is required in order for it to be validly considered as the underlying mechanism of the PFH.

DO MWM TECHNIQUES CORRECT POSITIONAL FAULTS?

There is a lack of quality studies as to the corrective effects of MWM on positional faults to enable any conclusion to be drawn in this regard. The comprehensive searches of databases, conference records and reference lists we have conducted in writing this book have returned two low quality papers that have specifically looked at this issue in living people. One of these papers was an extended conference abstract[42] that reported a study of eight recently sprained ankles and the other a single case study of a chronically injured thumb[43] with both utilising MRI to measure bony positions before and after MWM.

Merlin et al[42] studied the effect of the fibular MWM (postero–superior glide of the lateral malleolus in relation to the tibia; see Chapter 19 for a detailed description of the technique and Chapter 3 [Table 3.6] for details of the study) on fibular position immediately following application. They took MRI scans while the ankle was positioned at 90° in a brace. It would appear from the brief explanation provided that the position of the fibula in three planes was measured relative to two water markers on the ankle brace (i.e. the fibula to tibia relationship was not actually evaluated). No information was provided on the reliability (especially the error associated with the removal and re-application of the brace) or the validity of the MRI measurement technique. Nevertheless, the authors report a 0.35 cm (95% CI: 0.12 to 0.58) cephalad displacement in the sagittal plane following the MWM. It is difficult to know if the size of this fibular displacement is a meaningful one or not, but the treatment did improve weight-bearing dorsiflexion by 1.6 cm (95% CI: 0.53 to 2.67) linear length of longest toe to wall measure and single leg stance balance with eyes closed by 9.6 second (95% CI: 6.27 to 12.93). No changes in any other direction or plane were reported.

The other study was a single case report that evaluated the effect of a MWM of the first metacarpophalangeal joint in a patient with chronic thumb pain 7 months after a fall onto an outstretched hand.[43] Hsieh et al[43] used MRI to investigate the position of the first proximal phalanx on the metacarpal pre-MWM, during the application of MWM in situ, and 4 weeks after commencing MWM treatment when the condition had fully resolved (see Chapter 14). On examination, the treating practitioner determined that a supination glide of the proximal phalanx made a substantial change to the limited and painful thumb flexion. The assessor imaging the joint and the practitioner administering treatment were blind to each other's data. A 4° pronation 'positional fault' of the proximal phalanx was noted after comparative MRIs of both the patient's hands at baseline. This fault was reversed during the application of a self-supination MWM. Although the program of MWM self-treatment over 3 weeks improved the condition, a follow-up MRI at 4 weeks revealed that the positional fault itself was unchanged. It must be remembered that this is a single case study and as such there is low validity in externalising the results. Nevertheless, the paper describes a likely scenario of the presence of a positional fault, the specificity of effect with selecting the correct direction of accessory movement glide for the MWM, and importantly that the positional fault need not be improved in the longer term for the patient's pain and disability to resolve.

One further relevant study was identified that evaluated the displacement characteristics of the humeral head of an instrumented cadaver when 10 different physiotherapists applied a MWM in an anterior–posterior direction during abduction (see also Chapter 12).[44] The MWM produced substantially greater posterior displacement of the humeral head than did abduction without the MWM applied. The need for further study of humeral head displacement in live people with active contractions against gravity is required to validate the hypothesis that MWM produces changes in joint position during its application.

A LESSON FROM THE EXPERIENCE OF PFPS AND MCCONNELL'S INNOVATIONS

Taping the patella to manage patellofemoral pain syndrome (PFPS), which was first described by McConnell in 1986[23] is an effective form of management.[45, 46] The initial premise underlying the McConnell approach for patellofemoral pain was that taping would correct the faulty position of the patella in the trochlear notch of the femur,[46] much the same as the proposition of MWM altering a positional fault.

Aminaka and Gribble[47] conducted a structured review of the effects of McConnell's patellar taping on pain, patellar alignment and neuromuscular control. They report that while there is evidence supporting the effects of this taping in managing patellofemoral pain, this is not the case in terms of its ability to change patellar position. They concluded that the mechanisms by which the pain-relieving effects came about remain to be elucidated. Since that review, Herrington[48] used MRI to investigate change in lateral patellar displacement (LPD; i.e. alignment of the patella in the frontal plane) at 0°, 10°, and 20° knee flexion before and after taping. The authors reported that the taping resulted in a statistically significant reduction in LPD of 0.4, 1.1 and 0.7 mm at 0°, 10° and 20° knee flexion, respectively.

However, the size of this change in the main did not eclipse the minimal detectable change (or measurement error of 0.83 mm), which further highlights an issue related to the measurement of positional faults and any changes in such faults with treatment. That is, the faults and their corrections are likely to be very small and problematic in terms of measurement technique accuracy/error. Herrington[24] hypothesised that these small changes might be sufficient to bring about the biological effects that result in a reduction in pain associated with patella taping, but this relationship remains to be explored. The ability of tape to continue to change patellar alignment after it has been removed also remains untested.

The salient lesson for MWM to be learnt from the history of the evolution of evidence for patellar taping; is that while both patellar taping and MWM appear to improve pain, impairment and disability, this may not be achieved through the short-term or permanent correction of positional faults. Two issues need to be borne in mind when considering the PFH and MWM. First, care must be taken when interpreting the success of a MWM because that success (as measured with pain, disability and global satisfaction scales) need not indicate that a positional fault existed and that it was corrected by the technique. Second, the presence of an initial or immediate change in bony position may not necessarily precede a long-term change in positional fault. This is not to say that positional faults are irrelevant in the clinical application of MWM, because there does appear to be preliminary evidence (albeit of a low level) that the most effective direction of the glide applied in the MWM will be in the opposite direction to any existing positional fault.

SUMMARY
The PFH evolved as Mulligan's explanation for his clinical observation that MWM improves joint movement, relieves pain and restores function. Elements of the PFH appear to be supported to a small extent by the literature; for example, there is some evidence that positional faults may exist at some joints and low-level evidence indicating that the most effective direction of a MWM is in the opposite direction to any positional fault. There is no evidence to support or refute that the PFH, in part or in full, explains the mechanism(s) by which MWM produces its clinical effects on pain, impairments and disability. The main issue to consider in the PFH is the difficulty in accurately measuring any positional faults. This clouds the current evidence on the existence, or not, of positional faults, though with the advent of improved and more sophisticated imaging technologies this problem may not be insurmountable, at least in the research laboratory initially, and portends further elucidation on the PFH in MWM. There are likely other mechanisms by which MWM produces its clinical effects and these are further explored in the following three chapters.

KEY POINTS

- The positional fault hypothesis (PFH) proposes that MWM corrects the minor bony incongruities, which putatively occur after an injury or with misuse and are responsible for ongoing symptoms and dysfunction.

- There is evidence that positional faults may indeed exist; for example, at the inferior tibiofibular, patellofemoral and shoulder joints.

- Measurement of positional faults is achieved largely through imaging techniques that are not readily available clinically to the practitioner of MWM.

- Though difficult to prove, it is hypothesised that positional faults lead to pain and impairment through abnormal joint mechanics and ensuing wear and tear of soft tissues.

- There is little research into the effects of MWM on positional faults.

- There is no evidence to support or refute that the PFH, in part or in full, explains the mechanism(s) by which MWM produces its clinical effects on pain, impairments and disability.

- There is low level, very preliminary evidence that indicates that the direction of a successful MWM may well be in the opposite direction to the positional fault.

- Amelioration of symptoms and restoration of function do not prove a positional fault existed.

References

1 Mulligan B. Manual Therapy: 'NAGS', 'SNAGS', 'PRP'S' etc. (1st edn). Wellington: Plane View Services Ltd 1989.

2 Mulligan B. Mobilisations with movement (MWM). The Journal of Manual & Manipulative Therapy. 1993;1(4):154–6.

3 Mulligan B. Mobilisations with movement (MWMs) for the hip joint to restore internal rotation and flexion. Journal of Manual and Manipulative Therapy. 1996;4(1): 35–6.

4 Mulligan B. Manual Therapy: 'NAGS', 'SNAGS', 'MWMS' etc. (6th edn). Wellington: Plane View Services Ltd 2006.

5 Folk B. Traumatic thumb injury management using mobilization with movement. Manual Therapy. 2001 Aug;6(3):178–82.

6 McKenzie R. The Lumbar Spine: Mechanical Diagnosis and Therapy. Waikanae, New Zealand: Spinal 1981.

7 Palmer DD. The Chiropractor's Adjuster: the Science, Art and Philosophy of Chiropractic. Portland: Portland Printing House 1910.

8 Hertel J. Functional Anatomy, Pathomechanics, and Pathophysiology of Lateral Ankle Instability. Journal Athletic Training. 2002 Dec;37(4):364–75.

9 Hetherington B. Lateral ligament strains of the ankle, do they exist? Manual Therapy. 1996 Dec;1(5):274–5.

10 Hubbard TJ, Hertel J, Sherbondy P. Fibular position in individuals with self-reported chronic ankle instability. Journal of Orthopaedic Sports Physical Therapy. 2006 Jan;36(1):3–9.

11 Hubbard TJ, Hertel J. Anterior positional fault of the fibula after sub-acute lateral ankle sprains. Manual Therapy. 2008 Feb;13(1):63–7.

12 Refshauge K, Gass E. Musculoskeletal Physiotherapy: Clinical Science and Evidence-based Practice (2nd edn). Oxford: Butterworth-Heinemann 2004.

13 LeBrun CT, Krause JO. Variations in mortise anatomy. The American journal of sports medicine. 2005 Jun 1;33(6):852–5.

14 Scranton P, McDermott J, Rogers J. The relationship between chronic ankle instability and variations in mortise anatomy and impingement spurs. Foot & Ankle International. 2000;21:657–64.

15 Mavi A, Yildirim H, Gunes H, Pestamalci T, Gumusburun E. The fibular incisura of the tibia with recurrent sprained ankle on magnetic resonance imaging. Saudi Medical Journal. 2002 Jul;23(7):845–9.

16 Brukner P, Khan K. Clinical Sports Medicine (3rd edn). Sydney: McGraw-Hill 2007.

17 Wilson T. The measurement of patellar alignment in patellofemoral pain syndrome: are we confusing assumptions with evidence? Journal of Orthopaedic Sports Physical Therapy. 2007 Jun;37(6):330–41.

18 Merchant A. Roentgenographic analysis of patellofemoral congruence. The Journal of Bone and Joint Surgery. 1974;56(7):1391–6.

19 Aglietti P, Insall JN, Cerulli G. Patellar pain and incongruence. I: measurements of incongruence. Clinical Orthopaedic Related Research. 1983 Jun(176):217–24.

20 Laurin CA, Levesque HP, Dussault R, Labelle H, Peides JP. The abnormal lateral patellofemoral angle: a diagnostic roentgenographic sign of recurrent patellar subluxation. Journal of Bone and Joint Surgery America. 1978 Jan;60(1):55–60.

21 Sheehan FT, Seisler AR, Alter KE. Three-dimensional in vivo quantification of knee kinematics in cerebral palsy. Clinical Orthopaedic Related Research. 2008 Feb;466(2):450–8.

22 McConnell J. The physical therapist's approach to patellofemoral disorders. Clinics in Sports Medicine. 2002 21(3):363–87.

23 McConnell J. The management of chondromalacia patellae: a long-term solution. The Australian Journal of Physiotherapy. 1986;32(4):215–23.

24 Herrington L. The difference in a clinical measure of patella lateral position between individuals with patellofemoral pain and matched controls. Journal of Orthopaedic Sports Physical Therapy. 2008;38(2):59–62.

25 Smith TO, Davies L, Donell ST. The reliability and validity of assessing medio-lateral patellar position: a systematic review. Manual Therapy. 2009 Aug;14(4):355–62.

26 Brossmann J, Preidler KW, Pedowitz RA, White LM, Trudell D, Resnick D. Shoulder impingement syndrome: influence of shoulder position on rotator cuff impingement — an anatomic study. American Journal of Roentgenology. 1996 Dec;167(6):1511–5.

27 Azzoni R, Cabitza P, Parrini M. Sonographic evaluation of subacromial space. Ultrasonics. 2004 Apr;42(1–9):683–7.

28 Azzoni R, Cabitza P. Sonographic versus radiographic measurement of the subacromial space width. La Chirurgia degli Organi di Movimento. 2004 Apr–Jun;89(2):143–50.

29 Cholewinski JJ, Kusz DJ, Wojciechowski P, Cielinski LS, Zoladz MP. Ultrasound measurement of rotator cuff thickness and acromio-humeral distance in the diagnosis of subacromial impingement syndrome of the shoulder. Knee Surgery Sports Traumatology Arthroscopy. 2008 Apr;16(4):408–14.

30 Hebert LJ, Moffet H, Dufour M, Moisan C. Acromio-humeral distance in a seated position in persons with impingement syndrome. Journal of Magnetic Resonance Imaging. 2003;18:72–9.

31 Graichen H, Bonel H, Stammberger T, Heuck A, Englmeier KH, Reiser M, et al. An MR-based technique for determination of the subacromial space width in subjects with and without shoulder muscle activity. Zeitschrift fur Orthopadie und ihre Grenzgebiete. 1999 Jan–Feb; 137(1):2–6.

32 Desmeules F, Minville L, Riederer B, Cote CH, Fremont P. Acromio-humeral distance variation measured by ultrasonography and its association with the outcome of rehabilitation for shoulder impingement syndrome. Clinical Journal of Sports Medicine. 2004 Jul;14(4):197–205.

33 McKenna L, Straker L, Smith A. The validity and intratester reliability of a clinical measure of humeral head position. Manual Therapy. 2009 Aug;14(4):397–403.

34 Dye SF. The knee as a biologic transmission with an envelope of function: a theory. Failed anterior cruciate ligament surgery. Clinical Orthopaedics and Related Research. 1996;325:10.

35 Dye SF. The pathophysiology of patellofemoral pain: a tissue homeostasis perspective. Clinical Orthopaedics and Related Research. 2005;436:100.

36 Sahrmann S. Diagnosis and Treatment of Movement Impairment Syndromes. St Louis: Mosby 2002.

37 White AA, Panjabi MM. Clinical Biomechanics of the Spine (2nd edn). Philadelphia: Lippincott 1990.

38 Zatsiorsky VM. Kinematics of human motion. Champaign, III: Human Kinematics 1998.

39 Gerber C, Matter P. Biomechanical analysis of the knee after rupture of the anterior cruciate ligament and its primary repair: an instant-centre analysis of function. Journal of Bone Joint Surgery British. 1983;65:391–9.

40 Frankel VH, Burstein AH, Brooks DB. Biomechanics of internal derangement of the knee: pathomechanics as determined by analysis of the instant centers of rotation. Journal of Bone Joint Surgery Am. 1971;53:945–62.

41 Comerford MJ, Mottram SL. Movement and stability dysfunction — contemporary developments. Manual Therapy. 2001 Feb;6(1):15–26.

42 Merlin DJ, McEwan I, Thom JM. Mulligan's mobilisation with movement technique for lateral ankle pain and the use of magnetic resonance imaging to evaluate the 'positional fault' hypothesis. XIV International Congress on Sports Rehabilitation and Traumatology 2005. Online. Available: www.isokinetic.com (accessed 27 April 2010).

43 Hsieh CY, Vicenzino B, Yang CH, Hu MH, Yang C. Mulligan's mobilization with movement for the thumb: a single case report using magnetic resonance imaging to evaluate the positional fault hypothesis. Manual Therapy. 2002 Feb;7(1):44–9.

44 Kai-Yu Ho, Hsu A-T. Displacement of the head of humerus while performing 'mobilization with movements' in glenohumeral joint: a cadaver study. Manual Therapy. 2009;14(2):160–6.

45 Gerrard B. The patello-femoral pain syndrome: A clinical trial of the McConnell program. The Australian Journal of Physiotherapy. 1989;35(2):71–80.

46 Crossley K, Cowan SM, Bennell KL, McConnell J. Patellar taping: is clinical success supported by scientific evidence? Manual Therapy. 2000 Aug;5(3):142–50.

47 Aminaka N, Gribble PA. A systematic review of the effects of therapeutic taping on patellofemoral pain syndrome. Journal of Athletic Training. 2005 Oct–Dec;40(4):341–51.

48 Herrington L. The effect of corrective taping of the patella on patella position as defined by MRI. Research in Sports Medicine. 2006;14(3):215–23.

Chapter 5
A new proposed model of the mechanisms of action of Mobilisation with Movement

Bill Vicenzino, Toby Hall, Wayne Hing and Darren Rivett

INTRODUCTION

As canvassed in Chapter 3, there is for some techniques an evolving body of evidence attesting to the claims made by practitioners regarding the clinical utility and benefits of those Mobilisation with Movement (MWM) techniques. That chapter also included a call for further clinical studies of higher quality to test the clinical efficacy of MWM generally for the range of different treatment techniques for a variety of musculoskeletal conditions. That endeavour focuses on addressing the question, *does MWM work*, whereas there is also another focus required in our consideration of MWM, and that is to answer the question, *how does MWM work*. This focus is more about the underlying mechanism(s) by which MWM exerts its clinical effects. Understanding the underlying mechanism(s) of action is likely to lead to advances in MWM and a better informed application of MWM, both as a sole intervention and as part of a multi-modal management approach.

In Chapter 4, we explored Mulligan's proposed positional fault hypothesis and concluded that evidence to support or refute it is lacking. In this chapter we propose a new model for the mechanism(s) of action through which MWM brings about its benefits. It is important to preface this with an understanding that the model deals with the processes that are stimulated with a single successful repetition of MWM; that is, one that produces a substantial (if not total) improvement in the client specific impairment measure (CSIM). For example, visualise that you have applied a lateral glide to the wrist and improved wrist extension from 15° to 60° at first onset of pain. An immediate question of *how did that happen* often springs to mind. This chapter proposes a model by which you the practitioner may conceptualise a response to this question. There is also some consideration given to the possible mechanisms underpinning the sustained effect gained with many repetitions of MWM, which leads on from the model for a single repetition. It assumes that the practitioner has conducted a thorough clinical examination and made some decisions regarding the underlying patho-anatomical and patho-physiological features of the condition being treated with the MWM treatment technique.

This chapter, along with Chapters 4, 6 and 7, seeks to present our thinking on possible mechanism(s) of action and effects of MWM, with evidence-informed consideration where possible.

BIOMECHANICAL AND NEUROSCIENCE PARADIGMS

The mechanism(s) underpinning the clinical efficacy of joint manipulation was initially conceived in simple terms of bony malposition and subluxations.[1] This likely originated at the clinical level on the basis of primary feedback experienced by the practitioner and/or pioneers of the field. That is, when applying a joint manipulation, the practitioner will have sensed a relative motion of the bony members of a joint and on another level the patient feeding back improvements in pain, function and capacity. It could be argued that the sensing of this joint motion is what the practitioner is aiming to achieve, possibly as an initial feedback of a successful manipulation. Certainly, much energy and time is spent in the training of manipulative therapists to sense such motion and bony displacements, with instructions focussed on positioning of the patient, the joint being manipulated, the therapist's body and therapist's hands, in order to optimise the bony displacement achieved during the manipulation.[1–6] These instructions form the basis of some of the foundation textbooks of joint manipulation. It is conceivable that when the practitioner witnessed both the local bone-joint changes and the accompanying improvement in the patient's condition, the practitioner would ascribe the patient's improvements in mechanical terms; that is, an underlying biomechanical mechanism of action. Consistent with this, it appears that much of the original written material on manipulation focussed on the hypotheses of underlying mechanisms of actions of joint manipulation that were biomechanical in nature (Figure 5.1), with the emphasis on stretching, tearing, straightening, and reducing a variety of proposed lesions of either bone, joint, muscles, nerves or blood vessels.[7–15] In relatively more recent times, with increasing research and data on the nervous system and in the pain-related sciences, came an increasing appreciation of how manipulation may evoke changes in the nervous system (Figure 5.1) [16–18] and bring about the clinically beneficial improvements in a patient's condition. The genesis of the biomechanical and neuroscience paradigms does not only have a historical basis but to some extent seems to have been reinforced by research laboratory set-ups, which have tended to reflect the scientific disciplines of the researchers; for example, biomechanics or neurophysiology.

A PROPOSED MODEL IN OVERVIEW

We propose to demonstrate that both biomechanical and neurophysiological mechanisms are implicated in the mechanism of action of MWM, and that furthermore they are likely interrelated in this model, as shown schematically in Figure 5.2. In brief, the proposition is that the practitioner skilfully applies a painless MWM force to a joint, paying careful attention to such aspects as location of application of force, direction of force and amount or level of force applied (see Chapter 2 for more detail), which produces a transient change in bone position that then allows a concomitant and substantial improvement in a previously painfully impaired physical task. Such a substantial improvement implies that the transient change in bone position is a critical element of an input into some body systems, likely to be the central nervous system. In regard to the central nervous system involvement, MWM has been shown to produce a non-opioid mechanical hypoalgesia,[25–28] which is regarded as evidence of central nervous system involvement. That is, the MWM, through its mechanical perturbations at the treated joint, is an effective stimulus to instantaneously trigger processes within the central nervous system, which are responsible for bringing about the clinical improvements. A large component of this central nervous system involvement appears to be the endogenous descending pain inhibitory system(s) (DPIS) (Figure 5.2), [29–31] though sensory and motor system mechanisms are yet to be explored to any great extent. It is important to keep in mind that MWM by definition must not be painful on application or afterwards.

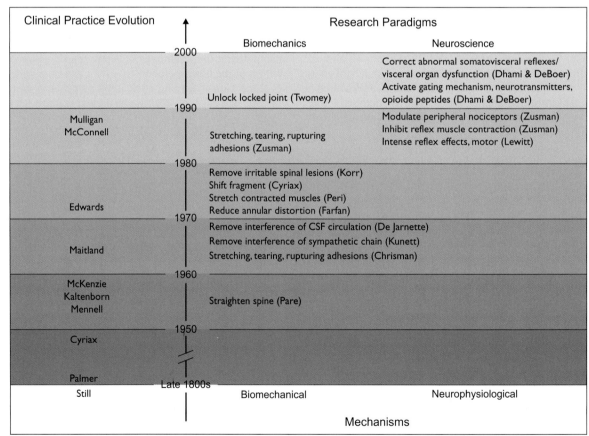

Figure 5.1 Timeline bringing together the timing of some of the works of key manual therapy practitioners, [3, 5, 8, 19–24] research paradigms and putative mechanisms of action

Note: By and large the evolution of our understanding of the mechanisms of action of manual therapy generically has gone from reasonably simplistic mechanical concepts[7–15] to more involved and sophisticated neuroscience.[16–18]

Biomechanical component

The predominant hypothesis of the mechanism underpinning MWM is the positional fault hypothesis (Chapter 4). It is interesting that such a proposition has been advanced for MWM, as it follows strongly that of many other manipulation approaches by proposing that a positional fault exists at the affected joint and that the mechanism of action underpinning the clinically observable improvements of MWM is in the treatment's correction of this fault. An exposition of the positional fault hypothesis is provided in Chapter 4 and the reader is referred there for more detail, whereas here we will focus on the only two case studies that we are aware of in which positional changes have been demonstrated during the application of joint manipulation, one a spinal manipulation technique on two fresh intact cadaveric spines and the other a MWM for thumb pain.

Gal et al performed a 3-D kinematic analysis of a unilateral posterior to anterior spinal manipulative thrust of T_{10-12} motion segments in two unembalmed 77-year-old human cadavers.[32] They ensured that their manipulation was within that which is clinically applied by measuring applied force and only including manipulations within the force levels shown to occur in clinic. In brief, their results indicated that manipulation produces short-term global displacement of vertebrae in the order of 6–12 mm, which decays to pre-manipulation levels within 10 minutes. Though not about MWM, this is one of the few studies that meticulously measured the input force and output displacements of joint manipulation, thereby verifying that clinical observations can be substantiated in a laboratory situation, albeit in cadavers.

Hsieh et al treated a 79-year-old female with persistent thumb pain of 7 months duration and showed that a MWM, which consisted of a supination glide of the proximal phalange of the thumb while the patient flexed the thumb, was able to reverse a positional fault as visualised on magnetic resonance imaging (MRI, see Chapter 14).[33] However, this only occurred while the MWM was in place, as the phalanx reverted to the pre-treatment pronated position on re-imaging when the patient had fully recovered. A salient feature of this case study was that of the glides of supination, pronation, lateral and medial glides that were tested, only the former proved able to immediately on application completely ameliorate the impaired thumb motion.

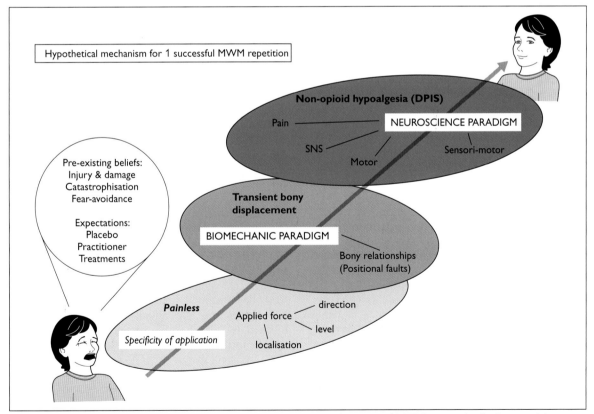

Figure 5.2 A mind map laying out the proposed mechanism of action of MWM on each single repetition
Note: In brief Figure 5.2 shows that specific forces applied to the body produce mechanical perturbations and changes in pain, motor, sensory and sympathetic nervous systems (SNS).

From a mechanistic perspective this may well be a preliminary insight into the relative importance of bony and joint displacements during MWM in that it would seem it is critical to the successful application of the MWM for the right direction to be selected. It is thus compelling to speculate that the reason for such specificity in joint glide direction is that it provides the most effective afferent input signal, which brings about an adequate level of stimulation of and response from the body's intrinsic self-reparative/protective mechanisms. Alternatively, in some joints the proposed reduction of entrapped meniscoids[34, 35] or synovial fringe may be the mechanism by which a specifically directed MWM glide brings about its clinically beneficial effects, possibly in those cases where only one repetition is required to bring about substantial and long lasting effects.

Neurophysiological component

The neurophysiological component covers a number of somewhat different areas of science, which in the main are the pain and motor control sciences related literature.

Pain sciences

There are several characteristics of the effects of MWM on the pain system, which have likely implications on the mechanisms of action underpinning the clinical outcomes from MWM. For example, it would appear that MWM produces a mechanical hypoalgesia that does not involve opioid peptides.[25–28] Several studies of the lateral glide MWM for tennis elbow have shown a significant moderate pooled effect (standardised mean difference [SMD] 0.49; 95% confidence interval [CI] 0.08 to 0.90, see Figure 3.3) on pressure pain thresholds over the lateral elbow. The postero–lateral glide at the glenohumeral joint for shoulder elevation MWM induces an effect on pressure pain threshold in the order of a SMD of 0.87 (95% CI: 0.28 to 1.47),[36] however this was not the case with the dorsiflexion MWM applied to sub-acute ankle sprains (SMD -0.22 [95% CI: -0.97 to 0.52]).[37] In stark contrast, MWM does not appear to have an effect on thermal pain thresholds with a study by Paungmali et al showing little difference between pre and post application of the lateral glide MWM in tennis elbow (0.3° [95% CI: -1.85 to 2.45]),[38] which is similar to studies of cervical spine lateral glide mobilisation grade III on this condition. [39–41] It may well be that conditions such as tennis elbow do not have thermal hypoalgesia and so there is a ceiling effect that masks any effect of MWM on thermal pain. This has not been studied in MWM, but a study of the cervical lateral glide technique applied to whiplash injured patients who had a 1.5° (95% CI: 0.11 to 2.89) deficit in thermal pain threshold reported no real change (mean difference: 0.2° [95% CI: -0.78 to 1.2]) following spinal manipulative therapy.[42] The exact implications of preferential effects on mechanical pain are not

yet clear, though it may be that the mechanical hypoalgesia is mediated through noradrenergic neurons emanating from medullopontine nuclei and thermal through more centrally located serotonergic raphe nuclei.[43–52] However this requires further work.

The pain-relieving effects of MWM and some other joint manipulation techniques are likely not to involve endogenous pain suppression mechanisms that are mediated by opioid peptides. Paungmali et al conducted the only studies on MWM that we are aware of and they were on the lateral glide MWM for tennis elbow.[25, 26] The details of one of these studies[25] are shown in Chapter 3 (Table 3.6), but in brief it used naloxone in an attempt to antagonise the pain relieving effects of MWM and reported that naloxone did not antagonise the MWM pain effects. This was interpreted as a lack of endogenous opioid in the pain-relieving effect of MWM. Other somewhat similar non-MWM techniques have been studied in a similar way with similar outcomes.[41, 53] Other methodologies have also been used to study the role of opioid peptides in joint manipulation, such as evaluating their presence in plasma and testing the endorphin mediated hypoalgesia characteristic of tolerance to repeated stimulation, [26, 30, 54–56] with the majority arriving at similar conclusions.

Interestingly, there are some experiments of joint manipulation in a rat animal model that may have relevance to the mechanisms of action for MWM.[57, 58] The rat model involves the injection of capsaicin into the ankle joint, which produces hyperalgesia in that paw. The measurement of mechanical hyperalgesia was through paw withdrawal to pressure from von Frey filaments, with a reduced paw pressure to elicit paw withdrawal indicating hyperalgesia. The joint manipulation was applied to the ipsilateral knee joint. It was a grade III mobilisation into extension with an anterior posterior accessory glide applied to the knee.[5] The coupling of a physiological movement and accessory glide taken to the end of range, albeit passive, bears some resemblance to that of a MWM that could potentially be applied to the knee in humans.

In their first set of experiments, this group demonstrated that the joint manipulation produced a robust and substantial reversal of the capsaicin induced mechanical hyperalgesia.[58] In their latter experiments, they demonstrated that the manipulation-induced hypoalgesia was substantially antagonised or totally blocked by intrathecally administered methysergide maleate and yohimbine, which are specific antagonists for serotonergic ($5-HT_1$ and $5-HT_2$) receptors or α_2-adrenergic receptors, respectively.[57] This was not the case following the administration of naloxone hydrochloride dihydrate and bicuculline methiodide, which are antagonists to opioid and γ-aminobutyric acid ($GABA_A$) receptors, respectively. The failure of naloxone to antagonise the manipulation-induced hypoalgesia parallels the findings from human research reported above, supporting the claim that the mechanism of action of MWM is probably not endorphin based. The application of the joint manipulation to the knee whilst measuring effects distally at the foot also tends to remove local changes at the site of the provoked hyperalgesia as an underlying mechanism of action for the joint manipulation. This leaves central nervous system mechanisms as likely candidates for mechanisms underpinning manipulation-induced hypoalgesia. Others have shown that stimulation of the Rostro-ventral Medulla (RVM) and periaqueductal gray (PAG) increase spinal release of serotonin and noradrenaline leading Skyba et al[57] to conclude that joint manipulation activates a descending inhibitory pathway, which is non-opioid mediated.

The conclusion from animal research that a descending pain inhibitory system is, at least in part, the mechanism of action of joint manipulation is supported by other human research of joint manipulation that has concurrently evaluated its effect on pain and the sympathetic nervous system.[29–31, 39] Paungmali et al have shown that the application of MWM mimics the initial effects of spinal manipulative therapy for which there appear to be concomitant effects in the sympathetic nervous system.[38] The work on spinal manipulative therapy has found that the initial effects on pain and the sympathetic nervous system are correlated, implying that the treatment technique triggered a mechanism that has some capacity to coordinate a response in both the endogenous pain control and sympathetic nervous systems. An hypothesis was proposed that this may well be a specific column of cells within the PAG, because when this column is stimulated in animal and human experiments there is a concurrent non-opioid hypoalgesia, sympathoexcitation and motor facilitation.[39, 59–61] The PAG-spinal connection is likely not direct, with relay sites for the endogenous pain inhibitory system and the pre-motor sympathetic cells being situated in the RVM, which could plausibly be another centre that is stimulated by the joint manipulation technique. These centres receive inputs from many areas of the central nervous system and so it is likely that the mechanism by which joint manipulation activates the PAG is complex, probably indirect and multifactorial. Nevertheless, when taken in conjunction with the animal studies above, there is a good basis for suggesting that joint manipulation, including MWM, brings about its clinical pain-relieving effects, at least in part, through activation of a descending pain inhibitory system, which is likely not opioid mediated.

Motor system

On a prima facie basis, the motor system plays a pivotal role in MWM, because many CSIMs involve impairments and dysfunction of the motor system.

The motor system here being defined in its broadest sense, from the passive structural level through to the more dynamic and complex control systems level. Despite the apparent inseparable relationship between motor system and MWM there is very little research that provides some insight into the underlying motor system processes that might be engaged in the mechanism(s) of action of MWM, especially in comparison to the research of the pain system. This section will explore possible motor system effects and mechanisms of MWM.

Interestingly, although relatively more research of manipulative therapy, including MWM, has focussed on the pain sciences, the impact of MWM appears greater on the motor system. For example, as outlined in Chapter 3, the lateral glide MWM for tennis elbow, which has been studied the most of all MWM techniques, seems to influence the motor system as it produces more of an effect on force generation as measured by pain-free grip strength (pooled SMD 1.28; 95% CI: 0.84 to 1.73) than directly on the pain system, as measured by pressure pain threshold (pooled SMD 0.49; 95% CI: 0.08 to 0.90). Pain-free grip strength is defined as the amount of grip force generated to the onset of pain; that is, it is primarily a motor action that is limited by perception of pain, so it is not inhibited by pain, but ceased by a cognitive decision by the patient who is driving the motor action of forming a grip with his/her hands against the dynamometer handles. The change in pain-free grip strength brought about by MWM exceeds that of a credible placebo in this laboratory situation and so the cognitive decision is likely not explained by the desire of the patient to please the practitioner.[27] It is salient to recall that the difference between the MWM and placebo in the studies of tennis elbow [25–27, 38] was in the location of the manual contact and the point of application of the lateral gliding force. In the placebo condition the hand producing the lateral glide was not only on the ulnar but also equally on the humerus and the stabilising hand was not only on the humerus but also on the lateral proximal forearm. The practitioner applying the placebo MWM exerted similar force and pressure to that of the MWM, but equally to the humerus and ulnar on medial and lateral sides. The differences between the MWM and the placebo are likely important in the underlying mechanisms of action. We propose that the difference is in the afferent input sensed by the central nervous system.

The example of MWM in tennis elbow in which motor system effects are relatively larger than pain system effects is somewhat similar to research in the ankle for which a dorsiflexion MWM of the talocrural joint improves dorsiflexion (pooled SMD: 1.2) in preference to pressure pain threshold (single study SMD -0.22; [95% CI: -0.97 to 0.52]), which was not influenced by the treatment technique.[37] However, there seems to be a degree of mechanism differentiation with different MWM techniques, because the postero–lateral glide applied to the glenohumeral joint during elevation of the arm only improves elevation in the scapular plane (SMD 0.99) marginally beyond relatively that of pressure pain threshold (SMD 0.87).[36] That is, the relative effects observed in motor and pain systems appear to be related to the CSIM and MWM technique being used, as well as the body region and condition being treated. Assuming that the mechanisms that bring about motor system effects are different to those that bring about pain system effects, then it is likely that a number of mechanisms of action underpin the clinical efficacy of different MWM techniques. It is compelling to speculate that these mechanisms are specifically determined by such factors as: the MWM technique; CSIM; treated body part; and the patient's condition.

It is possible that the motor system mechanism of action for MWM could be linked with the PAG mediated descending pain inhibitory system outlined above in the pain sciences section of this chapter. The column of the PAG responsible for the coordinated non-opioid analgesia and sympathoexcitation also produces concomitant motor facilitation.[59–61] It is plausible that the pain-free grip strength effects of the lateral glide MWM for tennis elbow are an expression of the motor facilitation arm of the tri-partite PAG response profile and that the observed preferential influence on pain-free grip strength arises from a combination of motor and pain system changes, because the end point criterion for this measure is pain onset. Other factors may also be at play.

An alternative motor system mechanism may involve the sensory motor system. There is some unpublished and preliminary evidence that MWM influences joint position sense in recurrent lateral ankle sprain by about 60% of the deficit (Vicenzino's laboratory, see Chapter 7 for more information). This was evident for joint position error in ankle inversion following an ankle dorsiflexion MWM performed in either weight-bearing or non-weight-bearing positions (Figure 5.3). This effect was not present on active weight-bearing dorsiflexion stretching even though both increased range of dorsiflexion to a similar degree. The effect on joint position sense is likely due to the difference between these MWM techniques and the dorsiflexion stretching, which was essentially the strong pressure and contact exerted to the distal posterior leg, as well as the plantar and dorsal foot surfaces by the treatment bed, treatment belt and the practitioner's hand or thigh during the application of the MWM (Figure 5.3). Possibly the MWM provides a re-integration of somatosensory input that allows more precise motion to occur. Research is required to follow up the sensory motor effects and likely related mechanisms.

PSYCHOLOGICAL SYSTEM

All interventions applied to patients with musculoskeletal pain will be influenced by a range of non-physical factors, such as the patient's and practitioner's pre-existing beliefs on injury, tissue damage and pain; as well as any tendency for the patient towards catastrophisation and fear-avoidance responses to the condition. From a mechanism of action perspective, it is readily apparent that many of these issues are brought to the patient–practitioner interaction prior to the MWM application, but very likely they are dealt with in quite a pragmatic way by the test-application-retest feature of MWM, which provides immediate feedback to both patient and practitioner. However, how these factors influence the underlying mechanisms of MWM is not known presently, prompting an urgent need for further research.

The patient's willingness to please (i.e. placebo) or not (i.e. nocebo)[62] is often linked to the psychological system. There are a number of things to consider with regard to placebo, such as the experimental design of studies into effects and mechanisms of MWM and the possible influence of placebo effects on mechanisms of action of MWM. Importantly, it is critical to remember that unlike the placebo pill it is very difficult to devise a credible placebo for a manual therapy treatment technique without any component parts of the treatment technique (especially when little is conclusively known about the specific active components of the treatment technique). This chapter has dealt with the initial effect of a MWM and as such in the studies reported herein there was a range of design features utilised in order to control for placebo effects. For example, many of the studies used naïve subjects who were led to believe that the study was evaluating some other aspect of physical therapy, such as manual handling and positioning of the patient and practitioners. The control conditions that were utilised sought to apply comparable forces to the general region being studied, while also endeavouring to avoid specifically gliding the joint as required for a successful MWM. In addition, the patient–practitioner interactions were kept minimal. This approach to the experiment design features is premised on the basis that a placebo intervention/condition has a negative connotation, being conceptualised as an inactive or even deceptive treatment. This has underpinned medical practitioners' belief that placebo responders were not valid patients, but rather somehow psychologically disturbed.[63] However, there are known physiological mechanisms by which pain relief may be produced by a placebo intervention[64] and there is a growing awareness of the beneficial effects of placebo.[63] It has become apparent that practitioner attitudes and postures, both vocalised and non-verbal, that express confidence in treatment being pain relieving and healing can engender physiological changes and should be used in the clinical interaction.[63] So it is very likely

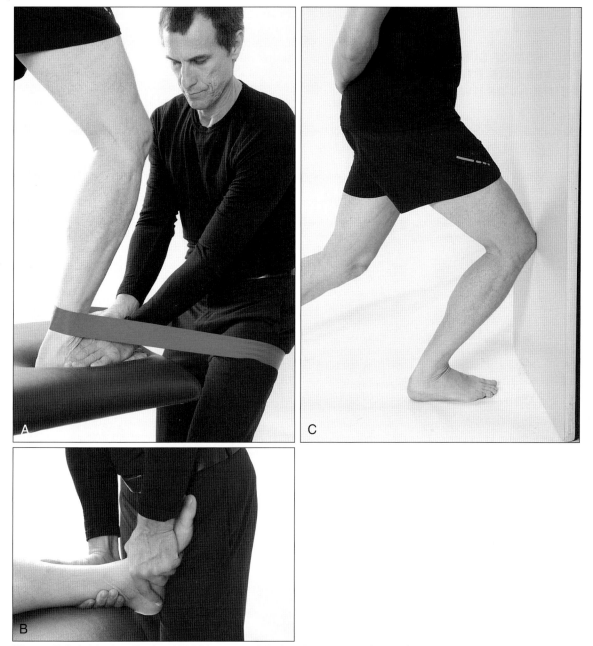

Figure 5.3 Ankle dorsiflexion MWM in non-weight-bearing and weight-bearing, showing the patient–practitioner interaction, by contrast to weight-bearing dorsiflexion only

that the mechanism of action underpinning a specific MWM application is modulated by a number of non-MWM factors.

MWM may engender psychological mechanisms of action. In the event that the MWM brought about a substantial improvement and further repetitions provide commensurate levels of improvement and sustainability of improvement, then there may well be a psychological mechanism(s) by which MWM brings about its clinically beneficial effects. That is, now that movement is possible without pain, the patient feels less averse to using that body part and implicitly it would be expected that fear-avoidance behaviours be ameliorated. In the event that on balance the patient is averse to the movement even with an MWM in place, then MWM would be contraindicated for further use and the question of psychological mechanisms in this case becomes redundant.

MECHANISM OF SUSTAINED IMPROVEMENTS WITH MANY REPETITIONS OF MWM

The model outlined in Figure 5.2 describes a proposed mechanism of action that is evoked at a single repetition of MWM. As indicated in Chapter 2, to gain long lasting improvement in most patients, there is a need to repeat MWM over several sessions, including self-treatment by the patient. To our knowledge there has been no research into the possible underlying mechanisms of the sustained effects of MWM. However, Zusman has proposed mechanisms of musculoskeletal physiotherapy[18] that may have utility in considering the sustained effects of MWM. While acknowledging the evidence for manipulative therapy evoking descending pain inhibitory systems, like that outlined above, he proposes that resourceful practitioners would then put the initial pain relief offered by this mechanism to functionally significant use by ongoing application of the technique to gain lasting improvements.[18] Of particular relevance is central learning theory and the physiological and behavioural mechanisms involved in extinction of aversive memories.[65] In brief, Zusman proposed that repeated application of musculoskeletal physiotherapy interventions extinguishes acquired aversive memories through a process of habitual non-associative learning, thereby leading to the learning of new presumably normal pain-free motor memories.[18]

Repeated MWMs not only allow motion without aversive connotation, but also may well improve internal feedback mechanisms (see above and Chapter 7 for preliminary data regarding joint position sense changes), which would be a critical element in the learning of normal pain-free movement.[18]

MWM requires the patient to be attentive to the treatment. This attention may well be critical in the long-term improvement gained with repeated MWM because there is evidence that selective attention to something other than pain produces physiological changes that modulate nociception.[66] For example, Longe et al have shown that selective attention to thermal pain while being treated with transcutaneous electrical nerve stimulation (TENS) is much less effective at suppressing the sensory perception of pain than if the patient focussed on the treatment and that this was associated with changes in functional brain images.[67] Perhaps repeated MWM engages this sort of mechanism.

SUMMARY
The model proposed herein requires further evaluation and testing, because although it relies on the best evidence to date, much of it is of a low level and in many cases raises questions that need to be answered in order to progress the development of an appropriate theoretical model.

One of the purposes of this chapter was to provide a source from which researchers and practitioners could progress the evidence and application of the evolving model. Nevertheless, with suitable caveats and care, practitioners may wish to use the current proposed model to better gain an understanding of MWM or, more likely, to explain to others how the MWM has brought about the clinically observed improvements in the patient's condition. For example, take the wrist lateral glide MWM case introduced at the outset of this chapter, in which the CSIM of wrist extension was improved from 15° to 60°. It is not uncommon for the practitioner to be then compelled to consider how this came about, often by way of an explanation to the patient or colleagues. The model proposed herein would dictate that the direction of the lateral glide along with the amount of force used (Chapter 2) is critical to stimulating some endogenous reparative or coping mechanism(s). Although there may have been a positional fault of the wrist at the outset, the limited data available (Chapter 4) seems to indicate that, although the patient will recover full pain-free function in the long term, the positional fault will likely remain. This may indicate that using the positional fault hypothesis may not entirely resolve the mechanism underpinning MWM clinical efficacy. Evidence from the neurosciences of both human and animal research has shown that specific non-opioid mediated descending pain inhibitory systems are likely responsible for the reduction in pain during and immediately following MWM application. Preliminary data may also reflect that MWM stimulates some sensorimotor system mechanisms, which may contribute to the observed improvements in movement (these will be dealt with in more detail in Chapters 6 and 7). In synopsis, the practitioner may well indicate that the MWM, when successfully applied, is an appropriate, adequate stimulus that activates pain, sensory and motor system mechanisms.

A salutary and fundamental characteristic of MWM is that it is not only pain-free but also requiring a sufficient level of force, which on prima facie grounds would generate forces within the tissues that are likely to stimulate large diameter afferent fibres (A beta). Interestingly, the stimulation of large diameter afferent fibres and immediate pain relief was reported when Melzack and Wall proposed their Gate Control Theory of pain.[68, 69] However, they used TENS as the means to stimulate large diameter afferent fibres. Notwithstanding these obviously apparent differences in input stimuli, it is then compelling to speculate that the MWM technique may well activate a similar gating mechanism as that proposed by Melzack and Wall.[68]

In other healthcare applications, the Gate Control Theory has been used to explain how manual pressure and mechanical vibration can reduce pain of injection to the dorsolateral gluteal region[70] and the oral cavity,[71] respectively. In a similar way the Gate Control Theory may be used to explain MWM. There is also further convergence of the mechanism of action of MWM and the Gate Control Theory through the descending pain inhibitory system because as outlined above joint manipulation appears to activate such a system and the Gate Control Theory of pain also encompasses similar descending systems.

The foregoing explanation would need to be clearly placed in context of this mechanism being present with a single repetition of the lateral glide MWM for the wrist. As presented in Chapter 2, when the MWM is able to substantially change the CSIM on a single repetition, then it is repeated in sufficient volume to ensure sustainability of the relief from the wrist pain and impairment. Thus, in explaining improvement in the wrist condition after a course of MWM treatment, which would include self-treatment and possibly taping, the practitioner may well consider that the treatment has engaged a process of habitual non-associative learning in restoring normal pain-free movement. That is, the previous memory of aversive wrist activity that is captured clinically in the form of the CSIM of pain-limited extension is increasingly and progressively extinguished with every repetition of a non-painful MWM.

KEY POINTS

- Historically, the mechanisms of action of manual therapy, including MWM, have been closely linked to joint subluxation, alignment and mechanical compromise of joint and associated structures.

- In more recent times an improved knowledge of the nervous system has lead to its consideration in manual therapy mechanisms.

- MWM evokes a non-opioid descending pain inhibitory system in bringing about its initial clinical effects.

- Resourceful practitioners may use the initial descending pain inhibitory effects of MWM in ongoing treatment to bring about lasting changes, possibly through learning mechanisms.

- Psychological factors need to be considered as playing a role in the mechanisms of action of MWM.

- The model presented herein explains that specific mechanical perturbations evoke neurophysiological mechanisms, which are likely distributed across a number of systems (e.g. sensory, motor, sympathetic).

References

1 Stoddard A. Manual of Osteopathic Practice (2nd edn). London: Hutchinson Books Ltd 1969.
2 Bergmann T, Peterson D. Chiropractic Technique: Principles and Procedures (2nd edn). Missouri: Mosby 2002.
3 Edwards B. Combined movements in the cervical spine (C2-7): their value in examination and technique choice. Australian Journal of Physiotherapy. 1980 Dec 5;26(5):165–71.
4 Gibbons P, Tehan P. Manipulation of the Spine, Thorax and Pelvis: An Osteopathic Perspective (3rd edn). Melbourne: Churchill Livingstone 2009.
5 Maitland G, Hengeveld E, Banks K, English K. Maitland's Vertebral Manipulation (7th edn). Sydney: Butterworths-Heinemann 2007.
6 Haldeman S. Principles and Practice of Chiropractic. Sydney: McGraw-Hill 2005.
7 Chrisman OD, Mittnacht A, Snook GA. A study of the results following rotatory manipulation in the lumbar intervertebral disc syndrome. Journal of Bone and Joint Surgery. 1964;46A:517–24.
8 Cyriax R. Textbook of Orthopedic Medicine (6th edn). London: Bailliere Tindall 1975.
9 DeJarnette B. The Philosophy, Art and Science of Sacro-Occipital Technique. Nebraska: B. DeJarnette 1967.
10 Farfan HF. Mechanical Disorders of the Low Back. Philadelphia: Lea & Febiger 1973.
11 Korr IM. The spinal cord as organizer of disease processes: some preliminary perspectives. Journal of the American Osteopathic Association. 1976;76:89–99.
12 Kunert W. Functional disorders of internal organs due to vertebral lesions. Ciba Symposium. 1965;13(3):85–6.
13 Perl ER. Pain: Spinal and peripheral factors. In: Goldstein M (ed.) The Research Status of Spinal Manipulative Therapy: NINCDS Monograph No. 15, DHEW Publication No. NIH 76-998, 1975:173–82.
14 Twomey LT. A rationale for the treatment of back pain and joint pain by manual therapy. Physical Therapy. 1992;72(12):885–92.
15 Zusman M. Spinal manipulative therapy: review of some proposed mechanisms, and a new hypothesis. The Australian Journal of Physiotherapy. 1986;32(2):89–99.
16 Dhami MSI, DeBoer KF. Systemic Effects of Spinal Lesions. In: Haldeman S (ed.) Principles and Practice of Chiropractic (2nd edn). Norwalk: Appleton & Lange 1992.
17 Lewit K. Manipulative Therapy in Rehabilitation of the Locomotor System. London: Butterworths 1985.
18 Zusman M. Mechanisms of musculoskeletal physiotherapy. Physical Therapy Reviews. 2004;Apr 29;9:39–49.
19 American Osteopathy Association. Biography of Andrew Taylor Still: Founder of Osteopathic Medicine. Online. Available: http://www.osteopathic.org/index.cfm?PageID=ost_still (accessed Jan 2010).
20 Kaltenborn F. Manual Mobilisation of the Extremity Joints, Basic Examination and Treatment Techniques. Norway: Olaf Norlis Bokhandel 1989.
21 McConnell J. The management of chondromalacia patellae: a long term solution. Australian Journal of Physiotherapy. 1986;32:215–33.
22 McKenzie R. The Lumbar Spine: Mechanical Diagnosis and Therapy. New Zealand: Waikanae 1981.

23 Mulligan B. Manual Therapy — 'NAGS', 'SNAGS', 'MWMS' etc. (5th edn). Wellington: Plane View Services 1999.

24 Palmer DD. The Chiropractor's Adjuster: the Science, Art and Philosophy of Chiropractic. Portland: Portland Printing House 1910.

25 Paungmali A, O'Leary S, Souvlis T, Vicenzino B. Naloxone fails to antagonize initial hypoalgesic effect of a manual therapy treatment for lateral epicondylalgia. Journal of Manipulative and Physiological Therapeutics. 2004 Mar–Apr;27(3):180–5.

26 Paungmali A, Vicenzino B, Smith M. Hypoalgesia induced by elbow manipulation in lateral epicondylalgia does not exhibit tolerance. Journal of Pain. 2003 Oct;4(8):448–54.

27 Vicenzino B, Paungmali A, Buratowski S, Wright A. Specific manipulative therapy treatment for chronic lateral epicondylalgia produces uniquely characteristic hypoalgesia. Manual Therapy. 2001 Nov;6(4):205–12.

28 Vicenzino B, Paungmali A, Teys P. Mulligan's mobilization-with-movement, positional faults and pain relief: current concepts from a critical review of literature. Manual Therapy. 2007 May 1;12(2):98–108.

29 Souvlis T, Vicenzino B. Efectos analgesicos de la terapia manual en la columna cervical. In: Cueco R (ed.) La Columna Cervical:Evaluacion Clinica y Aproximacinoes Terapeuticas Principios anatomicos y funcionales, explorracion clinica y tecnicas de tratamiento. Spain: Editoral Medica Panamericana 2008:303–18.

30 Souvlis T, Vicenzino B, Wright A. The neurophysiological mechanisms of spinal manual therapy. In: Boyling G, Jull G (eds) Grieves' Modern Manual Therapy (3rd edn). Edinburgh: Elsevier Churchill Livingstone 2005:367–79.

31 Vicenzino B, Souvlis T, Sterling M. Neurophysiologic effects of spinal manipulation. In: Fernandez-de-las-Penas C, Gerwin R (eds) Tension-Type and Cervicogenic Headache Pathophysiology, Diagnosis and Management. USA: Jones and Bartlett Publishers 2008:213–20.

32 Gal JM, Herzog W, Kawchuk GN, Conway PJ, Zhang YT. Movements of verterbrae during manipulative thrusts to unembalmed human cadavers. Journal of Manipulative and Physiological Therapeutics. 1997;20(1):30–40.

33 Hsieh CY, Vicenzino B, Yang CH, Hu MH, Yang C. Mulligan's mobilization with movement for the thumb: a single case report using magnetic resonance imaging to evaluate the positional fault hypothesis. Manual Therapy. 2002 Feb;7(1):44–9.

34 Mercer S, Bogduk N. Intra-articular inclusions of the cervical synovial joints. Rheumatology. 1993 August 1;32(8):705–10.

35 Mercer S, Rivett D. Meniscoids and manual therapy of the ankle. In: Magarey M (ed.) More Than Skin Deep: Proceedings of the 12th Biennial Conference of Musculoskeletal Physiotherapy Australia; 2001 21–24 November; Adelaide, South Australia: Musculoskeletal Physiotherapy Australia: A National Special Group of the Australian Physiotherapy Association; 2001. p 18.

36 Teys P, Bisset L, Vicenzino B. The initial effects of a Mulligan's mobilization with movement technique on range of movement and pressure pain threshold in pain-limited shoulders. Manual therapy. 2008 Oct 25;13(1):37–42.

37 Collins N, Teys P, Vicenzino B. The initial effects of a Mulligan's mobilization with movement technique on dorsiflexion and pain in sub-acute ankle sprains. Manual Therapy. 2004 May;9(2):77–82.

38 Paungmali A, O'Leary S, Souvlis T, Vicenzino B. Hypoalgesic and sympathoexcitatory effects of mobilization with movement for lateral epicondylalgia. Physical Therapy. 2003 Apr;83(4):374–83.

39 Vicenzino B, Collins D, Benson H, Wright A. An investigation of the interrelationship between manipulative therapy induced hypoalgesia and sympathoexcitation. Journal of Manipulative & Physiological Therapeutics. 1998;21(7):448–53.

40 Vicenzino B, Collins D, Wright A. The initial effects of a cervical spine manipulative physiotherapy treatment on the pain and dysfunction of lateral epicondylalgia. Pain. 1996 Nov;68(1):69–74.

41 Vicenzino B, O'Callaghan J, Kermode F, Wright A. The influence of Naloxone on the initial hypoalgesic effect of spinal manual therapy. In: Devor M, Rowbotham M, Wiesenfeld-Hallin Z (eds) Proceedings of the 9th World Congress on Pain. Seattle: IASP Press 2000:1039–44.

42 Sterling M, Pedler A, Chan C, Puglisi M, Vuvan V, Vicenzino B. Cervical lateral glide increases nociceptive flexion reflex threshold but not pressure or thermal pain thresholds in chronic whiplash associated disorders: A pilot randomised controlled trial. Manual Therapy. 2009 Oct 31.

43 Cameron AA, Khan IA, Westlund KN, Willis WD. The efferent projections of the periaqueductal gray in the rat: a Phaseolus vulgaris-Leucoagglutinin study. II. Descending projections. Journal of Comparative Neurology. 1995;351(4):585–601.

44 Clark FM, Proudfit HK. Projections of neurons in the ventromedial medulla to pontine catecholamine cell groups involved in the modulation of nociception. Brain Res. 1991;540(1–2):105–15.

45 Lakos S, Basbaum A. An ultrastructural study of the projections from the midbrain periaqueductal gray to spinally-projecting serotonin immunoreactive neurons of the medullary raphe magnus in the rat. Brain Research. 1988;443:383–8.

46 Lovick T. Interactions between descending pathways from the dorsal and ventrolateral periaqueductal gray matter in the rat. In: Depaulis A, Bandler R (eds) The Midbrain Periaqueductal Gray Matter. New York: Plenum Press 1991:101–20.

47 Lovick T, Li P. Integrated function of neurones in the rostral ventrolateral medulla. Progress in Brain Research. 1989;81:223–32.

48 Lovick T, West C, Wolstencroft J. Responses of raphe-spinal and other raphe neurones to stimulation of the periaqueductal grey matter in the cat. Neuroscience Letters. 1978;8:45–9.

49 Lovick TA. Ventrolateral medullary lesions block the antinociceptive and cardiovascular responses elicited by stimulating the dorsal periaqueductal grey matter in rats. Pain. 1985;21(3):241–52.

50 Proudfit H. Pharmacologic evidence for the modulation of nociception by noradrenergic neurones. In: Fields H, Besson J (eds) Pain Modulation. Amsterdam: Elsevier Science 1988:357–70.

51 Takeshige C, Sato T, Mera T, Hisamitsu T, Fang J. Descending pain inhibitory system involved in acupuncture analgesia. Issn: 0361-9230. 1992;29:617–34.

52 Van Bockstaele E, Aston-Jones G, Peribone V, Ennis M, Shipley M. Subregions of the periaqueductal gray topographically innervate the rostral ventral medulla in the rat. Journal of Comparative Neurology. 1991;309(3):305–27.

53 Zusman M, Edwards B, Donaghy A. Investigation of a proposed mechanism for the relief of spinal pain with passive joint movement. Journal of Manual Medicine. 1989;4:58–61.

54 Sanders GE, Reinert O, Tepe R, Maloney P. Chiropractic adjustive manipulation on subjects with acute low back pain: visual analog pain scores and plasma beta-endorphin levels. Journal of Manipulative Physiological Therapy. 1990;13(7):391–5.

55 Christian G, Stanton G, Sissons D, How H, Jamison J, Alder B, et al. Immunoreactive ACTH, beta-endorphin, and cortisol levels in plasma following spinal manipulative therapy. Spine 1988;13(12):1411–7.

56 Richardson D, Kappler R, Klatz R, Tarr R, Cohen D, Bowyer R, et al. The effect of osteopathic manipulative treatment on endogenous opiate concentration. Journal of the American Osteopathic Association. 1984;84(1):127.

57 Skyba DA, Radhakrishnan R, Rohlwing JJ, Wright A, Sluka KA. Joint manipulation reduces hyperalgesia by activation of monoamine receptors but not opioid or GABA receptors in the spinal cord. Pain. 2003 Nov;106(1–2):159–68.

58 Sluka KA, Wright A. Knee joint mobilization reduces secondary mechanical hyperalgesia induced by capsaicin injection into the ankle joint. European Journal of Pain — London. 2001;5(1):81–7.

59 Fanselow MS. The midbrain periaqueductal gray as a coordinator of action in response to fear and anxiety. In: Depaulis A, Bandler R (eds) The Midbrain Periaqueductal Gray Matter. New York: Plenum Press 1991:151–73.

60 Morgan M. Differences in antinociception evoked from dorsal and ventral regions of the caudal periaqueductal gray matter. In: Depaulis A, Bandler R (eds) The Midbrain Periaqueductal Gray Matter. New York: Plenum Press 1991:139–50.

61 Bandler R, Carrive P, Depaulis A. Emerging principles of organisation of the midbrain periaqueductal gray matter. In: Depaulis A, Bandler R (eds) The Midbrain Periaqueductal Gray Matter. New York: Plenum Press 1991:1–10.

62 Wall P. The placebo and the placebo response. In: Wall P, Melsack R (eds) Textbook of Pain (3rd edn). Edinburgh: Churchill Livingstone 1994:1297–308.

63 Roche P. Pain and placebo analgesia: two sides of the same coin. Physical Therapy Reviews. 2007;12(3): 189–98.

64 Fields H, Basbaum A, Heiricher M. CNS mechanisms of pain modulation. In: McMahon S, Koltzenburg M (eds) Textbook of Pain. London: Elsevier 2006:125–43.

65 Myers KM, Davis M. Behavioral and neural analysis of extinction. Neuron. 2002 Nov 14;36(4):567–84.

66 Villemure C, Bushnell MC. Cognitive modulation of pain: how do attention and emotion influence pain processing? Pain. 2002 Feb 1;95(3):195–9.

67 Longe SE, Wise R, Bantick S, Lloyd D, Johansen-Berg H, McGlone F, et al. Counter-stimulatory effects on pain perception and processing are significantly altered by attention: an MRI study. Neuroreport. 2001 Jul 3;12(9):2021–5.

68 Melzack R, Wall PD. Pain mechanisms: a new theory. Science. 1965 Nov 19;150(699):971–9.

69 Dickensen A. Editorial I: Gate Control Theory of pain stands test of time. British Journal of Anaesthesia. 2002 Dec 4;88(6):755–7.

70 Barnhill BJ, Holbert MD, Jackson NM, Erickson RS. Using pressure to decrease the pain of intramuscular injections. Journal of Pain and Symptom Management. 1996 Jul 1;12(1):52–8.

71 Nanitsos E, Vartuli R, Forte A, Dennison P, Peck C. The effect of vibration on pain during local anaesthesia injections. Australian Dental Journal. 2009;54(2): 94–100.

Chapter 6
Pain and sensory system impairments that may be amenable to Mobilisation with Movement

Michele Sterling and Bill Vicenzino

INTRODUCTION

Historically there has been a tendency for the clinical assessment of musculoskeletal pain conditions to be geared around the identification of the patho-anatomical source/s of the patient's reported symptoms; for example, in the case of low back pain.[1, 2, 3] This approach has had limited success as a patho-anatomical diagnosis is not possible in the vast majority of patients with common musculoskeletal pain conditions[4, 5] nor does such a diagnosis necessarily shed light on the most optimal intervention for a specific condition or patient. As a consequence, there has been a growing focus in recent years towards attempting to identify the underlying mechanisms or processes of the patient's pain syndrome.[6] The purpose of this pain-specific diagnosis in the classification of musculoskeletal pain syndromes is to help tailor interventions toward identifiable underlying processes in order to optimise treatment outcomes, particularly in some of the more recalcitrant conditions.

The presence of injury and inflammation either as a consequence of frank injury or as a result of more insidious onset microtrauma are known to have profound effects on both peripheral and central pain-processing mechanisms. The explosive growth in the understanding of mechanisms responsible for pain and nociception has been a result of investigation in animal models. Direct extrapolation to humans should be made with caution. However, by using quantitative sensory testing that utilises a variety of stimuli to detect changes in sensory function, an appreciation of underlying disturbances in pain processing can be made.[7] Using such methods, advances have been made in the understanding of disturbances in pain-processing mechanisms in musculoskeletal conditions commonly managed with Mobilisation with Movement (MWM) techniques, including osteoarthritis, lateral epicondylalgia and spinal pain.[8–11] In addition to interpreting responses with sensory testing, the nature of symptoms and signs reported by the patient may also allude to processes underlying the condition and assist in treatment direction.[12]

In broad terms the sensory characteristics found to be present to varying degrees in musculoskeletal pain conditions include mechanical hyperalgesia, thermal hyperalgesia, hypoaesthesia (increased detection thresholds), heightened motor responses following sensory stimulation and sympathetic nervous system (SNS) changes and certain pain processes may be inferred from these various presentations. In tandem with this research, recent investigation of manual therapy (MT) has focused not only on the efficacy of such interventions in the management of musculoskeletal pain but also to establish possible mechanisms of action. Research of the latter may assist in determining the types of patient presentations that may benefit from such a treatment approach. Much investigation of MT and more recently MWM treatments has demonstrated a likely neurophysiological effect of these approaches manifested by their influence on pain, sensory characteristics and the SNS.[13, 14]

This chapter will present a synthesis of data pertaining to pain and sensory system impairments common to many musculoskeletal conditions, and also data demonstrating the capacity or potential capacity of MWM to modulate these presentations. The chapter approaches the biological evidence surrounding MWM and musculoskeletal pain through a different perspective to that taken in the preceding mechanisms chapter (Chapter 5), yet it is nonetheless intended to complement the information in that chapter so as to better inform the clinical reasoning process and possibly further research in this field.

SELF-REPORTED PAIN

MT in general has been shown to have an analgesic effect in terms of producing a reduction in the level of pain reported by the patient usually determined via VAS scales of current pain intensity at rest.[13] With respect to the application of MWM techniques, such analgesic effects have been shown to occur following treatment of a variety of painful musculoskeletal conditions involving various body areas, including the cervical spine, shoulder, elbow, lumbar spine, ankle and knee.[15–19] Most studies have investigated MWM as the sole intervention but some have combined this approach with additional modalities such as exercise and shown beneficial effects on pain.[18]

Some studies have reported improvements in function as well as pain. This may be in the relatively simple form of less pain with certain activities such as grip-strength testing[20] and active movements.[21] Improved function measured via validated questionnaires has not been commonly investigated probably since most studies have utilised only a pre- to immediately post-study design[1, 5, 12] where such tools (that may include items about daily activity, sport, sleep) are not able to be used. It is also not clear whether MWM treatment can change symptoms other than pain; for example, anaesthesia and paraesthesia. Further investigation of this area may be useful since these types of symptoms have been suggested to assist in gauging underlying mechanisms of the condition, namely a neuropathic pain component.[12] Nevertheless the data indicate that MWM is a useful intervention to decrease reported pain and improve function with certain activities in various musculoskeletal conditions (see Chapter 3).

MECHANICAL HYPERALGESIA

Common musculoskeletal conditions that are frequently managed with MWM techniques demonstrate mechanical hyperalgesia either locally over the involved area or additionally in more widespread body regions.[22] This phenomenon can be detected via sensory testing usually using pressure or pin prick stimuli but may also be obvious during manual examination of the patient.[23] Possible pain mechanisms underlying the condition being assessed can be inferred from the results of testing. The presence of local mechanical hyperalgesia may represent areas of primary hyperalgesia resulting from sensitised peripheral nociceptors within injured musculoskeletal structures.[24]

Manual therapy techniques, including MWM, have also been shown to exhibit hypoalgesic effects to mechanical stimuli (i.e. reduction in mechanical hyperalgesia) with most studies demonstrating effects on local hyperalgesia.[14] Specific MWM techniques applied to the glenohumeral joint of individuals with shoulder pain increased pressure pain thresholds (hypoalgesia) measured over the anterior aspect of the shoulder.[21] MWM techniques applied to the elbow joint of people with lateral epicondylalgia showed a similar effect on pressure pain thresholds measured over the lateral epicondyle.[20] However, not all studies have demonstrated a positive influence on local mechanical hyperalgesia. Collins et al[25] were not able to demonstrate a change in pressure pain thresholds over the anterior talofibular ligament following MWM to the talocrural joint of patients with sub-acute ankle sprains. Furthermore, in a study where pain was experimentally induced in the extensor carpi radialis brevis muscle, pressure pain thresholds at the elbow remained unchanged following a MWM intervention.[26] Taken together these findings suggest that MWM may exert a superior local hypoalgesic effect in conditions of more longstanding duration with lesser effects in acute and sub-acute conditions.

However, the local hyperalgesia seen in more chronic or longstanding conditions may represent mechanisms other than local peripheral nociceptor sensitisation. In many cases of musculoskeletal pain, a specific local musculoskeletal or neurological disease process is not clearly discernible. Examples of this scenario include neck pain where no patho-anatomical lesion is apparent with imaging techniques[27] and lateral epicondylalgia where evidence of acute inflammation is lacking.[28] In these and other examples, it has been suggested that the hyperalgesic areas may in fact represent areas of secondary hyperalgesia present as a result of augmented central nervous system pain processes.[29, 30] If this is the case then it would appear that MWM may have the capacity to modulate augmented or hyper-excitable central nervous system activity.

Additionally, mechanical hyperalgesia in widespread areas remote to the area of injury or involvement are found in some musculoskeletal conditions and are believed to be also indicative of alterations in the neurobiological processing of nociception within the central nervous system.[31, 32] An example of this phenomenon can be found in the investigation of whiplash associated disorders where mechanical hyperalgesia occurs not only in cervical spine areas but also in the upper and lower limbs.[24] These widespread sensory disturbances are likely important for the clinician to consider in their patient assessment because they have been associated with poor functional recovery,[24] greater reported pain severity, and prevalence of other symptoms such as depression, some aspects of coping, life satisfaction and general health.[33]

MWM treatment appears to demonstrate similar neurophysiological effects as other spinal manipulative therapy (SMT) interventions including characteristics indicative of non-opioid mediated endogenous mechanisms (non-naloxone reversible and no tolerance to repeated applications), hypoalgesia and sympatho-excitation (see Chapter 3).[14] The apparent activation of endogenous pain inhibitory mechanisms suggests that MWM treatment may be of benefit in the modulation of more generalised mechanical hyperalgesia. The effects of MWM techniques or SMT in general on these more generalised sensory disturbances have not been well investigated. A recent study of SMT (lateral glides) applied to the cervical spine in individuals with chronic whiplash showed some immediate modulatory effects on pressure pain thresholds of the upper limb but no effects at lower limb sites.[34] The capacity of MWM techniques to decrease widespread mechanical hyperalgesia requires further investigation.

THERMAL HYPERALGESIA

Thermal hyperalgesia is also a common feature of many musculoskeletal conditions. Heat hyperalgesia may reflect sensitisation of C-nociceptors and a corresponding sensitisation of second order neurons [35] and has been shown to be present in conditions such as whiplash[24], non-traumatic neck pain,[10] cervical radiculopathy,[36] low back pain[9] and in the referred forearm and hand pain in lateral epicondylalgia.[37] Interestingly, while MWM treatment (and MT) has consistently been shown to have a hypoalgesic effect for mechanical hyperalgesia, a similar consistency for a lack of effect on heat pain thresholds has also been demonstrated. Paungmali et al[38] demonstrated no effect of MWM applied to the elbow on heat pain thresholds also measured at the elbow and Collins et al[25] showed no effect with MWM to the talocrural joint of participants with sub-acute ankle sprain. Consistently similar results have been demonstrated for MT techniques other than MWM in various conditions including neck pain, lateral epicondylalgia and in healthy asymptomatic participants.[39–41] The only exception to these findings comes from a recent study of high velocity thrust manipulation of the lumbar spine in healthy asymptomatic participants where a positive effect on heat pain thresholds was found.[42] However, the obvious differences between manipulative and MWM techniques suggest that different mechanisms would likely be evoked and this may be one reason for these disparate findings.

Cold hyperalgesia or increased cold pain threshold is usually considered as a consistent feature of neuropathic pain conditions.[43] Recent evidence indicates that it is also a feature of some musculoskeletal conditions including whiplash,[24] cervical radiculopathy,[36] knee osteoarthritis[44] and following immobilisation.[45] In the case of whiplash, the presence of cold hyperalgesia is both predictive of poor functional recovery[46, 47] and associated with non-responsiveness to physical interventions predominantly comprising of exercise.[48] For these reasons, it would seem important to identify treatment interventions that may be able to modulate cold hyperalgesia and potentially improve outcomes for these patients. Recent data indicate that high velocity spinal manipulation may exert some influence on cold pain thresholds in asymptomatic participants[42] but other preliminary data of SMT failed to show an effect on these sensory thresholds in individuals with chronic whiplash.[34] It may well transpire that MWM and MT is not indicated where there is cold hyperalgesia. However, the specific effects, if any, of MWM techniques on cold pain thresholds have not been investigated in either patient or asymptomatic groups but would seem an important avenue for further investigation. Some data indicate a moderate correlation between cold hyperalgesia and psychological distress[49] indicating that psychological and cognitive interventions in addition to physical treatments may be required.

NEURAL PROVOCATION TESTS AND HEIGHTENED MOTOR RESPONSES

In addition to positive sensory responses to various stimuli, heightened motor responses have also been demonstrated following provocation in musculoskeletal pain conditions. Clinicians will be well aware of such motor responses in their use of assessment techniques of neural provocation including the brachial plexus provocation test (also known as the upper limb tension test) and the straight leg raise test.[50] In these tests, mechanical stimulation in the form of movement is performed and a response from the patient is measured (range of movement and associated pain). The loss of range of movement is a motor response that has been likened to a heightened flexor withdrawal response.[11, 51] It has also been argued to represent a motor correlate of central sensitisation.[23]

Oscillatory manual therapy techniques have demonstrated capacity to improve range of movement and decrease pain associated with neural provocation tests in participants with neck/arm pain,[52] lateral epicondylalgia[41] and in asymptomatic individuals.[53] MWM techniques appear to demonstrate similar modulatory effects on patient responses to these tests (e.g. see Chapter 18). Increased range of shoulder movement with a radial nerve biased neural provocation test following MWM techniques applied to the elbow in patients with lateral epicondylalgia has been demonstrated.[20] Hall et al[16] demonstrated improved range of straight leg raise movement and decreased pain following MWM treatment in patients with low back pain. Interestingly, these responses were more apparent at 24 hours post-intervention, which is in contrast to most other studies that have assessed only immediate outcomes. Nevertheless, these findings indicate that MWM interventions may have the capacity to decrease heightened motor responses associated with positive neural provocation tests in painful musculoskeletal conditions, which provides some level of support for the capacity of these techniques to decrease augmented central pain-processing mechanisms.

Nerve tissue provocation tests have been proposed to be an indirect correlate of the flexor withdrawal response.[11, 51] A more direct measure of this response can be achieved in the laboratory using the nociceptive flexion reflex (NFR), a spinal reflex where threshold muscle reflex activity is measured following electrical stimulation to the sural nerve at the ankle.[54] The NFR is a measure of spinal cord excitability that (unlike pain threshold tests and clinical neural provocation tests) does not rely on a cognitive response from participants.[54] We have recently shown that oscillatory MT applied to the cervical spine of patients with chronic whiplash increases the NFR threshold, thus decreasing spinal cord excitability, at least in the short term.[34] This is probably the first direct evidence of SMT's potential to modulate central nervous system pain processes and warrants further investigation. Due to the similar effects of MWM to those demonstrated with SMT, a modulatory influence of MWM of spinal cord activity could be expected and requires further investigation.

Hypoaesthetic sensory changes

The majority of research of sensory disturbances in musculoskeletal conditions has focused on positive symptoms such as allodynia, hyperalgesia (decreased pain thresholds) and other heightened responses to stimulation. Perhaps somewhat paradoxically, negative sensory changes or hypoaesthesia (increased detection thresholds) seem to occur concurrently with hypersensitivity in many musculoskeletal conditions. Hypoaesthesia to various stimuli including vibration, heat, cold and electrical current has been shown to be present in various chronic conditions including patellofemoral pain,[55] cervicobrachial pain,[56] whiplash,[57] low back pain[58] and cervical radiculopathy.[36] Similar changes have also been found in patients with acute whiplash[59] but are not so apparent in individuals with idiopathic neck pain, indicating that it is not a universal phenomenon. Most authors feel that the hypoaesthetic changes reflect central plasticity induced by activation of the nociceptive system via central inhibition of non-painful processing in the spinal cord or the brain.[60]

The relevance of these hypoaesthetic changes to patient outcomes is not clear but they do seem to be related to pain and disability levels. Chien et al[59] showed that hypoaesthesia to vibration, cold and electrical stimuli resolved in parallel with decreasing pain and disability levels in recovering individuals following acute whiplash injury. Additionally the changes are not present or are less apparent in conditions with lower levels of pain and disability.[61, 62] In light of this association with levels of pain, it is hypothetically feasible that MWM treatment may modulate hypoaesthesia in tandem with its analgesic effect. Further investigation of the influence of MWM intervention on this aspect of the sensory manifestations of musculoskeletal pain is warranted and may further improve understanding of its mode of action and indications for use.

Sympathetic nervous system activity

There is increasing interest about the possible involvement of the sympathetic nervous system (SNS) in initiation and maintenance of chronic musculoskeletal pain conditions of different aetiology. Epidemiological data show that stresses of a different nature (e.g. work related, psychosocial, etc), typically characterised by SNS activation, may be a co-factor in the development of some pain syndromes and/or negatively affect its time course.[63] Both systemic changes such as disturbances in cardiovascular function[63] and peripheral changes such as decreased vasoconstrictive responses[24] have

been demonstrated in conditions such as low back pain, whiplash, frozen shoulder, lateral epicondylalgia and fibromyalgia.[24, 64–67] The reasons for the involvement of SNS disturbance in musculoskeletal pain are not clear and both stress-related models[63, 68] and models involving central and peripheral pain-processing mechanisms[69] have been proposed.

While SNS changes have been demonstrated in various musculoskeletal conditions, it has not yet been established whether or not they relate to autonomic type symptoms reported by some patients, although these certainly do occur.[63] It is also not clear whether there is a decrease or increase in SNS activity as both have been reported to occur.[24, 64] However, there is some evidence from investigation of whiplash associated disorders that shows impaired sympathetic vasoconstriction is associated with poor functional recovery in the long term,[70] thus suggesting SNS changes may play a role in the transition from acute to chronic pain.

There has been much investigation of the effects of MT and MWM on SNS activity. MWM treatment applied to the elbow of patients with lateral epicondylalgia has demonstrated sympathoexcitatory effects of increased heart rate, blood pressure and skin conductance and decreased peripheral blood flow[38] that were similar to effects demonstrated with spinal MT.[39, 41] However, the authors cautioned that the magnitude of effects on SNS function was small and this is likely not of clinical relevance.[38] In fact most studies of MT have explored their effect on SNS activity more to determine a possible mechanism of action rather than determining any therapeutic effects on SNS function. Nevertheless, it is becoming clear that SNS disturbance likely plays a role in the maintenance of musculoskeletal pain but the precise nature of SNS activity requires further elucidation before it could be speculated that MWM may influence this system in a way that could be realised as therapeutic.

SUMMARY

Musculoskeletal pain conditions commonly managed with MWM treatment demonstrate varied sensory characteristics including hyperalgesia (mechanical and thermal), hypersensitive motor responses, hypoaesthesia and SNS disturbances. There is strong evidence that MWM treatment has a neurophysiological capacity to decrease pain, exert hypoalgesic effects and excite the SNS. With respect to hypoalgesia, MWM seems to preferentially modulate mechanical but not thermal hyperalgesia and can modulate heightened motor responses. This would suggest that this form of intervention could play an important role in modulating common features of musculoskeletal pain that likely reflect augmented pain-processing mechanisms and improve the outcome of these conditions. Although further investigation is required, MWM may have lesser effect on more widespread and generalised mechanical hyperalgesia as well as heat and cold hyperalgesia. Additional or different intervention strategies may be required to address these changes. The effects of MWM on SNS activity are apparent but their translation to improved patient outcomes is unclear. This also is an area for future research as the role of the SNS in musculoskeletal pain is becoming more apparent.

KEY POINTS

- Musculoskeletal pain presents with a range of sensory deficits, which may manifest as mechanical and thermal hyperalgesia, hypoaesthesia, heightened motor responses to sensory stimulation and changes in SNS function.

- Early after an injury local peripheral nociceptors are sensitised whereas in long-term chronic problems other nervous system changes predominate (e.g. widespread deficits at a distance to the injured area).

- Presence of cold hyperalgesia tends to signal poor response to manual therapy.

- MWM appears to target mechanical hyperalgesia predominantly.

References

1 Kent P, Keating JL. Classification in nonspecific low back pain: what methods do primary care clinicians currently use? Spine. 2005 Jun 15;30(12):1433–40.

2 Kent PM, Keating JL, Buchbinder R. Searching for a conceptual framework for nonspecific low back pain. Manual Therapy. 2009 Aug 1;14(4):387–96.

3 Kent PM, Keating JL, Taylor NF. Primary care clinicians use variable methods to assess acute nonspecific low back pain and usually focus on impairments. Manual Therapy. 2009 Feb 1;14(1):88–100.

4 Kokkonen SM, Kurunlahti M, Tervonen O, Ilkko E, Vanharanta H. Endplate degeneration observed on magnetic resonance imaging of the lumbar spine — Correlation with pain provocation and disc changes observed on computed tomography diskography. Spine. 2002 Oct;27(20):2274–8.

5 Videman T, Battie MC, Gibbons LE, Maravilla K, Manninen H, Kaprio J. Associations between back pain history and lumbar MRI findings. Spine. 2003 Mar;28(6):582–8.

6 Max M. Is Mechanism-based pain treatment attainable? Clinical Trial Issues. The Journal of Pain. 2000;1:2–9.

7 Jensen TS, Baron R. Translation of symptoms and signs into mechanisms in neuropathic pain. Pain. 2003 Mar;102(1–2):1–8.

8 Farrell M, Gibson S, McMeeken J, Helme R. Pain and hyperalgesia in osteoarthritis of the hands. Journal of Rheumatology. 2000;27(2):441–7.

9 Giesecke T, Gracely RH, Grant MA, Nachemson A, Petzke F, Williams DA, et al. Evidence of augmented central pain processing in idiopathic chronic low back pain. Arthritis Rheumatology. 2004 Feb;50(2):613–23.

10 Scott D, Jull G, Sterling M. Widespread sensory hypersensitivity is a feature of chronic whiplash-associated disorder but not chronic idiopathic neck pain. Clinical Journal of Pain. 2005 Mar–Apr;21(2):175–81.

11 Wright A, Thurnwald P, O'Callaghan J, Smith J, Vicenzino B. Hyperalgesia in tennis elbow patients. Journal of Musculoskeletal Pain. 1994;2(4):83–97.

12 Rasmussen PV, Sindrup SH, Jensen TS, Bach FW. Symptoms and signs in patients with suspected neuropathic pain. Pain. 2004 Jul;110(1–2):461–9.

13 Schmid A, Brunner F, Wright A, Bachmann LM. Paradigm shift in manual therapy? Evidence for a central nervous system component in the response to passive cervical joint mobilisation. Manual Therapy. 2008 Oct;13(5):387–96.

14 Vicenzino B, Paungmali A, Teys P. Mulligan's mobilization with movement, positional faults and pain relief: Current concepts from a critical review of literature. Manual Therapy. 2007;12:98–108.

15 O'Brien T, Vicenzino B. A study of the effects of Mulligan's mobilization with movement treatment of lateral ankle pain using a case study design. Manual Therapy. 1998;3(2):78–84.

16 Hall T, Hardt S, Schafer A, Wallin L. Mulligan bent leg raise technique — a preliminary randomized trial of immediate effects after a single intervention. Manual Therapy. 2006 May;11(2):130–5.

17 Reid SA, Rivett DA, Katekar MG, Callister R. Sustained natural apophyseal glides (SNAGs) are an effective treatment for cervicogenic dizziness. Manual Therapy. 2007 Oct 19:357–66.

18 Bisset L, Beller E, Jull G, Brooks P, Darnell R, Vicenzino B. Mobilisation with movement and exercise, corticosteroid injection, or wait and see for tennis elbow: randomised trial. British Medical Journal. 2006 September 29, 2006:bmj.38961.584653.AE.

19 Hall T, Chan HT, Christensen L, Odenthal B, Wells C, Robinson K. Efficacy of a C1–C2 self-sustained natural apophyseal glide (SNAG) in the management of cervicogenic headache. Journal of Orthopaedic Sports Physical Therapy. 2007 Mar;37(3):100–7.

20 Paungmali A, O'Leary S, Souvlis T, Vicenzino B. Naloxone fails to antagonise initial hypoalgesic effect of a manual therapy treatment for lateral epicondylalgia. Journal of Manipulative and Physiological Therapeutics. 2004;27(3):180–5.

21 Teys P, Bisset L, Vicenzino B. The initial effects of a Mulligan's mobilization with movement technique on range of movement and pressure pain threshold in pain-limited shoulders. Manual Therapy. 2008 Oct 25:37–42.

22 Arendt-Nielsen L, Graven-Nielsen T. Muscle pain: sensory implications and interaction with motor control. Clinical Journal of Pain. 2008 May;24(4):291–8.

23 Sterling M, Kenardy J. Physical and psychological aspects of whiplash: Important considerations for primary care assessment. Manual Therapy. 2008 May;13(2):93–102.

24 Sterling M, Jull G, Vicenzino B, Kenardy J. Sensory hypersensitivity occurs soon after whiplash injury and is associated with poor recovery. Pain. 2003 Aug;104(3):509–17.

25 Collins N, Teys P, Vicenzino B. The initial effects of a Mulligan's mobilization with movement technique on dorsiflexion and pain in sub-acute ankle sprains. Manual Therapy. 2004 May;9(2):77–82.

26 Slater H, Arendt-Nielsen L, Wright A, Graven-Nielsen T. Effects of a manual therapy technique in experimental lateral epicondylalgia. Manual Therapy. 2006 May;11(2):107–17.

27 Ronnen HR, de Korte PJ, Brink PR, van der Bijl HJ, Tonino AJ, Franke CL. Acute whiplash injury: is there a role for MR imaging? — a prospective study of 100 patients. Radiology. 1996 Oct;201(1):93–6.

28 Coombes BK, Bisset L, Vicenzino B. An integrative model of lateral epicondylalgia. British Journal of Sports Medicine. 2008 Dec 2:252–8.

29 Sheather-Reid RB, Cohen ML. Psychophysical evidence for a neuropathic component of chronic neck pain. Pain. 1998;75:341–7.

30 Vicenzino B. Lateral epicondylalgia: a musculoskeletal physiotherapy perspective. Manual Therapy. 2003 May;8(2):66–79.

31 Curatolo M, Petersen-Felix S, Arendt-Nielsen L, Giani C, Zbinden AM, Radanov BP. Central hypersensitivity in chronic pain after whiplash injury. Clinical Journal of Pain. 2001 Dec;17(4):306–15.

32 O'Neill S, Manniche C, Graven-Nielsen T, Arendt-Nielsen L. Generalized deep-tissue hyperalgesia in patients with chronic low-back pain. European Journal of Pain. 2007 May;11(4):415–20.

33 Peolsson M, Borsbo B, Gerdle B. Generalized pain is associated with more negative consequences than local or regional pain: A study of chronic whiplash-associated disorders. Journal of Rehabilitation Medicine. 2007;39:260–8.

34 Sterling M, Pedler A, Chan C, Puglisi M, Vuvan V, Vicenzino B. Cervical lateral glide increases nociceptive flexion reflex but not pressure or thermal pain threshold in chronic whiplash associated disorder. Manual Therapy. 2010;15(2):149–53.

35 Jensen TS, Gottrup H, Sindrup SH, Bach FW. The clinical picture of neuropathic pain. European Journal of Pharmacology. 2001 Oct 19;429(1–3):1–11.

36 Chien A, Eliav E, Sterling M. Whiplash (grade II) and cervical radiculopathy share a similar sensory presentation: an investigation using quantitative sensory testing. Clinical Journal of Pain. 2008d Sep;24(7):595–603.

37 Leffler AS, Kosek E, Hansson P. The influence of pain intensity on somatosensory perception in patients suffering from sub-acute/chronic lateral epicondylalgia. European Journal of Pain — London. 2000;4(1):57–71.

38 Paungmali A, O'Leary S, Souvlis T, Vicenzino B. Hypoalgesic and sympathoexcitatory effects of mobilization with movement for lateral epicondylalgia. Physical Therapy. 2003 Apr;83(4):374–83.

39 Sterling M, Jull G, Wright A. Cervical mobilisation: concurrent effects on pain, sympathetic nervous system activity and motor activity. Manual Therapy. 2001 May;6(2):72–81.

40 Vicenzino B. An investigation of the effects of spinal manual therapy on forequarter pressure and thermal pain threshold and sympathetic nervous system activity in asymptomatic subjects: A preliminary report. In: M Shacklock (ed.) Moving in on Pain. Adelaide: Butterworth-Heinemann 1995:185–93.

41 Vicenzino B, Collins D, Benson H, Wright A. An investigation of the interrelationship between manipulative therapy-induced hypoalgesia and sympathoexcitation. Journal of Manipulative and Physiological Therapeutics. 1998 Sep;21(7):448–53.

42 George SZ, Bishop MD, Bialosky JE, Zeppieri G, Jr., Robinson ME. Immediate effects of spinal manipulation on thermal pain sensitivity: an experimental study. BMC Musculoskelet Disord. 2006;7:68.

43 Wasner G, Naleschinski D, Binder A, Schattschneider J, McLachlan EM, Baron R. The effect of menthol on cold allodynia in patients with neuropathic pain. Pain Medicine. 2008 Apr;9(3):354–8.

44 Moss P, Knight E, Wright A. Subjects with knee osteoarthritis exhibit widespread mechanical and cold, but not heat, hyperalgesia. ISAP 12th World Congress on Pain. Glasgow: ISAP. 2008:PW046.

45 Terkelsen AJ, Bach FW, Jensen TS. Experimental forearm immobilization in humans induces cold and mechanical hyperalgesia. Anesthesiology. 2008 Aug;109(2):297–307.

46 Sterling M, Jull G, Kenardy J. Physical and psychological factors maintain long-term predictive capacity post-whiplash injury. Pain. 2006 May;122(1–2):102–8.

47 Williams M, Williamson E, Gates S, Lamb S, Cooke M. A systematic literature review of physical prognostic factors for the development of Late Whiplash Syndrome. Spine. 2007 Dec 1;32(25):E764–80.

48 Jull G, Sterling M, Kenardy J, Beller E. Does the presence of sensory hypersensitivity influence outcomes of physical rehabilitation for chronic whiplash? — A preliminary RCT. Pain. 2007 May;129(1–2):28–34.

49 Sterling M, Pettiford C, Hodkinson E, Curatolo M. Psychological factors are related to some sensory pain thresholds but not nociceptive flexion reflex threshold in chronic whiplash. Clinical Journal of Pain. 2008;24;124–30.

50 Butler D. Mobilisation of the Nervous System. Melbourne: Churchill Livingstone 1991.

51 Hall T, Pyne E, Hamer P. Limiting factors of the straight leg raise test. Singer K (ed.) 8th Biennial Conference MPAA Perth: MPAA. 1993:32–9.

52 Coppieters MW, Stappaerts KH, Wouters LL, Janssens K. The immediate effects of a cervical lateral glide treatment technique in patients with neurogenic cervicobrachial pain. Journal of Orthopaedic Sports Physical Therapy. 2003 Jul;33(7):369–78.

53 Saranga J, Green A, Lewis J, Worsfold C. Effect of a cervical lateral glide on the upper limb neurodynamic test 1. A blinded placebo-controlled investigation. Physiotherapy. 2003;89(11):678–84.

54 Emery CF, France CR, Harris J, Norman G, Vanarsdalen C. Effects of progressive muscle relaxation training on nociceptive flexion reflex threshold in healthy young adults: a randomized trial. Pain. 2008 Aug 31;138(2):375–9.

55 Jensen R, Kvale A, Baerheim A. Is pain in patellofemoral pain syndrome neuropathic? Clinical Journal of Pain. 2008 Jun;24(5):384–94.

56 Tucker AT, White PD, Kosek E, Pearson RM, Henderson M, Coldrick AR, et al. Comparison of vibration perception thresholds in individuals with diffuse upper limb pain and carpal tunnel syndrome. Pain. 2007 Feb;127(3):263–9.

57 Chien A, Eliav E, Sterling M. Hypoaesthesia occurs with sensory hypersensitivity in chronic whiplash: further evidence of a neuropathic condition. Manual Therapy. 2009;14(2): 138–46.

58 Freynhagen R, Rolke R, Baron R, Tolle TR, Rutjes AK, Schu S, et al. Pseudoradicular and radicular low-back pain — a disease continuum rather than different entities? Answers from quantitative sensory testing. Pain. 2008 Mar;135(1–2):65–74.

59 Chien A, Eliav E, Sterling M. Hypoaesthesia occurs in acute whiplash irrespective of pain and disability levels and the presence of sensory hypersensitivity. Clinical Journal of Pain. 2008a Nov–Dec;24(9):759–66.

60 Geber C, Magerl W, Fondel R, Fechir M, Rolke R, Vogt T, et al. Numbness in clinical and experimental pain — a cross-sectional study exploring the mechanisms of reduced tactile function. Pain. 2008 Sep 30;139(1):73–81.

61 Chien A, Sterling M. Hypoaesthesia is a feature of chronic whiplash but not idiopathic neck pain. Manual Therapy. 2010;15(1): 48–53.

62 Johnston V, Jimmieson N, Jull G, Souvlis T. Quantitative sensory testing measures distinguish office workers with varying levels of neck pain and disability. Pain. 2008;137:257–65.

63 Passatore M, Roatta S. Influence of sympathetic nervous system on sensorimotor function: whiplash associated disorders (WAD) as a model. European Journal of Applied Physiology. 2006 Nov;98(5):423–49.

64 Gockel M, Lindholm H, Niemisto L, Hurri H. Perceived disability but not pain is connected with autonomic nervous function among patients with chronic low back pain. Journal of Rehabilitation Medicine. 2008 May;40(5):355–8.

65 Mani R, Cooper C, Kidd BL, Cole JD, Cawley MI. Use of laser Doppler flowmetry and transcutaneous oxygen tension electrodes to assess local autonomic dysfunction in patients with frozen shoulder. Journal of Royal Society of Medicine. 1989;82(9):536–8.

66 McLean SA, Williams DA, Clauw DJ. Fibromyalgia after motor vehicle collision: evidence and implications. Traffic Injury Prevention. 2005 Jun;6(2):97–104.

67 Smith RW, Papadopolous E, Mani R, Cawley MI. Abnormal microvascular responses in a lateral epicondylitis. British Journal of Rheumatology. 1994 Dec;33(12):1166–8.

68 McLean SA, Clauw DJ, Abelson JL, Liberzon I. The development of persistent pain and psychological morbidity after motor vehicle collision: integrating the potential role of stress response systems into a biopsychosocial model. Psychosomatic Medicine. 2005a Sep–Oct;67(5):783–90.

69 Huge V, Lauchart M, Forderreuther S, Kaufhold W, Valet M, Azad SC, et al. Interaction of hyperalgesia and sensory loss in complex regional pain syndrome type I (CRPS I). PLoS ONE. 2008;3(7):e2742.

70 Sterling M, Jull G, Vicenzino B, Kenardy J, Darnell R. Physical and psychological factors predict outcome following whiplash injury. Pain. 2005 Mar;114(1–2):141–8.

Chapter 7
Motor and sensorimotor deficits and likely impact of Mobilisation with Movement

Paul Hodges and Bill Vicenzino

INTRODUCTION

Movement is changed by pain and there is increasing evidence that rehabilitation of movement is an important component of recovery from symptoms. Movement is coordinated by a complex system than involves not just the joint arthrokinematics guided by passive elements such as structural bone and joint mechanisms and muscle contraction, but the sensory system that provides information of the current status of the body (e.g. position, orientation to gravity, etc) and information about the effect of internal and external disturbances, and the nervous system that considers the requirements of a movement or position and plans a strategy to meet an intended objective, whether it be the maintenance of the current position or the intention to move. When a person presents with musculoskeletal pain, movement is altered and this may have begun prior to the onset of pain and contributed to its development, or begun as a result of an adaptation due to pain and/or injury. Regardless of the mechanism of onset it may be a factor in the recurrence or persistence of pain and/or injury.

A range of physical therapies aim to change movement to relieve pain and prevent persistence or recurrence of pain. Mobilisation with Movement (MWM), which by definition aims to facilitate normal movement (Chapter 2), is one potentially potent intervention to change movement. This chapter aims to discuss how movement changes in pain, to present new ideas of the underlying mechanisms for movement to change in pain, and to postulate a range of mechanisms that involve multiple components of the movement system that may underlie how MWM leads to pain relief. It aims to complement the information and concepts presented in the preceding chapters on possible underlying mechanisms of action of MWM (Chapters 4 and 5) as well as the chapter on pain and sensory system impairment (Chapter 6).

MECHANISMS FOR CHANGES IN MOVEMENT WITH PAIN AND INJURY

Interpretation of the changes in movement with pain requires consideration of the time-course. In the acute situation movement and pain/injury are inextricably linked. If the nervous system determines that there is threat to the tissues (thermal, mechanical or chemical) then movement changes to protect the painful part. Such changes occur at multiple levels of the nervous system, from simple flexor withdrawal reflexes to more complex adaptations in movement pattern, such as walking with an externally rotated lower limb to reduce the requirement for ankle dorsiflexion after an acute ankle sprain.

Theories of motor adaptation to acute pain

Several simple theories have been developed to explain motor system changes in acute pain. The most notable were the 'vicious cycle' theory and the 'pain adaptation' theory. The vicious cycle theory proposed that muscle activity increases in association with pain/injury and the accompanying build up of metabolites due to contraction-related ischaemia contributes to the perpetuation of pain.[1] The pain adaptation theory posits a more variable response with reduced excitability or inhibition of muscles that produce a painful movement (agonist muscles) and increased excitability of muscles that oppose a painful movement (antagonist muscles) with the effect to reduce the amplitude and velocity of movement of the painful segment.[2] Although attractive and helpful for the interpretation of some of the observations that accompany acute pain/injury, there are numerous observations that do not fit the predictions of these models. First, when pain is induced in a muscle, there is neither uniform inhibition nor excitation of the motoneuron pool.[3] Although numerous studies of whole muscle recordings report evidence of decreased activity of agonist muscles,[4, 5] there are at best variable changes in antagonist muscles[6] and studies of activity of single motor units (the smallest functional unit of the motor system that includes the motoneuron at all the muscle fibres it innervates) provide a different explanation.[7]

When pain is induced in a muscle and the participant is required to generate the same force before and during pain, rather than uniform reduction in activity of that muscle, there is a redistribution of activity

93

within and between muscles.[3, 7] This suggests that the nervous system does not simply inhibit or facilitate muscle activity, but establishes a new solution to generate force. This solution may be a strategy to meet the goal of the task, but with protection of the painful or injured part. A further problem with the pain adaptation theory is that although this theory appears logical for voluntary movement (reduced activity of the muscle that produces a painful movement to limit the displacement and velocity of that movement) the theory makes no predictions of the effect of pain on postural control. In this case, if activity of a muscle was inhibited, movements/moments that result from internal (e.g. reactive moments from voluntary movements) and external forces (e.g. perturbation from unexpectedly applied load) could lead to increased displacement and/or velocity. Finally, neither theory can explain the variability in adaptation identified in many people with clinical pain.[6, 8] Although both theories predict stereotypical changes, data of whole muscle behaviour show huge individual variation in response to pain. For instance, although acute back pain is associated with an overall increase in trunk muscle activity, no two individuals respond in an identical manner.[8]

An alternative theory of adaptation in acute pain is required. In the acute phase it is hypothesised that the nervous system identifies a solution that is protective of the painful or injured part by redistribution of activity within (between regions within a muscle) and between muscles,[3, 7, 8] but this is not stereotypical.[8, 9] This adaptation changes the mechanical properties (for protection)[10] that may involve decreased or modified motion of a segment and less variation in motion. Although this protective adaptation implies a 'decision' by the nervous system to protect the painful part, it is important to recognise that there are multiple underlying effects that will influence the resultant change in movement, and this is likely to explain some of the variability of the change in movement and muscle activity. Pain and injury can affect movement at many levels of the motor system (Figure 7.1).

Mechanisms underlying the motor adaptation to pain

On the sensory side, injury can affect the mechanoreceptors in muscle, ligament, joint capsule and skin that provide input to the nervous system about the position of a body segment or its movement. This can either be due to direct injury of the mechanoreceptor or trauma or inflammation of the structure that contains the mechanoreceptor. Such changes may be the result

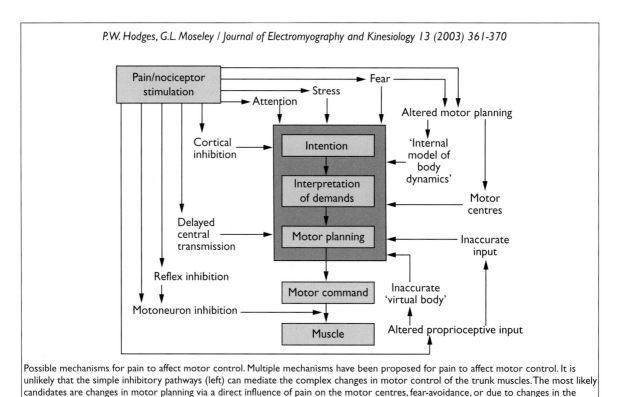

P.W. Hodges, G.L. Moseley / Journal of Electromyography and Kinesiology 13 (2003) 361-370

Possible mechanisms for pain to affect motor control. Multiple mechanisms have been proposed for pain to affect motor control. It is unlikely that the simple inhibitory pathways (left) can mediate the complex changes in motor control of the trunk muscles. The most likely candidates are changes in motor planning via a direct influence of pain on the motor centres, fear-avoidance, or due to changes in the sensory systems.

Figure 7.1 Pain and injury can influence the motor system at many different levels. Reproduced with permission from Hodges and Moseley[9]

of repeated loading of the structure[11] as opposed to frank trauma. Alternatively, pain is associated with changed processing or interpretation of sensory information. For instance, despite availability of information from the back muscles in people with back pain, this information is often ignored.[12] In chronic pain there is reorganisation of the sensorimotor cortex and the extent of reorganisation is related to the duration of pain.[13] Any of these changes in sensory function would mean that the nervous system has corrupted input or interpretation of sensory information. This has two major impacts on the control of movement. First, interpretation of the position of the body segments and any perturbation would be corrupted. Second, the internal representation of the body that is used by the nervous system to interpret and plan movement would be built on the basis of incorrect information of movement and position of the body segments. In either case, movement is based on inaccurate interpretation of body position and displacement and cannot be ideal. The consequence is likely to involve either poorly controlled motion or adaptation by the nervous system to protect the part by adopting more stereotypical movement or a strategy of co-contraction.

On the motor side, changes have been identified at multiple levels from the muscle to the higher centres of the nervous system. Muscle can adapt to disuse and altered neural input by atrophy and fatty infiltration[14-17] and this can initiate rapidly.[17] At the spinal cord, injury to joint structures can cause reflex inhibition, particularly of extensor muscles.[18, 19] This leads to inhibition of motoneurons, the nerve cells that innervate muscle. As indicated above, pain leads to increased and decreased excitability of the motoneurons.[3, 20] Higher in the motor pathway, pain increases and/or decreases excitability of cells at the motor cortex[21, 22 (Tsao, unpublished data)] and in more persistent pain states, the organisation of the motor cortex is changed.[23] As many regions of the nervous system contribute to control of movement, other changes are likely. Furthermore, as discussed earlier, there is also evidence that the nervous system selects a new strategy during pain, to protect the body segment that is injured or painful or has the potential to be painful or injured. These multiple effects on the motor system can be additive, competitive or synergistic.

In summary, the nervous system appears to adopt a protective strategy in acute pain that involves redistribution of activity within and between muscles and leads to changes in mechanical behaviour (stiffening or modified movement), and is mediated by changes at multiple levels of the nervous system. A critical issue is that although the adaptation has potential benefits in the short term (for protection of pain and/or injury or potential pain and/or injury) there are potential long-term consequences if the adaptation is maintained in the long term.

The complexity of motor adaptation in chronic or recurrent musculoskeletal pain

Changes in movement in chronic conditions are more difficult to explain than the adaptation in acute pain. There are three main scenarios. A first scenario is that the peripheral source of nociception may still be relevant with nociceptor input from peripheral structures still continuing to signal information to the central nervous system regarding mechanical or chemical threat to the tissues and also the communication of nociceptive information may be heightened by sensitisation of the pain system through, for example, peripheral sensitisation and changes in the dorsal horn (also see Chapter 6). In this case, restoration of ideal movement control to optimise the loading of the irritated peripheral structure is required. Although the initial adaptation may be beneficial in the short term to protect the painful/injured structure, this may not be ideal in the long term (see below).

A second scenario is the patient who recovers from the initial acute pain episode, but continues to experience episodes of pain. Data from patients during remission from symptoms in back pain and other conditions, suggest that adaptations in motor control persist during remission.[24] It is hypothesised that this adaptation may predispose an individual to recurrence of pain/injury.

A third scenario is the case where biological changes in the nervous system contribute to the perpetuation of pain experience, irrespective of the peripheral nociceptor inputs. It is critical to remember that pain is generated by the nervous system in response to information regarding threat that is conveyed by the nociceptors and moderated by a person's experiences and beliefs about pain. In a chronic state the combination of biological changes in the central nervous system and a person's beliefs can perpetuate the experience of pain.[25, 26] In this case the peripheral factors may be less relevant for the persistence of pain, but the adaptation to movement may lead to further problems. An important consideration is that there is interaction between motor control and psychology. A person's attitudes and beliefs about pain may influence the adaptation and their ability to change an adaptation.

Consequences of the adaptation in motor behaviour

Although adaptation in motor behaviour may be protective in the short term by reduction of movement or modified loading via changes in movement, it may have consequences, and may in fact contribute to the persistence or recurrence of pain. This may be due to increased loading from co-contraction, or increased activity for protection, or as a result of a less ideal movement strategy due to reduced activity of some parts of the motor system, decreased or altered movement, or decreased movement variability. For similar reasons an initial onset of pain may arise from any other factor that changes movement; for example, disuse, habitual movement patterns and postures, etc.

Redistribution of activity between and within muscles has several mechanical consequences that are unlikely to be ideal. First, protective strategies that involve increased activity and co-contraction increase load on joint structures. For instance, when people with back pain lift a mass there is greater load on the spine as a result of the muscle activation strategies.[27] Although some load is good, increased load over a sustained period is likely to have negative consequences. Second, co-contraction reduces movement. Movement is important for shock absorption, particularly for weight-bearing joints. Third, reduced contribution of some muscles to joint control (e.g. transversus abdominis and multifidus in low back pain), is likely to lead to less than optimal control.[9] Fourth, redistribution of activity will change movement path or load distribution on joint structures. Although load sparing may be helpful in the short term, in the long term the quality of unloaded structures may be compromised, and the structures with increased or more consistent load may undergo changes.

Variability in movement is important. When movement is too variable this implies lack of control, but some variability is important. When movement is variable every repetition of a movement loads different structures and loading is distributed over joint surfaces and between structures. If there is too little variation in movement the same structures are loaded in the same manner with every repetition of a task.[28] Variability is also important for learning. It is by trying new alternatives that the nervous system identifies new solutions. Variation is critical for this process. New non-linear analysis methods have revealed that several clinical conditions are characterised by reduced variation[28] and lack of variation has been associated with lack of resolution of an adaptation after recovery of an acute pain episode.[29]

In summary, although adaptation may be beneficial in the short term, and some adaptation may be required if there is disruption of osseoligamentous structures, if this is maintained in the long term this is likely to have consequences for the tissues in the painful region. This may contribute to the persistence of symptoms, contribute to the recurrence of symptoms, or contribute to the development of secondary changes and symptoms. Clinical strategies are required to restore optimal movement. This may involve restoration of movement to a preclinical state by reducing reliance on some strategies, increased activity of other muscles, modified movement path, or optimised variation.

MWM SENSORIMOTOR SYSTEM AFFECTS: POSSIBLE MECHANISMS

MWM aims to facilitate normal movement. By manual guidance of joint position, movement and muscle contraction, MWM is likely to provide a potent stimulus that provides novel sensory input, novel muscle activation strategies, and exposes the nervous system to new movement solutions. These mechanisms have been hypothesised and some have initial experimental support. Each is outlined below.

Sensory affects of MWM

Sensory input from large diameter afferents (non-nociceptive mechanoreceptors) may have multiple effects on interpretation and processing of nociceptive information and motor output. First, sensory input from mechanoreceptors in skin, ligament and joint capsule changes muscle activity. Electrical stimulation of the anterior cruciate ligament leads to excitation of the quadriceps[30] and electrical stimulation of the annulus fibrosis of an intervertebral disc,[31] or mechanical stretch of the supraspinous ligament,[32] facilitate activity of the lumbar multifidus muscles. This activity of the multifidus is related to the region of disc that is stimulated.[33] Similarly, discharge of mechanoreceptors in the skin of the hand is associated with modulation of activity of muscles in the region[34] and stretch of the skin over the patella changes activity of the vasti muscles of the knee.[35] This latter finding was specific to the direction of stretch of the skin. Taken together these data imply that specific mechanical stress to joint structures or skin, as would be applied in a MWM, could change the activity of muscles around the joint. This could lead to improved arthrokinematics and control of the joint. This hypothesis requires further investigation.

Second, several studies report the effect of MWM on indices of sensory function and imply improved capacity to perceive motion. Although the underlying mechanisms for the improvement in sensation remain unclear, improved movement could be mediated by improved sensory acuity and function. Most studies of sensory function have tested error in repositioning a joint. There is preliminary evidence that joint position error is improved by MWM. The effects of a weight-bearing MWM for ankle dorsiflexion (see Chapter 5, Figure 5.3) on joint position error as measured with a pedal goniometer[36] was evaluated in a pilot study of 23 people with recurrent lateral ankle sprain and a joint position error deficit of 4° (SD: 1.3). Joint position error was improved by 2.4° (1.5 to 3.3) after application of the MWM. This amplitude of improvement is larger than the standard error of the measurement of 1.7° (Vicenzino, unpublished data) and may be considered as a clinically meaningful improvement. These findings were not supported by a recent study of the traction straight leg raise (SLR) MWM in 23 asymptomatic people with limited SLR (mean 44.4° [SD: 11.3]). Although this study showed that the MWM improved straight leg raise by ~7°[37] and confirmed the findings of others[38–40], there was no significant change in joint position error of the hip in non-weight-bearing and weight-bearing test positions (Vicenzino et al[41]). However, subjects reported significant changes in the perception and sensation of stretch at endpoint (e.g. reduced sensation of stretch or felt as if the SLR went higher). These differences may be due to a number of factors, such as: (1) the latter study evaluated the MWM in subjects who did not have a deficit in joint position error, but rather had a deficit in range of straight leg raise; and (2) the ankle and leg raise MWM techniques are quite different techniques. Either of these differences may be significant in the treatment effect produced by MWM.

Balance effects of MWM

Evidence of improved sensorimotor function has also been derived from studies of balance control. However, it is difficult to disentangle whether these improvements are due to changes in the sensory or motor function. Balance is a complex function that involves sensory information of the status of body (joint positions, orientation relative to gravity), sensory information regarding perturbation, interpretation of the sensory information, planning of a motor response (from simple reflex responses mediated by spinal cord circuits to complex whole body responses orchestrated by higher centres), and generation of the movement (which depends on the generation of the motor command and the ability of the muscles to enact the command).[42] Thus, due to the complexity of balance control it is difficult to determine *how* MWM leads to improved balance, but these data provide further evidence that MWMs change movement.

Merlin et al[43] studied the effect of three sets of 10 repetitions of posterior-cephalad glide of the lateral malleolus during plantar-flexion/inversion movements in eight patients who had recently injured their lateral ligament complex (see Chapter 19 for technique description in full). The fibular glide MWM produced a mean improvement (95% confidence interval [CI]) of 9.6 seconds (6.27 to 12.93) in the eyes closed Rhomberg single leg stance test as well as a mean increase in the range of motion (ROM) of dorsiflexion in a weight-bearing position of 1.6 cm (0.53 to 2.67), but not the pain experienced with the latter. Although a preliminary and small study, these findings may implicate a direct influence of MWM on the motor and/or sensorimotor systems. Merlin et al[43] also studied 30 uninjured subjects (note: we were unable to obtain this data in order to calculate point estimates of effect) and reported no change in any of the measures, implying that MWM may only serve a

purposeful clinical utility when there are pre-existing impairments.

Hopper et al[44] evaluated the effects on balance of the fibular taping technique which is designed to replicate the MWM technique studied by Merlin et al[43] in 20 recreational athletes with unilateral chronic ankle instability. They reported that the taping technique did not change static or dynamic balance measures under rested or fatigued conditions.[44] Although this finding contrasts those of Merlin et al[43], this may reflect differences between the manually applied MWM and the taping analogue. However, the cohort evaluated by Hopper et al[44] had a Functional Ankle Disability Index (FADI) of 84.2% (SD± 9.4), which is indicative of minimally impaired chronic ankle instability. Thus, this group may have had a limited potential for an effect of the magnitude required to be measured accurately.

Reid et al[45] evaluated the effect of a cervical MWM for cervical dizziness, referred to as a sustained natural apophyseal glide (SNAG), on the sway pattern measured through four foot force plates when the person stood in quiet standing with eyes open, closed and cervical spine extended. Seventeen patients were treated with the SNAG and 17 with a placebo. At 12 weeks post-treatment there was a between-groups mean difference (90% CI) of 3.7 (0.3 to 7.1) and 2.6 (0.1 to 5.1) in sway pattern index with eyes closed and cervical spine extended, respectively.[45] The SNAG also reduced the frequency of dizziness and cervical pain with a mean 8.5° (95% CI: 1.4 to 18.3) increase in cervical extension ROM to a greater extent than the placebo treatment.

As mentioned above, it is difficult to extract the underlying mechanism for the improvement in balance function reported in these studies. One interesting observation from the studies of Merlin et al[43] and Reid et al[45] is that both studies reported increased ROM at the treated regions. This raises the possibility that there is some association between changes in sensorimotor function and ROM. It would be tempting to speculate that the MWM produces a direct mechanical effect on the underlying joints, increasing ROM (see below), which then leads to improved sensorimotor function, not only locally at the treated motion segments, but also more globally distributed as measured through the balance tests. However, equally plausible is that the afferent input from the MWM leads to changes to either pain or motor systems that result in increased ROMs.

Motor/movement effects of MWM

MWM is used to change parameters of movement such as ROM (e.g. see Chapters 3, 8–12 and 14–19). The underlying mechanism for these changes could be sensory as highlighted in the earlier discussion. However, other motor effects are possible. One key motor change could be the exposure, via the manual application of a MWM, of the patient to movement without pain. In this manner the MWM may provide a stimulus for motor learning. Changes in motor control or the learning of new movement solutions is dependent on trials of multiple options and this depends on movement variability. A healthy nervous system has some variability and a major benefit of such variation is the experience of different movement options. As mentioned in an earlier section, pain is often associated with reduced variation in movement[29, 46] and this may not only lead to repeated loading of joint structures, but also limit a person's potential to trial new solutions. Application of a MWM may provide such exposure, and with repetition the patient may learn the new pain-free movement solution. This new solution may involve changes in the balance of activity between muscles or change the distribution of activity between motor units within a muscle.

Another observation is increased strength following MWM. Several studies have shown improved grip force after elbow MWM in people with lateral epicondylalgia (Chapter 13).[47, 48] Slater et al[49] suggested that the phenomenon of post-exercise facilitation might be one means by which MWM improves strength. Merton et al[50] reported an increase in the size of the responses in a muscle evoked by transcutaneous magnetic stimulation of the motor cortex after a voluntary isometric muscle contraction and terms this effect 'post-exercise facilitation'. Later this facilitation was shown to last after the preceding muscle contraction had ceased.[51] Slater et al[49] hypothesised that the repeated isometric muscle contractions that are part of a MWM, such as that used for lateral epicondylalgia (see Chapter 13), may be sufficient to facilitate improved muscle contraction post-MWM and thereby constitute a mechanism through which MWM produces its beneficial effects. However, notwithstanding the inherent differences between the demonstrated motor facilitation and force generation, the evidence to date does not support such a hypothetical mechanism. As post-exercise facilitation is not limited to people with pain, if this effect underlies the improvement in force after MWM this could be expected after application of a technique to a non-painful segment as well. However, Abbott et al[47] and Vicenzino et al[48] did not find augmented grip force during or following the application of a lateral glide MWM to the *unaffected* elbow of patients with unilateral lateral epicondylalgia. Instead they showed a slight decrement in force output (~5%) following the MWM on the unaffected elbow and a significant effect on the affected elbow in the order of 20–50% of pre-MWM baseline. Furthermore, Slater et al[49] were unable to demonstrate any effect of the same MWM on experimentally induced lateral elbow pain. Alternatively, increased force after MWM may be explained by improved efficiency of force

generation secondary to changed distribution of activity within the muscle (changes in force direction due to redistribution of activity within a muscle during pain are thought to be less efficient), due to effects secondary to reduced pain (e.g. reduced inhibition) or due to reduced effects of fear or anticipation of pain.

An important observation is that motor effects are not only restricted to the treated joint. Abbott[52] described the effect of a lateral glide MWM in a study of 23 patients with lateral epicondylalgia and reported that the elbow MWM not only improved grip force of the affected limb, but also significantly increased internal rotation ROM at the shoulder of the affected limb by 16.7° (95% CI: 7.4 to 26.0) and the unaffected side by 11.1° (95% CI: 1.9 to 20.4). The author also reported significant improvements in external rotation of 7.4° on the affected side and 3.9° on the unaffected side with one-tailed t-tests. The author postulated that the bilateral effect at a joint not being treated was likely due to neurophysiological effects changing muscle tone at the shoulder. This highlights a possible broad-based effect of MWM on the motor system.

SUMMARY

As highlighted in the preceding discussion, there are multiple mechanisms that could underlie the efficacy of MWM for the improvement of function and reduction of pain. These mechanisms could involve both motor and sensory components, and a combination is likely. Pain and injury have potent effects on the motor system and MWM could interject at many levels. Although further work is clearly required to clarify the underlying mechanisms, there is mounting evidence that MWMs change movement. Further clarification of the mechanisms is likely to aid refinement of techniques and contribute to identification of those patients for whom the techniques may be most effective.

KEY POINTS

- Movement is affected when pain is present and the underlying mechanisms appear to be time dependent; that is, different mechanisms early after an injury or pain onset versus chronic presence of pain.
- The classic 'vicious cycle' and 'pain adaptation' theories do not satisfactorily explain the likely mechanisms of altered movement in those who have pain.
- Recent evidence indicates that at multiple levels, the nervous system adopts a protective strategy in acute pain, which involves redistribution of activity within and between muscles.
- Motor adaptation in chronic musculoskeletal pain is complex.

- With chronic musculoskeletal pain there is altered activity within and between muscles, which leads to impaired control of movement and changes in load distribution across joint structures.
- MWM, with its fine tuning of specific glide direction, may well be an appropriate modulator of the imbalanced activity within and between muscles and imbalanced loading of joints.
- There is preliminary evidence that MWM may directly influence the sensori-motor nervous system in bringing about improved movement.
- Further research is needed to understand how MWM improves movement.

References

1 Roland M. A critical review of the evidence for a pain–spasm–pain cycle in spinal disorders. Clinical Biomechanics. 1986;1:102–9.

2 Lund JP, Donga R, Widmer CG, Stohler CS. The pain-adaptation model: a discussion of the relationship between chronic musculoskeletal pain and motor activity. Canadian Journal of Physiology and Pharmacology. 1991;69(5):683–94.

3 Tucker K, Butler J, Graven-Nielsen T, Riek S, Hodges P. Motor unit recruitment strategies are altered during deep-tissue pain. Journal of Neuroscience. 2009 Sep 2;29(35):10820–6.

4 Arendt-Nielsen L, Graven-Nielsen T, Svarrer H, Svensson P. The influence of low back pain on muscle activity and coordination during gait: a clinical and experimental study. Pain. 1996;64(2):231–40.

5 Farina D, Arendt-Nielsen L, Merletti R, Graven-Nielsen T. Effect of experimental muscle pain on motor unit firing rate and conduction velocity. Journal of Neurophysiology. 2004 Mar;91(3):1250–9.

6 van Dieen JH, Selen LP, Cholewicki J. Trunk muscle activation in low-back pain patients, an analysis of the literature. Journal of Electromyography and Kinesiology. 2003 Aug;13(4):333–51.

7 Tucker KJ, Hodges PW. Motoneuron recruitment is altered with pain induced in non-muscular tissue. Pain. 2009 Jan;141(1–2):151–5.

8 Hodges PW, Moseley GL, Gabrielsson A, Gandevia SC. Experimental muscle pain changes feedforward postural responses of the trunk muscles. Experimental Brain Research. 2003 Jul;151(2):262–71.

9 Hodges PW, Moseley GL. Pain and motor control of the lumbopelvic region: effect and possible mechanisms. Journal of Electromyography and Kinesiology. 2003 Aug;13(4):361–70.

10 Hodges P, van den Hoorn W, Dawson A, Cholewicki J. Changes in the mechanical properties of the trunk in low back pain may be associated with recurrence. Journal Biomechanics. 2009 Jan 5;42(1):61–6.

11 Solomonow M, Zhou BH, Baratta RV, Lu Y, Harris M. Biomechanics of increased exposure to lumbar injury caused by cyclic loading: Part 1. Loss of reflexive muscular stabilization. Spine. 1999;24(23):2426–34.

12 Brumagne S, Cordo P, Verschueren S. Proprioceptive weighting changes in persons with low back pain and elderly persons during upright standing. Neuroscience Letters. 2004 Aug 5;366(1):63–6.

13 Flor H, Braun C, Elbert T, Birbaumer N. Extensive reorganization of primary somatosensory cortex in chronic back pain patients. Neuroscience Letters. 1997;224(1):5–8.

14 Herbison GJ, Jaweed MM, Ditunno JF. Muscle atrophy in rats following denervation, casting, inflammation, and tenotomy. Archives of Physical Medicine and Rehabilitation. 1979 Sep;60(9):401–4.

15 Hides JA, Stokes MJ, Saide M, Jull GA, Cooper DH. Evidence of lumbar multifidus muscle wasting ipsilateral to symptoms in patients with acute/subacute low back pain. Spine. 1994;19(2):165–77.

16 Hodges PW, Galea MP, Holm S, Holm AK. Corticomotor excitability of back muscles is affected by intervertebral disc lesion in pigs. European Journal of Neuroscience. 2009 Apr;29(7):1490–500.

17 Hodges PW, KaigleHolm A, Hansson T, Holm S. Rapid atrophy of the lumbar multifidus follows experimental disc or nerve root injury. Spine. 2006;31(25):2926–33.

18 Spencer JD, Hayes KC, Alexander IJ. Knee joint effusion and quadriceps reflex inhibition in man. Archives of Physical Medicine and Rehabilitation. 1984;65:171–7.

19 Stokes M, Young A. The contribution of reflex inhibition to arthrogenous muscle weakness. Clinical Science. 1984;67:7–14.

20 Le Pera D, Graven-Nielsen T, Valeriani M, Oliviero A, Di Lazzaro V, Tonali PA, et al. Inhibition of motor system excitability at cortical and spinal level by tonic muscle pain. Clinical Neurophysiology. 2001 Sep;112(9):1633–41.

21 Martin PG, Weerakkody N, Gandevia SC, Taylor JL. Group III and IV muscle afferents differentially affect the motor cortex and motoneurons in humans. Journal of Physiology. 2008 Mar 1;586(5):1277–89.

22 Valeriani M, Restuccia D, Di Lazzaro V, Oliviero A, Profice P, Le Pera D, et al. Inhibition of the human primary motor area by painful heat stimulation of the skin. Clinical Neurophysiology. 1999;110(8):1475–80.

23 Tsao H, Galea MP, Hodges PW. Reorganization of the motor cortex is associated with postural control deficits in recurrent low back pain. Brain. 2008 Aug;131(Pt 8):2161–71.

24 Richardson C, Hodges P, Hides J. Therapeutic Exercise for Lumbopelvic Stabilization (2nd edn). Edinburgh; New York: Churchill Livingstone 2004.

25 Foster N. Beliefs and preferences: do they help determine the outcome of musculoskeletal problems? Physical Therapy Reviews. 2007;12(3):199–206.

26 Leeuw M, Goossens M, Linton S, Crombez G, Boersma K, Vlaeyen J. The fear-avoidance model of musculoskeletal pain: current state of scientific evidence. Journal of Behavioral Medicine. 2007;30(1):77–94.

27 Marras WS, Ferguson SA, Burr D, Davis KG, Gupta P. Spine loading in patients with low back pain during asymmetric lifting exertions. The Spine Journal. 2004;4:64–75.

28 Hamill J, van Emmerik RE, Heiderscheit BC, Li L. A dynamical systems approach to lower extremity running injuries. Clinical Biomechanics (Bristol, Avon). 1999 Jun 1;14(5):297–308.

29 Moseley GL, Hodges PW. Reduced variability of postural strategy prevents normalisation of motor changes induced by back pain — a risk factor for chronic trouble? Behavioral Neuroscience. 2006;120(2):474–6.

30 Miyatsu M, Atsuta Y, Watakabe M. The physiology of mechanoreceptors in the anterior cruciate ligament. An experimental study in decerebrate-spinalised animals. Journal of Bone Joint Surgery, Br. 1993 Jul;75(4):653–7.

31 Indahl A, Kaigle A, Reikeras O, Holm S. Electromyographic response of the porcine multifidus musculature after nerve stimulation. Spine. 1995;20(24):2652–8.

32 Solomonow M, Zhou BH, Harris M, Lu Y, Baratta RV. The ligamento-muscular stabilizing system of the spine. Spine. 1998;23(23):2552–62.

33 Holm S, Indahl A, Solomonow M. Sensorimotor control of the spine. Journal of Electromyography Kinesiology. 2002;12(3):219–34.

34 McNulty PA, Macefield VG. Modulation of ongoing EMG by different classes of low-threshold mechanoreceptors in the human hand. Journal of Physiology. 2001;537(Pt 3):1021–32.

35 Macgregor K, Gerlach S, Mellor R, Hodges PW. Cutaneous stimulation from patella tape causes a differential increase in vasti muscle activity in people with patellofemoral pain. Journal of Orthopaedic Research. 2005 Mar;23(2):351–8.

36 Boyle J, Negus V. Joint position sense in the recurrently sprained ankle. Australian Journal of Physiotherapy. 1998;44(3):159–63.

37 Vicenzino B, unpublished data.

38 Hall T, Anuar K, Darlow B, Gurumoorthy P, Ryder M. The effect of Mulligan Traction Straight Leg Raise in participants with short hamstrings. Annals of the Academy of Medicine. 2003 Jan 1.

39 Hall T, Beherlein C, Hansson U, Teck Lim H, Odermark M, Sainsbury D. Mulligan Traction SLR: a pilot study to investigate effects on range of motion in patients with low back pain. Journal of Manual and Manipulative Therapy. 2006 Jul 22;14(2):95–100.

40 Hall T, Cacho A, McNee C, Riches J, Walsh J. Effects of the Mulligan Traction Straight Leg Raise Technique on Range of Movement. Journal of Manual and Manipulative Therapy. 2001 Jan 2;9(3):128–33.

41 Vicenzino B, unpublished data.

42 Shumway-Cooke A, Woollacott MH. Motor Control. Baltimore: Williams and Wilkins 1995.

43 Merlin D, McEwan I, Thom J. Mulligan's mobilisation with movement technique for lateral ankle pain and the use of magnetic resonance imaging to evaluate the 'positional fault' hypothesis. Isokenetic: Education Research Department. 2005. Online. Available: www.isokinetic.com/index.cfm?page=centro_studi/congressi/congresso_2005 (accessed 20 May 2010).

44 Hopper D, Samsson K, Hulenik T, Ng C, Hall T, Robinson K. The influence of Mulligan ankle taping during balance performance in subjects with unilateral chronic ankle instability. Physical Therapy in Sport. 2009;10(4): 125–30.

45 Reid S, Rivett D, Katekar M, Callister R. Sustained natural apophyseal glides (SNAGs) are an effective treatment for cervicogenic dizziness. Manual Therapy. 2008;13(4): 357–66.

46 Madeleine P, Mathiassen SE, Arendt-Nielsen L. Changes in the degree of motor variability associated with experimental and chronic neck-shoulder pain during a standardised repetitive arm movement. Experimental Brain Research. 2008 Mar;185(4):689–98.

47 Abbott JH, Patla CE, Jensen RH. The initial effects of an elbow mobilization with movement technique on grip strength in subjects with lateral epicondylalgia. Manual Therapy. 2001;6(3):163–9.

48 Vicenzino B, Paungmali A, Buratowski S, Wright A. Specific manipulative therapy treatment for chronic lateral epicondylalgia produces uniquely characteristic hypoalgesia. Manual Therapy. 2001 Nov;6(4):205–12.

49 Slater H, Arendt-Nielsen L, Wright A, Graven-Nielsen T. Effects of a manual therapy technique in experimental lateral epicondylalgia. Manual Therapy. 2006 May 1;11(2):107–17.

50 Merton P, Morton H, Hill D, Marsden C. Scope of a technique for electrical stimulation of human brain, spinal cord, and muscle. The Lancet. 1982;320(8298): 597–600.

51 Nørgaard P, Feldbæk Nielsen J, Andersen H. Post-exercise facilitation of compound muscle action potentials evoked by transcranial magnetic stimulation in healthy subjects. Experimental Brain Research. 2000;132(4):517–22.

52 Abbott JH. Mobilization with movement applied to the elbow affects shoulder range of movement in subjects with lateral epicondylalgia. Manual Therapy. 2001 Aug 1;6(3):170–7.

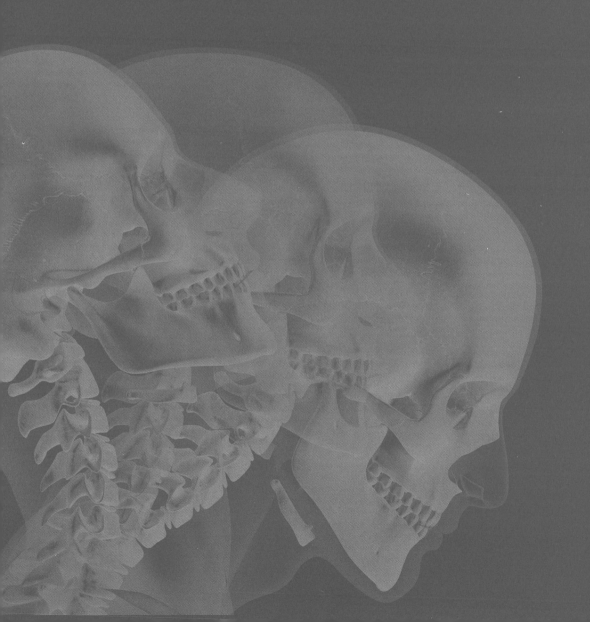

SECTION FOUR

Case studies

PREFACE TO CASE STUDIES

This section consists of 12 case studies that report on real-life clinical encounters as documented by eminent clinicians experienced in the application of Mobilisation with Movement (MWM) principles and techniques. These practitioners have been selected on the basis of their international clinical reputation, as well as their teaching expertise and publication record in the area of the Mulligan Concept.

There are a number of complementary reasons for devoting a major section of the book to these cases. In particular, the case studies are designed to:

1 Demonstrate to the reader how MWM can be seamlessly integrated into existing contemporary neuromusculoskeletal clinical practice, both as part of the assessment but more importantly as a treatment intervention. A variety of mechanical disorders covering most body regions are used to illustrate the utility and adaptability of this approach.

2 Provide guidance on how to select, apply and evaluate MWM techniques in the absence of comprehensive higher-level empirical evidence of efficacy (see Chapter 3) and established clinical prediction rules or evidence-based guides. Although the evidence base for MWM is rapidly growing, the cases highlight that the clinician still needs to employ advanced skills in clinical reasoning (as detailed generically in Chapter 2) to make appropriate clinical decisions.

3 Foster the development of clinical reasoning skills in the reader as they compare their thinking with that of the case contributor as the clinical findings gradually unfold. Clinical reasoning is the process that enables the scientific evidence for MWM (Chapters 4 to 7) to be applied in the unique context and for the individual presentation of any given patient.

4 Provide low-level evidence for the effectiveness of MWM as a treatment for a variety of musculoskeletal problems. It is largely from case studies which document contemporary clinical practice that the rationale for undertaking experimental studies (such as randomised controlled trials) arises.

The thought processes of the clinician have been exposed in each case study through the intermittent use of retrospective stimulus questions designed to highlight their clinical reasoning and application of the underpinning evidence base for the chosen MWM technique. The reader should propose their own answer to each question before comparing to that of the contributing clinician. Commentary is offered by the authors at the conclusion of each case study to enable the reader to consider additional viewpoints and relevant information on the application of MWM for the illustrated problem and similar presentations, in addition to

highlighting key learning messages from the chapter. At times, the commentary looks to promote thinking beyond traditional boundaries, consistent with the overall approach of Mulligan. Importantly, it also links the clinician's clinical reasoning in regard to the application of MWM in that particular case to the clinical reasoning framework established in Chapter 1.

Clinical reasoning in the various case studies is discussed in the paradigm of Sackett et al's 'evidence-based practice'[1] as elaborated in Chapters 1 and 3. The empirical and biological evidence for MWM explored in Chapters 3 to 6 provides a foundation to help inform the clinical reasoning discussed in the clinician's responses to the questions posed by the authors and the commentary on the clinician's reasoning offered by the authors at the conclusion of each case chapter. Given that clinical reasoning should be informed by the scientific evidence, rather than dictated, the term 'evidence-informed clinical reasoning' is used. The overall aim of the case studies is consistent with that of Sackett et al; that is, an integration of best research evidence with clinical expertise and the patient's values and preferences.[1]

The reader should be aware that the case studies are not designed to detail every possible available item of clinical data for a given patient. There would undoubtedly be other questions that could be asked in the patient history and other physical tests that could be performed, but what clinical information is presented in these case studies constitutes the relevant findings obtained by the expert practitioner at the actual time of the clinical encounter(s). The case studies are real-life examples of clinical practice, with the information and actions presented reflective of the available time and actual context of the clinical encounter (such as accessibility of physical measurement equipment) and the unique clinical approach and individual reasoning processes of the contributing expert clinician. Therefore, while there are broad similarities in structure between cases, variations in presentation have been preserved to help capture each clinician's usual practice.

The reader is encouraged to explore each case with an open but critical frame of mind. It is anticipated that the case studies will help facilitate the translation of the reader's understanding of MWM from a conceptual and theoretical basis to actual clinical application. It is also expected that they will help to integrate the evidence base for MWM within the reader's existing overarching clinical reasoning approach.

Reference

1 Sackett DL. Evidence based medicine: what it is and what it isn't. BMJ, 1996;312:71–2.

Chapter 8
A headache that's more than just a pain in the neck

Toby Hall and Kim Robinson

HISTORY

Norm is a 38-year-old schoolteacher, with a 20-year history of headaches. He is a reasonably active, fit individual who enjoys swimming at least 3 days per week. His headaches do not restrict his work or sporting activity but they do cause him to seek medical help due to their frequency, intensity and duration. When asked what he thought was causing the headachs, he suggested there 'could be something wrong with my neck'. When asked what he thought manual therapy could offer, he suggested there 'may be some exercises I could do to help my neck'.

Current history

Norm described that the headache tended to start with a feeling of neck stiffness and discomfort mainly on the right side of his neck before spreading to the occiput, top of his head and right eye (Figure 8.1). The pain was predominantly right sided, but with some spread to the whole head. There was no warning or aura prior to the onset of headaches. Norm also described a feeling of nausea and some watering of his right eye when the pain was severe. At no time did the headache change side or did he vomit during the headache attack.

The frequency of his headache was reported as an average of twice per week, with the symptoms lasting approximately 1–2 days. The duration of symptoms partly depended on the intensity of the headache at the time. Headache intensity varied according to the particular activity Norm was undertaking, but at worst reached 8/10 on a visual analogue scale (VAS). Norm reported no symptoms in his upper limbs.

The headache, although chronic, had been exacerbated over the previous 18 months by a change in Norm's work practice. He had changed jobs from a sedentary one to his current job, which involved writing on a whiteboard in front of a class of students. He found holding his arm in elevation with his neck in extension and rotation aggravated his headaches. Norm had seen his medical practitioner who had referred him to a neurologist for a specialist medical opinion. The neurologist diagnosed the headache as migraine and he was prescribed indomethacin,

which had not provided significant benefit and he had stopped taking it.

Of his own accord Norm had sought relief from an acupuncturist and a chiropractor. Both had given some short-term, temporary relief, but the headache kept on returning. His next step, if manual therapy was unsuccessful, was to see a pain specialist.

Previous history

Norm could not think of any specific incident of onset 20 years ago when the headaches began. Since then the headaches had gradually increased to a frequency of approximately one per week, with a further increase in frequency about 18 months ago. Over the 20 years there had been periods when his headaches had waxed and waned, but there appeared to be no specific activity that correlated with this. In the past he had tried various forms of treatment from his medical practitioner, mainly medication, and from allied health professionals, but these treatments had not been successful.

Symptom behaviour

Aggravating activities and postures included working on the computer for more than an hour, sleeping in prone lying position and writing on a whiteboard in front of his students continuously for more than 20 minutes. Once initiated, the headache usually subsided in 24 hours if he could avoid the provocative activities. Norm did not experience pain associated with rising from lying or standing up from forward bending.

Easing factors essentially were to avoid the computer and whiteboard and any awkward positions of the neck; for example, falling asleep in a chair with the head unsupported or holding the neck out of the neutral position for a prolonged period (such as when watching a movie or TV from an angle). He also found that resting quietly on his bed gave some relief, as did taking aspirin at the onset of symptoms. Norm had no difficulty sleeping but woke in the morning with headache if he had been sleeping in a prone lying position or if his head was in an awkward position on the pillow. Over a typical 24-hour period there appeared to be no

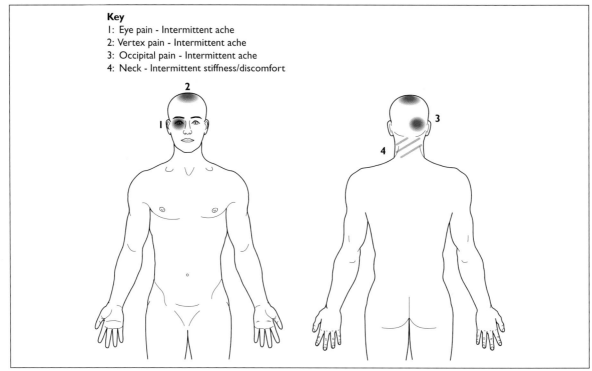

Key
1: Eye pain - Intermittent ache
2: Vertex pain - Intermittent ache
3: Occipital pain - Intermittent ache
4: Neck - Intermittent stiffness/discomfort

Figure 8.1 Body chart indicating area of patient's headache and neck pain

pattern to his pain unless he undertook the described provocative activities.

The Headache Disability Inventory (HDI) is an easy-to-administer, internally valid, reliable and stable instrument, which measures self-perceived disability related to headache.[1, 2] The HDI scores 25 items that evaluate the functional and emotional effects of headache on everyday life. Each activity is rated from 0 to 4, with a maximum total score of 100 and the minimum score being 0. The higher the score, the greater the disability caused by headache. Norm scored 36/52 for the emotional aspects, and 28/48 for the functional aspects, which gave a combined score of 64/100. While there are no published reference data for normal, these scores do serve as useful baseline measures for re-evaluation. The 95% confidence interval for test-retest change is reported as 29 points, which implies that a change of ± 29 points is required to reflect a true change in headache impact.[2]

Medical history and investigations

There was no evidence of other health issues including vertebrobasilar insufficiency. Norm's general health was good and he reported no recent weight loss. Radiographs showed minor narrowing of the C5-C6 disc space. His medical practitioner had also referred him for a computed tomography scan of the brain, the results of which were normal.

EVIDENCE-INFORMED CLINICAL REASONING

1 At the end of the history, what were your thoughts or hypotheses regarding the source of Norm's headache?

Clinician's response

Current evidence suggests manual therapy is only effective for some forms of headache. Bronfort et al[3] reviewed the evidence for non-invasive physical treatments for five types of headache: migraine, tension-type, cervicogenic headache (CGH), a mix of migraine and tension-type and post-traumatic headache. They found evidence that manual therapy was effective for CGH. In contrast, their review did not support the use of manual therapy for the long-term management of other headache forms. It therefore follows that correct classification of the headache disorder is very important so that appropriate treatment can be given.

Headache has been classified by the International Headache Society (IHS) into 14 major categories.[4] CGH is one sub-group of headache defined by the IHS, which accounts for up to 18% of all headaches[5] with a prevalence of 4.5%.[6] This form of headache is often misdiagnosed due to the similarity of symptoms between migraine, tension-type headache and common daily headache. Indeed, studies have shown that an incorrect headache diagnosis may occur in more than 50% of cases.[7] Diagnosis is essentially based on the presenting symptoms, together with the clinical physical examination findings.[8] Similarities of signs and symptoms between the many forms of headache[9] undoubtedly contribute to the challenge of differentiating between some headache types, whereas those headaches with unique characteristics are more readily identified. The diagnostic challenge is particularly difficult in a significant proportion of patients who have mixed features of CGH, migraine, tension-type headache or other headache forms.

A recent study may prove helpful however, in that it has revealed differences in headache profile between sufferers of relatively 'pure' CGH and 'pure' migraine.[6, 10] Migraine sufferers are more likely to be female, and more frequently report nausea, photophobia, phonophobia and throbbing pain. In addition, migraine headache onset is in the anterior head and is only infrequently brought on by mechanical provocative activity (such as sustained or awkward neck positioning), but is exacerbated by a change in spatial orientation (for example, standing up from lying or moving from forward bending to an upright position).[10]

At this stage, Norm appears to suffer from CGH. The diagnostic challenge is to differentiate CGH from migraine.[11] Norm's case history supports the CGH hypothesis as the patient is male, does not report photophobia or phonophobia, and does not describe throbbing pain. Moreover, his pain also starts in the posterior neck and spreads to his head and is brought on by physical activity and awkward head positioning, but not by a change in spatial orientation. Taken as a whole, the information obtained in the history supports the possible involvement of the cervical spine in Norm's headache pathogenesis. Physical tests are now required to test the CGH hypothesis and confirm the diagnosis.

2 Did you have any treatment hypotheses under consideration at this early stage? If so, what factors in the patient's history, based on your experience and the scientific evidence, support your treatment hypothesis?

Clinician's response

At this early stage, although there were factors in the history suggestive of a diagnosis of CGH, this was still not certain. The physical examination is needed to confirm the diagnosis. Furthermore, it is recognised that CGH may arise from dysfunction within the articular, neural and myofascial systems.[12] Hence any hypotheses regarding treatment would be very preliminary. However, Norm has provided some information that may be of assistance in identifying potential treatments. For example, he believed there was something wrong with his neck (although this notion might have

been conditioned by previous treating practitioners) and he was willing to undertake exercise to correct any dysfunction in this area. In addition, Norm had been receiving chiropractic treatment (neck manipulation) that had been of only short-term benefit. This might suggest an articular disorder secondary to poor motor control. Manipulation providing short-term improvement in headache and movement that is quickly lost may indicate poor functioning of the craniocervical muscles, but may also indicate the presence of other headache forms. Impairments in strength and endurance of the craniocervical muscles appear to be one of the defining features of CGH.[13] This is one aspect that has not been addressed by his previous therapy and might be a potential avenue for management. Certainly, according to Norm, no form of exercise had been prescribed in previous therapy.

PHYSICAL EXAMINATION

Posture

In standing, Norm had a 'sway back', with his pelvis located forwards in relation to the shoulder girdle. The thoracic spine was increased in kyphosis, and the head was displaced forward with a forward chin posture. The scapulae were protracted, depressed and medially rotated. In sitting, his pelvis was posteriorly tilted and he had a marked lumbar and thoracic spine kyphosis with forward chin posture. Manually correcting his pelvic posture in both sitting and standing improved his overall posture.

Active and passive physiological movements

In sitting, active cervical spine range of motion (ROM) was mildly restricted but not painful in right rotation and flexion. Extension was not limited in range but was poorly controlled, particularly upper cervical extension. Overpressure of right rotation reproduced mild pain on the right side of the neck in the same area as from which the headache symptoms usually originated. Isolating rotation above C2 by fixation of the C2 vertebra revealed a marked difference in passive movement between left and right rotation; right rotation was grossly restricted to only approximately 5° and Norm reported moderate pain during this movement. Similarly, active upper cervical flexion with the lower cervical spine maintained in a neutral position was also restricted to half the expected range and provoked mild upper neck pain on overpressure.

Neural tissue provocation tests

In view of the upper cervical spine restriction, screening tests for upper cervical neural tissue mechanosensitivity were carried out. This consisted of passive upper cervical flexion in long sitting, as well as passive upper cervical flexion with both shoulders abducted to 90° in supine lying.[14, 15] No difference in upper cervical flexion range was detected with the addition of either neural tissue sensitising manoeuvre so further testing for neural tissue mechanosensitivity was not pursued.

Passive segmental mobility tests

Passive physiological intervertebral motion testing revealed substantial right rotation hypomobility at the C1–C2 motion segment. Postero-anterior (PA) pressure applied on the right articular pillar at C2, and to a lesser extent C1, provoked neck pain and was significantly tender. With the cervical spine rotated 45° to the right, right-sided unilateral PA pressure on C2 was markedly more painful, but the response to pressure on the C1 vertebra was unchanged.

The flexion-rotation test was significantly restricted in right rotation (Figure 8.2) with much greater limitation than the cut-off value of 32° for a positive test for C1–C2 joint dysfunction.[16] In this test procedure the patient lies supine and the cervical spine is passively flexed to end of range. The therapist then rotates the head to the left and the right. Cervical flexion is thought to block movement at all levels apart from C1–C2, which due to its anatomy has the unique ability to rotate in any cervical posture. As movement at other cervical segments would be restricted by this end-range position, movement is isolated to the C1–C2 segment. Norm had an almost complete absence of right rotation in flexion, only 5°, with minimal limitation of left rotation. When this test was performed the neck was carefully maintained at end-range flexion to avoid a false-negative result.

Muscle function

There was evidence of poor postural control in sitting and standing. Furthermore, there was a notable prominence of the sternocleidomastoid muscles bilaterally. The control of cervical active movement into extension was poor, with most movement occurring in the

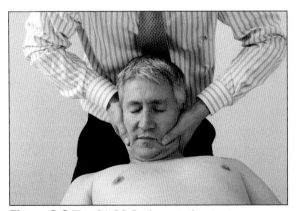

Figure 8.2 The C1-C2 flexion-rotation test

high cervical spine region. The sub-occipital muscles were tight on palpation and muscle length testing. Testing craniocervical flexion for function of the deep neck flexors revealed significant dysfunction, with marked inability to flex the high cervical spine without overactivity of the sternocleidomastoid muscles.[13] Norm could only flex the upper cervical spine by a few degrees and hold this position for 5 seconds without superficial neck muscle activity. In addition to the neck muscle dysfunction there was evidence of poor scapular control.

Other tests

There was no evidence of vertebrobasilar insufficiency and all other tests were negative.

EVIDENCE-INFORMED CLINICAL REASONING

1 After the physical examination, was your hypothesis of CGH confirmed? What clinical findings were most relevant in coming to this decision?

Clinician's response

The majority of headache forms are not directly relevant to the manual therapist, other than in differential diagnosis for exclusion. As each form of headache has a different pathological basis, incorrect differential diagnosis will most likely lead to treatment failure. This is of particular importance for manual therapy interventions as they are unlikely to be effective for the majority of headache forms. It should also be noted that different forms of headache may co-exist[17], presenting a greater challenge for differential diagnosis and management.

Characteristics of CGH according to the Cervicogenic Headache International Study Group[8, 18] are shown in Table 8.1. Vincent and Luna[19] examined the validity of these diagnostic criteria in patients with a mix of headache forms. Patients with CGH met significantly more criteria than tension-type headache or migraine. However, 30% of patients with CGH met the IHS criteria for migraine, whereas only 3% of patients with CGH met the criteria for tension-type headache, while the remaining two-thirds of patients could not be classified. Antonaci et al[11] reported that at least five of the Cervicogenic Headache International Study Group diagnostic criteria must be present in order to establish a diagnosis of CGH. Furthermore, Vincent[20] has shown that if all criteria are present, then CGH can be distinguished from migraine and tension-type headache with a high level of sensitivity and a moderate level of specificity.

Norm presented with generally poor spinal posture. The link between forward head posture and disorders of the cervical spine remains controversial.[21] Some studies have found a significant relationship[22–24]

Table 8.1 Cervicogenic Headache International Study Group diagnostic criteria for cervicogenic headache[8]

Major criteria	I. Symptoms and signs of neck involvement
	  (a) precipitation of comparable symptoms by:
	    (1) neck movement and/or sustained, awkward head positioning, and/or
	    (2) external pressure over the upper cervical or occipital region
	  (b) restriction of range of motion in the neck
	  (c) ipsilateral neck, shoulder or arm pain.
	II. Confirmatory evidence by diagnostic anaesthetic block
	III. Unilaterality of the head pain, without side shift

Head pain characteristics	IV. Moderate–severe, non-throbbing pain, usually starting in the neck (a) episodes of varying duration, or fluctuating, continuous pain.

Other characteristics of some importance	V. Only marginal or lack of effect of indomethacin
	  (a) only marginal or lack of effect of ergotamine and sumatriptan
	  (b) female gender
	  (c) not infrequent history of head or indirect neck trauma, usually of more than medium severity.

Other features of lesser importance	VI. Various attack-related phenomena, only occasionally present, and/or moderately expressed when present
	  (a) nausea
	  (b) phonophobia and photophobia
	  (c) dizziness
	  (d) ipsilateral 'blurred vision'
	  (e) difficulty swallowing
	  (f) ipsilateral oedema, mostly in the periocular area.

while others have not.[15, 25–27] Nevertheless forward head posture may indicate an abnormality of the upper cervical spine region involving a disturbance of control of the deep neck flexor muscles, as well as articular or neural dysfunction, hence further examination is required.

Restricted ROM of the neck is considered one of the key diagnostic criteria for CGH.[18] Some[15, 28, 29] but not all[25, 30] studies have reported diminished cervical ROM in patients with CGH, with limitation of active movement in the sagittal plane, in particular extension, as the major loss. In Norm's case, there was limitation of cervical movement in flexion and rotation, in particular right rotation of the upper cervical spine region, consistent with the criteria for CGH as proposed by the Cervicogenic Headache International Study Group.[8]

CGH is thought to arise primarily from dysfunction in the upper three cervical segments.[31] Zito et al[15] report that the presence of upper cervical joint dysfunction determined by manual examination is the most crucial criteria for the identification of patients with CGH. More recently Jull et al[28] condensed the manual examination for CGH to include only tests of palpation. Identification of a pain response, rather than joint hypermobility or hypo-mobility, simplifies the identification of cervical dysfunction and reduces the skill required. However, this information on its own is not sufficient to provide adequate sensitivity and specificity to identify CGH; other forms of assessment are required.[28] In Norm's case there was evidence on manual examination of upper cervical joint dysfunction with significant pain provocation on palpating the C2 vertebra.

The flexion-rotation test (Figure 8.2), is a simplified form of manual examination used within the Mulligan Concept to identify patients with C1–C2 joint dysfunction and CGH.[32] Range of rotation during the flexion-rotation test is normally 40–44° to each side.[30, 33] In contrast, patients with C1–C2 joint dysfunction have significantly less movement,[16, 30, 34, 35] and a range limited to 32° or less may be considered positive.[16] Using this test highly trained manual therapists have high sensitivity (91%) and specificity (90%) in differentiating patients with CGH from asymptomatic controls or patients with migraine with aura.[34]

Similar values (diagnostic accuracy = 89%, kappa = 0.85, positive cut-off value = 33°) have been reported when the flexion-rotation test was evaluated in a more heterogenous sample, including patients with CGH arising from levels other than C1–C2.[35] Although inexperienced examiners record a larger range of motion for the flexion-rotation test, the sensitivity (>83%), specificity (>83%) and agreement (kappa >0.67) are still acceptable. Another advantage of the flexion-rotation test is that it is independent of other factors including sleeping posture, age, gender, and hand-dominant recreation or occupation (activity involving repetitive use of one side of the body).[36] Consequently the test has utility regardless of the age, gender or lifestyle of the patient.

The restriction of rotation in the flexion-rotation test observed in Norm's case was greater than the results reported in published studies. The range of rotation was only 5° toward the restricted side, much less than the mean values of 28° reported by Hall and Robinson,[30] and 20° reported by Ogince et al.[37] Norm's range is also markedly restricted compared to the range available in patients without headache, reported as approximately 44° in each direction.[30, 38] This range is similar to the 40° recorded in patients with migraine headache.[37] While it would have been ideal to provoke the headache during the assessment to corroborate the cervical spine origin of the headache symptoms, unfortunately as is common in clinical evaluation of headache, this was not possible.

When considering Norm's case it is apparent that all the Cervicogenic Headache International Study Group criteria for CGH are fulfilled except for confirmatory evidence by diagnostic anaesthetic block. Such procedures are more suited to headache research rather than general clinical practice. Furthermore, Jull et al[28] demonstrated that collectively restricted neck movement in association with pain on palpation of the upper cervical joints and impairment in the deep neck flexors as identified by the craniocervical flexion test, had 100% sensitivity and 94% specificity in identifying CGH. On this basis, Norm's headaches appear to be almost purely cervicogenic in nature, with no features of either migraine or tension-type headache.

2 What were your primary hypotheses with respect to treatment and management? Was the Mulligan Concept indicated and, if so, why?

Clinician's response

The disorder was chronic, static and had not been helped by a range of previous interventions given by the patient's medical practitioner, neurologist and other health professionals. This might be partly due to the incorrect diagnosis of migraine. Being able to strictly classify the disorder as a relatively 'pure' CGH form suggests it is likely that an appropriate manual therapy intervention, targeting the specific dysfunctions, may be effective. Previous studies support the use of manual therapy for CGH[39, 40] but not for migraine or other headache forms.[41] The working hypothesis was a chronic but stable C1–C2 movement impairment associated with poor craniocervical muscle function. Due to the chronic nature of the CGH symptoms, the relative isolation of the segmental dysfunction to C1–C2, the gross limitation of motion on the flexion-rotation test, and the pattern of short-term relief with manipulations but with a poor long-term response to treatment in the past, a Mulligan C1–C2 rotation self-SNAG was determined to be the treatment technique of choice in the first instance. This technique was chosen because it provides a powerful mobilisation of the C1–C2 segment that can be easily performed outside the clinic as a self-mobilisation procedure, hence ensuring an adequate volume of MWM treatment. Self-treatment appears to be the missing aspect of previous intervention. Manipulation failed to give long-term relief. One reason for this may have been inadequate follow-up or

insufficient volume of treatment, which a self-mobilisation can provide. Patients with similar headache characteristics and examination findings have been shown to respond very favourably to this Mulligan mobilisation including self-treatment with good short-term and long-term effects (see Chapter 3).[42]

The presence of craniocervical muscle dysfunction suggests that the long-term management should also incorporate interventions to improve deep neck flexor function. A randomised controlled trial of physical therapies for CGH of high methodological quality has shown that a combination of exercise to re-educate cervical and axio-scapular muscle function, together with manual therapy for articular dysfunction, provides an optimal outcome in the long term.[39]

TREATMENT AND MANAGEMENT

Treatment 1

The C1–C2 self-SNAG[40] was selected for treatment on the first visit. This technique can be used in the clinic and is also suitable as a self-treatment (see Table 8.2 for details of application). This is potentially an aggressive mobilisation technique, so it is important to follow the guidelines carefully. With Norm, a self-SNAG was first performed in the direction of right rotation only twice; the direction of mobilisation being determined by the flexion-rotation test. The immediate effect of the self-SNAG was a gain in range of active rotation in sitting, so that rotation was now full range and symmetrical to the left and right. Furthermore, on reassessing the flexion-rotation test, right rotation had improved to approximately half the normal range. Clinically it is not uncommon to gain full range of active rotation motion but still find a marked reduction in the range of the flexion-rotation test. While changes in measures of physical impairment have been shown to be less responsive than pain and disability measures in the overall outcome of low back pain,[43] intra-session changes in pain and ROM have been shown to predict a positive outcome to manual therapy.[44]

Norm was instructed to do two repetitions of the self-SNAG, twice each day with a cervical self-SNAG strap (Figure 8.3). He was asked to keep a note of any change in his headache symptoms over the ensuing 3-day period. On this occasion it was decided not to add any other form of intervention, so that the effect of the home exercise could be determined. The patient was, however, advised to avoid prone sleeping, which he had not been previously advised.

Treatment 2

Norm returned for re-evaluation and treatment 3 days later. He reported a mild headache in the evening after the first treatment session. Norm had also had a headache the next day, which was not quite as severe and did not last as long as it normally might have done.

Table 8.2	Rotation SNAG for loss of rotation at C1–C2	
Indication	**Cervicogenic headache or neck pain together with loss of movement at C1–C2 demonstrated on the flexion-rotation test**	
Positioning	Patient	Patient sitting in a chair with their torso supported against the back of the chair. A cervical self-SNAG strap is placed around the posterior aspect of the patient's neck. Each of the two handles of the strap are held, one in each hand, by the patient. The upper end of the strap, which is held by the hand that is contralateral to the side of headache, is wrapped around the C1 segment and the other end is held across the patient's chest.
	Treated body part	Cervical spine in neutral position.
	Therapist	The therapist: (a) stands behind the patient; (b) maintains the strap in position with gentle finger pressure until the movement commences; and (c) also ensures that the strap is maintained at the correct angle so that the patient applies the force, with the strap, in the correct direction.
	Therapist's hands	As the patient essentially applies the technique as a self-treatment, the therapist's hands are used only to assist the patient in keeping the strap at the correct angle and in the correct position. Once the patient learns how to apply the self-treatment safely and correctly, the patient is advised to use the technique at home.
Application guidelines	• Ensure that firm and not excessive force is applied through the self-SNAG strap. Excessive force may cause discomfort or pain in the patient's neck. • The force generated through the self-SNAG strap must be directed along the facet joint plane, which in the high cervical spine is in a horizontal direction with the neck in neutral. To ensure the correct application of the gliding force, the patient should ensure that the upper end of the strap is always maintained horizontally, placed no higher than the zygomatic arch. • Once the correct set-up of the technique is achieved, the patient applies a firm force directly forwards with the upper end of the strap, maintaining a counter force with the lower end of the strap across the chest. • No pain or other symptoms should be experienced at any stage of the technique. Should the patient experience any pain or other symptoms the technique should be stopped and modified. • Maintaining a horizontal force with the strap, the patient slowly rotates the head in the painful and/or limited direction. As this is done, the patient keeps the upper end of the strap directly in front of the face. • If the technique is indicated, the patient will be able to achieve full range active rotation in the problematic direction without pain. • If pain or other symptoms are experienced, the technique is temporarily ceased so that the therapist can ensure that the direction of the force application is horizontal and that the cervical spine is in the neutral position in the sagittal plane. Modifications can then be made as necessary so that the technique is rendered pain-free. • If pain persists, even after modifications are considered, the technique should not be used. • Repeat the movement twice only, once pain-free movement is achieved. • If full range and pain-free active rotation can be achieved by the patient, the therapist then applies gentle, passive, rotation overpressure to the patient for 1–2 seconds. This should also be pain-free. • Subsequent reassessment should reveal a significant improvement in pain-free ROM. • If after the initial application there is improvement in the range of movement and a reduction in pain, the patient is advised to use the technique as a home treatment. • The patient should apply two repetitions of the self-SNAG, twice per day.	
Comments	• Be careful to ensure that the force is applied correctly with the strap. • Maintain the force with the strap throughout the entire rotation movement until the patient actively returns to the starting position. • It is important to encourage the patient to achieve the maximum end-range position.	

On physical examination, the range of active movement in rotation was symmetrical to the left and right and overpressure to right rotation was no longer painful. Active upper cervical flexion had also improved to full range and was no longer painful on overpressure. In sitting with the C2 vertebra fixed, range of rotation to the right had increased to approximately 10°. The flexion-rotation test was now showing approximately 30° rotation to the right. At first glance these results might seem inconsistent, but based on clinical observation the normal range for the sitting C1–C2 rotation test is 15–20°. Hence both tests for C1–C2 rotation showed more than half range but still some limitation. Re-testing the deep neck flexors demonstrated some improved function. Norm was able to flex his neck by 5° and hold a steady position without superficial muscle activity for 3 sets of 10 seconds. This improvement might be partly explained by the increase in the available range of upper cervical flexion and resultant increase in extensibility of the sub-occipital muscles following the mobilisation of the hypomobile C1–C2 segment.

In view of the positive sustained response to the first treatment session the C1–C2 self-SNAG was repeated.

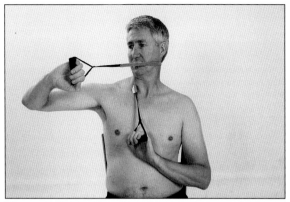

Figure 8.3 C1–C2 self-SNAG technique using a cervical self-SNAG strap

In addition, a re-education program for the deep neck flexor muscles was commenced. Norm was taught to perform upper cervical flexion, without over-activation of the superficial neck flexor muscles. He could only initiate a very small upper cervical flexion movement using this method, so he was instructed to carry out this low level of activation for five repetitions each held for 10 seconds, twice per day. At the end of the session the flexion-rotation test was only mildly restricted, with right rotation now 40°. In view of the intermittent nature of the headache, a follow-up session was scheduled for 1 week so as to clearly determine any change in headache frequency.

Treatment 3

Norm reported a significant reduction in his headache symptoms. He had experienced just one headache over the preceding week and this had been present for only 3 hours. He had been on half-term break from his students, which meant less time at the whiteboard but more time on the computer. The one episode of headache had started after sitting in front of the computer for 4 hours.

The flexion-rotation test was still mildly restricted at 40° of right rotation and had not changed since the previous session. On examining Norm's self-mobilisation it became apparent that he was not engaging another person (practitioner in clinic or wife at home) in assisting him with overpressure as he had been instructed at the first session. The C1–C2 self-SNAG was then repeated with overpressure and full range of right rotation during the flexion-rotation test was subsequently achieved. Norm was strongly encouraged to ask his wife to apply rotation overpressure during the C1–C2 self-SNAG as this was demonstrably a very important part of the technique.

Deep neck flexor muscle function was also improved. Norm could now achieve approximately half the normal range of upper cervical flexion without overactivity

of the sternocleidomastoid muscles. Deep neck flexor exercises were progressed in range. The number of repetitions was also to be gradually ramped up every second day until 10 repetitions were being performed at a time. In addition, postural re-education for the scapulae and spine was commenced.

Treatment 4

Two weeks later Norm reported further improvement. Headache frequency was approximately once per week but the headache was much less severe (2/10) and only lasted about 3 hours, even though he continued to use the whiteboard at work.

On physical examination, right rotation during the flexion-rotation test was now full range at approximately 45° and without pain. Deep neck flexor muscle function had also improved and the patient was able to hold at half the range of upper cervical flexion without over-activity of the sternocleidomastoid muscles for 10 seconds and repeat this 10 times.

In view of the significant improvement in headache symptoms Norm was instructed to continue with his current exercise program. The C1–C2 self-SNAG was to be carried out only once each day to maintain mobility. Deep neck flexor exercises were to be gradually progressed, gaining in range of upper cervical flexion. Furthermore, an exercise to improve cervical extension dynamic control was also commenced. This was to improve his control of upper cervical extension when writing on a whiteboard.

Treatment 5

Four weeks later Norm reported he had not experienced any headaches in the previous 2 weeks. He had continued to exercise as instructed. On reassessment, the cervical flexion-rotation test was full range and pain-free. Deep neck flexor muscle function was good at three-quarters of the range of upper cervical spine flexion. Postural control and deep neck flexor exercises were progressed.

In light of the evident substantial improvements the patient was discharged. Norm was contacted by telephone 4 months later, and he reported only mild headache approximately once per month which appeared to coincide with sustained work on the computer. Reassessment of the HDI revealed an improvement of 44 points, which is greater than that required to detect a true change in headache impact.[2]

AUTHORS' MWM COMMENTARY

A C1–C2 rotation self-SNAG was successful in the management of this particular case of CGH. Pain, ROM and physical disability all improved as a direct result of the intervention used.

The self-SNAG technique used to treat Norm has been shown to be effective in the management of CGH where a positive finding on the flexion-rotation test is the primary inclusion criteria.[45] In that study, 32 patients with CGH who were all positive on the flexion-rotation test, were treated either with the C1–C2 rotation self-SNAG or a placebo exercise. Both exercises were carried out twice each day. Follow-up assessment of headache symptoms, based on headache frequency, intensity and duration,[46] was carried out at 4 weeks and again at one year. Range of movement during the flexion-rotation test increased by 15° on the first day for the C1–C2 self-SNAG group (p < 0.001). This was significantly more than the 5° increase recorded for the placebo exercise group (p < 0.001) and is greater than the reported 6° minimal detectable change required for this test.[47] In addition, headache index scores were substantially less in the self-SNAG group compared to the placebo exercise group at 4 weeks (p<0.001) and 12 months (p<0.001), with an overall reduction of 54% for the self-SNAG group. While in Norm's case there was a more dramatic improvement in headache symptoms, this might, in part, be explained by the addition of exercises to improve motor control dysfunction. Motor control dysfunction is a significant factor for patients with CGH.[28] Furthermore, it has been shown that exercises designed to improve motor control have significant positive benefits for patients with CGH.[41] Indeed, a combination of motor control retraining and manual therapy has been shown to produce a 10% better response in long-term patient outcomes than when these interventions are used in isolation.[41]

This case illustrates that a simple pain-free mobilisation technique can have positive benefits in reduction of pain and disability in a patient with CGH. A number of studies have shown manual therapy to be effective in the management of CGH,[41, 48–52] but this is the first case to illustrate the use of a SNAG technique in conjunction with motor control exercises. The present case has demonstrated an effective self-management program for CGH requiring minimal therapist assistance. In a cost-driven society, self-management must be seen as a desirable goal and this case provides an example in this respect.

Possible mechanisms by which the C1–C2 rotation self-SNAG may have reduced headache symptoms are covered in other chapters (e.g. Chapters 4–7). Mobilisation is known to cause alteration in the resting excitability of the motor neuron pool in the spinal cord (producing facilitatory and inhibitory effects).[53] Muscle tone changes at the C1–C2 segment may explain the lack of rotation range during the flexion-rotation test and the subsequent rapid response to mobilisation using the C1–C2 self-SNAG.

Perhaps a less plausible explanation for the increase in cervical rotation range on the flexion-rotation test is that the C1–C2 self-SNAG decreased joint stiffness. Mobilisation is thought to break down adhesions in some instances and stretch surrounding tissues. That the improvement in rotation range was immediate, with subsequent further progression occurring more gradually, suggests that the effect of the C1–C2 self-SNAG technique is principally related to a neurophysiological change in pain modulation and segmental muscle tone, with perhaps minor effects on joint stiffness. Additional proposed mechanical effects of this mobilisation technique include changing minor bony positional faults of the vertebra,[42] correcting mal-tracking problems[54–56] and changes to the axes of motion of the functional spinal unit.[57] It is not known which if any of these proposed effects are the basis for the improvements seen with the C1–C2 self-SNAG, as no studies have yet investigated this specifically. Clearly studies are required to specifically identify the mechanisms of action for the C1–C2 self-SNAG.

References

1 Jacobson GP, Ramadan NM, Aggarwal SK, Newman CW. The Henry Ford Hospital Headache Disability Inventory (HDI). Neurology. 1994 May;44(5):837–42.

2 Jacobson GP, Ramadan NM, Norris L, Newman CW. Headache disability inventory (HDI): short-term test-retest reliability and spouse perceptions. Headache. 1995 Oct;35(9):534–9.

3 Bronfort G, Nilsson N, Haas M, Evans R, Goldsmith CH, Assendelft WJ, et al. Non-invasive physical treatments for chronic/recurrent headache. Cochrane Database Syst Rev. 2004(3):CD001878.

4 International Headache Society. The International Classification of Headache Disorders (2nd edn). Cephalalgia. 2004;24 Suppl 1:9–160.

5 Nilsson N. The prevalence of cervicogenic headache in a random population sample of 20–59 year olds. Spine. 1995;20:1884–8.

6 Sjaastad O, Bakketeig LS. Prevalence of cervicogenic headache: Vaga study of headache epidemiology. Acta Neurologica Scandinavica. 2007 Nov 20.

7 Pfaffenrath V, Kaube H. Diagnostics of cervicogenic headache. Functional Neurology. 1990 Apr–Jun;5(2):159–64.

8 Sjaastad O, Fredriksen TA, Pfaffenrath V. Cervicogenic headache: diagnostic criteria. The Cervicogenic Headache International Study Group. Headache. 1998 Jun;38(6):442–5.

9 Nicholson GG, Gaston J. Cervical headache. Journal of Orthopaedic & Sports Physical Therapy. 2001 Apr;31(4):184–93.

10 Sjaastad O, Bakketeig LS. Migraine without aura: comparison with cervicogenic headache. Vaga study of headache epidemiology. Acta Neurologica Scandinavica. 2007 Nov 20.

11 Antonaci F, Ghirmai S, Bono G, Sandrini G, Nappi G. Cervicogenic headache: evaluation of the original diagnostic criteria. Cephalalgia. 2001 Jun;21(5):573–83.

12 Hall TM, Briffa K, Hopper D. Clinical evaluation of cervicogenic headache. Journal of Manual and Manipulative Therapy. 2008;16(2):73–80.

13 Jull G, Barrett C, Magee R, Ho P. Further clinical clarification of the muscle dysfunction in cervical headache. Cephalalgia. 1999 Apr;19(3):179–85.

14 Hall TM, Elvey RL. Management of mechanosensitivity of the nervous system in spinal pain syndromes. In: Boyling G, Jull G (eds) Grieves Modern Manual Therapy (3rd edn). Edinburgh: Churchill Livingstone 2005:413–31.

15 Zito G, Jull G, Story I. Clinical tests of musculoskeletal dysfunction in the diagnosis of cervicogenic headache. Manual Therapy. 2006;11(2):118–29.

16 Ogince M, Hall T, Robinson K, Blackmore AM. The diagnostic validity of the cervical flexion-rotation test in C1/2-related cervicogenic headache. Manual Therapy. 2007 Aug;12(3):256–62.

17 Fishbain DA, Cutler R, Cole B, Rosomoff HL, Rosomoff RS. International Headache Society headache diagnostic patterns in pain facility patients. Clinical Journal of Pain. 2001 Mar;17(1):78–93.

18 Sjaastad O, Fredriksen TA, Pfaffenrath V. Cervicogenic headache: diagnostic criteria. Headache. 1990 Nov;30(11):725–6.

19 Vincent MB, Luna RA. Cervicogenic headache: a comparison with migraine and tension-type headache. Cephalalgia. 1999 Dec;19 Suppl 25:11–6.

20 Vincent M. Validation of criteria for cervicogenic headache. Functional Neurology. 1998 Jan–Mar;13(1):74–5.

21 Jull G, Niere K. The cervical spine and headache. In: Boyling G, Jull G (eds). Grieves Modern Manual Therapy (3rd edn). Edinburgh: Churchill Livingstone 2005:291–309.

22 Griegel-Morris P, Larson K, Mueller-Klaus K, Oatis CA. Incidence of common postural abnormalities in the cervical, shoulder, and thoracic regions and their association with pain in two age groups of healthy subjects. Physical Therapy. 1992 Jun;72(6):425–31.

23 Watson D, Trott P. Cervical headache: an investigation of natural head posture and upper cervical flexor muscle performance. Cephalalgia. 1993:2782–284.

24 Yip CH, Chiu TT, Poon AT. The relationship between head posture and severity and disability of patients with neck pain. Manual Therapy. 2007 Mar 14.

25 Dumas JP, Arsenault AB, Boudreau G, Magnoux E, Lepage Y, Bellavance A, et al. Physical impairments in cervicogenic headache: traumatic vs. nontraumatic onset. Cephalalgia. 2001 Nov;21(9):884–93.

26 Hanten WP, Olson SL, Russell JL, Lucio RM, Campbell AH. Total head excursion and resting head posture: normal and patient comparisons. Archives of Physical Medicine and Rehabilitation. 2000 Jan;81(1):62–6.

27 Treleaven J, Jull G, Atkinson L. Cervical musculoskeletal dysfunction in post-concussional headache. Cephalalgia. 1994 Aug;14(4):273–9; discussion 57.

28 Jull G, Amiri M, Bullock-Saxton J, Darnell R, Lander C. Cervical musculoskeletal impairment in frequent intermittent headache. Part 1: Subjects with single headaches. Cephalalgia. 2007 Jul;27(7):793–802.

29 Zwart JA. Neck mobility in different headache disorders. Headache. 1997 Jan;37(1):6–11.

30 Hall T, Robinson K. The flexion-rotation test and active cervical mobility — a comparative measurement study in cervicogenic headache. Manual Therapy. 2004 Nov;9(4):197–202.

31 Bogduk N. Headache and the neck. In: Goadsby P, Silberstein S (eds). Headache (17th edn). Melbourne: Butterworth-Heinemann 1997:369–81.

32 Dvorak J, Herdmann J, Janssen B, Theiler R, Grob D. Motor-evoked potentials in patients with cervical spine disorders. Spine. 1990 Oct;15(10):1013–6.

33 Amiri M, Jull G, Bullock-Saxton J. Measuring range of active cervical rotation in a position of full head flexion using the 3D Fastrak measurement system: an intra-tester reliability study. Manual Therapy. 2003;8(3): 176–9.

34 Ogince M, Hall T, Robinson K. The diagnostic validity of the cervical flexion-rotation test in C1/2 related cervicogenic headache. Manual Therapy. 2007;12:256–62.

35 Hall T, Robinson K, Fujinawa O, Kiyokazu A. Inter-tester reliability and diagnostic validity of the cervical flexion-rotation test in cervicogenic headache. Journal of Manipulative & Physiological Therapeutics. 2008;31:293–300.

36 Smith K, Hall T, Robinson K. The influence of age, gender, lifestyle factors and sub-clinical neck pain on cervical range of motion. Manual Therapy. 2008; 13:552–9.

37 Ogince M, Hall T, Robinson K. The diagnostic validity of the cervical flexion-rotation test in C1/2 related cervicogenic headache. Manual Therapy. 2007;12(3):256–62.

38 Dvorak J, Antinnes JA, Panjabi M, Loustalot D, Bonomo M. Age and gender related normal motion of the cervical spine. Spine. 1992 Oct;17 Suppl 10:S393–8.

39 Jull G, Trott P, Potter H, Zito G, Niere K, Shirley D, et al. A randomized controlled trial of exercise and manipulative therapy for cervicogenic headache. Spine. 2002;27(17):1835–43.

40 Mulligan BR. Manual Therapy: 'NAGS', 'SNAGS', 'MWMS' etc. (5th edn). Wellington, New Zealand: Plane View Services 2004.

41 Bronfort G, Haas M, Evans RL, Bouter LM. Efficacy of spinal manipulation and mobilization for low back pain and neck pain: a systematic review and best evidence synthesis. Spine. 2004;4(3):335–56.

42 Hall T, Ho Tak Chan B, Christensen L, Odenthal B, Wells C, Robinson K. Efficacy of a C1/2 self-SNAG (sustained natural apophyseal glide) in the management of cervicogenic headache. Journal of Orthopaedic & Sports Physical Therapy. 2007;37(3):100–7.

43 Pengel LH, Refshauge KM, Maher CG. Responsiveness of pain, disability, and physical impairment outcomes in patients with low back pain. Spine. 2004 Apr 15;29(8):879–83.

44 Tuttle N. Do changes within a manual therapy treatment session predict between-session changes for patients with cervical spine pain? Australian Journal of Physiotherapy. 2005;51(1):43–8.

45 Hall TM, Chan H, Christensen L, Odenthal B, Wells C, Robinson K. Efficacy of a C1-2 Self-sustained natural apophyseal glide (SNAG) in the management of cervicogenic headache. Journal of Orthopaedic and Sports Physical Therapy. 2007;37(3):100–7.

46 Niere K, Robinson P. Determination of manipulative physiotherapy treatment outcome in headache patients. Manual Therapy. 1997;2(4):199–205.

47 Hall TM, Briffa K, Hopper D, Robinson KW. Intratester reliability and minimal detectable change of the cervical flexion-rotation test. Journal of Orthopadic & Sports Physical Therapy. 2010;40(4):225–9.

48 Jensen O, Nielsen F, Vosmar L. An open study comparing manual therapy with the use of cold packs in the treatment of post concussional headache. Cephalalgia. 1990;10:241–9.

49 Li C, Zhang XL, Ding H, Tao YQ, Zhan HS. Comparative study on effects of manipulation treatment and transcutaneous electrical nerve stimulation on patients with cervicogenic headache. Zhong Xi Yi Jie He Xue Bao. 2007 Jul;5(4):403–6.

50 Nilsson N, Christensen H, Hartvigsen J. The effect of spinal manipulation in the treatment of cervicogenic headache. Journal of Manipulative & Physiological Therapeutics. 1997;20(5):326–30.

51 Schoensee H, Jensen G, Nicholson G, Gossman M, Katholi C. The effect of mobilisation on cervical headaches. Journal of Orthopaedic and Sports Physical Therapy. 1995;21:181–96.

52 Whorton R, Kegerreis S. The use of manual therapy and exercise in the treatment of chronic cervicogenic headache. Journal of Manual & Manipulative Therapy. 2000;8:193–203.

53 Dishman JD, Ball KA, Burke J. First Prize: Central motor excitability changes after spinal manipulation: a transcranial magnetic stimulation study. Journal of Manipulative & Physiological Therapeutics. 2002 Jan;25(1):1–9.

54 Mulligan B. Extremity joint mobilisations combined with movements. The New Zealand Journal of Physiotherapy. 1992;20:28–9.

55 Petty N, Moore A. Neuromusculoskeletal Examination and Assessment: A Handbook for Therapists. London: Churchill Livingstone 1998.

56 Wilson E. Mobilisation with movement and adverse neural tension: an exploration of possible links. Manipulative Physiotherapist. 1995;27:40–6.

57 Hearn A, Rivett D. Cervical SNAGS: a biomechanical analysis. Manual Therapy. 2002;7(2):71–9.

Chapter 9
A diagnostic dilemma of dizziness

Sue Reid and Darren Rivett

HISTORY

Howard was referred for physiotherapy assessment and treatment by a neurologist whom he had consulted about his longstanding dizziness. Howard is a 71-year-old retired store manager whose hobby is topiary hedging. Besides caring for his own garden, he also maintains his next-door neighbour's extensive garden and two other formal gardens in his neighbourhood for a small fee. He is also a keen swimmer but has not been able to swim for about 18 months because of his dizziness. Howard's wife passed away about 6 years ago and their adult son lives with him.

Symptoms

Currently Howard suffers from daily episodes of dizziness that are usually of moderate intensity. He describes his dizziness as feeling unsteady or having poor balance. Although he hasn't had a fall, he often feels that he might. On questioning, Howard stated the dizziness was never a spinning sensation and he did not get it rolling over in bed, but he did feel nauseous when the dizziness was more marked. He also complained of generalised neck stiffness, postero–superior neck pain, and an intermittent dull occipital headache (Figure 9.1). Howard often felt fullness in his right ear, sometimes experienced tinnitus, and had a feeling of sinus fullness which was worse on the right side of his face. There was no pain or other symptoms reported in the upper limbs, thoracic or lumbar spinal areas, nor any other symptoms suggestive of vertebrobasilar insufficiency (VBI).

Self-report measures

Howard was asked to complete three self-report forms. The first was the Dizziness Handicap Inventory (DHI) which assesses the impact of dizziness on the functional, emotional and physical aspects of everyday life.[1] The highest possible score is 100, indicating maximum self-perceived handicap. On assessment Howard's score was 34, indicating a moderate handicap.[2] The second was a visual analogue scale (VAS) for dizziness consisting of a 10 cm line anchored at one end with the words 'no dizziness' and at the other end with 'worst dizziness imaginable'; he rated it as

5.2 out of 10. The final self-report measure was a VAS for neck pain and headache consisting of a 10 cm line anchored at one end with the words 'no pain' and at the other end with 'worse pain imaginable'; he rated it as 3.4 out of 10. Both ratings were an average level over the previous few days.

Symptom behaviour

The main activity to bring on Howard's dizziness was hanging the washing out to dry on a clothesline. If he looked up at the clothesline he lost balance and 'did an Irish jig'. He usually pegged the clothes by feeling the line and avoided looking up. Howard also experienced unsteadiness if he looked up while hedging a topiary tree. Furthermore, he was no longer able to change light bulbs and had to ask his son to do that as he was now wary of looking up and avoided ladders. Similarly, if he went to buy groceries he could not get things off the top shelf and had to ask someone to do that for him. Over the last year, Howard noticed it was becoming more difficult to reverse the car. His dizziness had become worse in the last 6 months and he was now feeling anxious when driving even short distances. It had reached the point where he didn't like to drive to the shops unless his son came with him. Relief from the dizziness and pain was obtained by lying still in a facedown position with the neck in neutral or on his back with his neck propped up on two pillows. There was no particular pattern to his symptoms over the course of the day, with the behaviour of symptoms simply related to activities.

Current history

Howard had been having physiotherapy treatment consisting of ultrasound and laser modalities for several months, but had not obtained any relief. He had not had manual therapy. The referring neurologist had eliminated central nervous system, cardiac, vestibular and psychiatric causes for Howard's dizziness. His assessment involved taking a history, followed by a physical examination that included tests for vestibulo-spinal function, the vestibulo-ocular system and disequilibrium, such as gait and balance testing, eye movement tests, Dix-Hallpike manoeuvre and caloric testing (caloric testing assesses whether the vestibular system

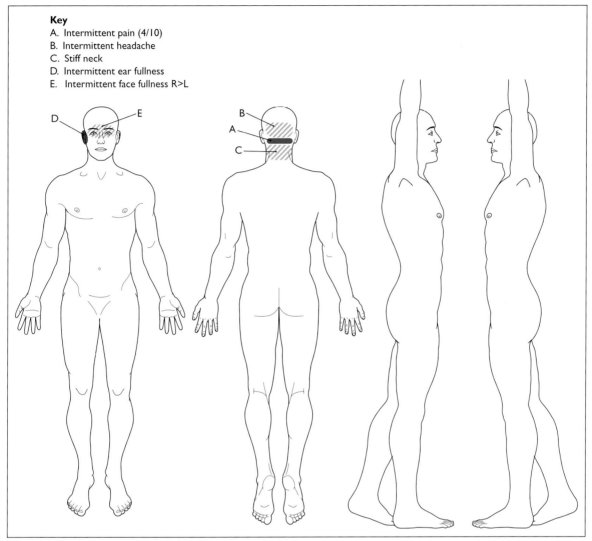

Key
A. Intermittent pain (4/10)
B. Intermittent headache
C. Stiff neck
D. Intermittent ear fullness
E. Intermittent face fullness R>L

Figure 9.1 Body chart depicting areas of patient's symptoms

is functioning normally; the inner ears are stimulated with warm and cold water and the eyes monitored for nystagmus). Because these tests were all normal and Howard had a stiff and painful neck, with movement of the same provoking his dizziness, the neurologist considered his dizziness was of cervical spine origin and referred him for manual therapy.

Previous history

Howard first noticed his dizziness about 3 years earlier after his usual Sunday morning swimming session. When he swims freestyle he breathes to the right. Around this time, he had also taken a night job packing grocery shelves. He found putting goods on the higher shelves was particularly difficult and produced some dizziness.

Howard had a motor vehicle accident 40 years ago, which resulted in a whiplash injury. He had experienced

episodes of neck pain and stiffness since the accident. X-rays showed some degenerative changes of the upper cervical spine (Figure 9.2). Howard's general health had been good and he was not taking any medication.

EVIDENCE-INFORMED CLINICAL REASONING

1 What were your initial thoughts regarding the cause of Howard's dizziness? What findings in the history tended to support or refute your hypothesis?

Clinician's response

Cervicogenic dizziness is dizziness described as a feeling of imbalance or disequilibrium (rather than a spinning sensation or vertigo), which is usually

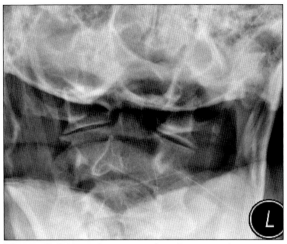

Figure 9.2 X-ray demonstrating degenerative changes in the upper cervical spine

brought on by neck positioning or movement.[3–6] It usually occurs in conjunction with cervical pain, stiffness or headache. There are several features in Howard's history consistent with a cervical spine cause for his dizziness, based both on the available research and clinical experience. Firstly, the dizziness was described as 'poor balance' and not a spinning sensation (that would suggest vertigo, which is usually due to a problem with the vestibular system). Secondly, he answered in the negative when questioned about experiencing dizziness when rolling over in bed. This is usually provocative for benign paroxysmal positional vertigo (BPPV), a common disorder of the inner ear.[6] In addition, the dizziness had been daily in frequency over 2–3 years, whereas BPPV tends to be episodic. Thirdly, the dizziness was accompanied by a stiff and painful neck. Finally, the initial onset of dizziness was after activities that involved cervical spine extension (packing high supermarket shelves) and right rotation (freestyle swimming). Similarly, current provocative activities involved cervical spine extension movements or positions, such as changing a light bulb and hanging the washing on the clothesline, as well as rotation (e.g. reversing the car).

Interestingly, the commencement of Howard's cervical spine problems began with his whiplash injury 40 years earlier following a car accident. The incidence of dizziness after whiplash has been variously reported as 20–58%,[7] 40–80%[8] and 80–90%,[9–11] although these were more immediate in reporting than in the present case. Nevertheless, it is likely that the degenerative changes in the upper cervical spine evident on the radiographs were related to the accident and may indeed have been related to the (delayed) onset of dizziness.

Conversely, it is not immediately apparent how the reported tinnitus relates to a mechanical cervical spine problem. However, there are reports of feelings of ear fullness, nausea, blurred vision, sweating and tinnitus associated with cervicogenic dizziness.[12, 13]

2 Did you consider VBI a possible cause for the dizziness?

Clinician's answer

Although Howard's dizziness was elicited by movements and positions of the cervical spine consistent with positional provocation of VBI (i.e. rotation or extension of the neck reducing vertebral artery blood flow leading to VBI),[14, 15] other causes of dizziness had been previously eliminated by the neurologist: cervicogenic dizziness is essentially a diagnosis of exclusion. That is, other causes of dizziness must first be excluded based on the history, physical examination and vestibular function tests[5, 7] before diagnosing cervicogenic dizziness. Moreover, there were no clear neurovascular symptoms or signs, and VBI is more typically associated with a feeling of vertigo.[15]

On the other hand, degenerative changes in the upper cervical spine may impinge on the vertebral artery, impeding blood flow to the hindbrain, although plain radiographs are inadequate to determine this. Nausea and tinnitus are commonly reported with VBI, although they are quite non-specific symptoms.[15, 16] Pain in the upper cervical spine and occiput has also been related to dissection of the vertebral artery, although it is typically more unilateral and of an intense, sharp and acute nature, previously unexperienced by the patient, as well as being of a shorter duration than in this case (i.e. days rather than years).[17]

All in all, VBI is an extremely unlikely cause.

PHYSICAL EXAMINATION

Observation

Howard adopted a forward head posture and sat in a 'slouched' position.

Cervical spine active movements

Howard was experiencing no pain or dizziness at rest, but his right ear felt 'blocked' and the right side of his face felt 'full'.

Gross cervical spine movements were assessed and measured with a Cervical Range-of-Motion (CROM) instrument (Performance Attainment Associates, St Paul, MN, USA):

- flexion: 40° and symptom-free
- extension: 40° and slight dizziness
- left rotation: 70° and symptom-free
- right rotation: 50° with some right-sided neck pain and a general feeling of stiffness
- left lateral flexion: 40° and symptom-free
- right lateral flexion: 40° and symptom-free.

Passive joint movements

A moderate movement restriction with local pain was found on central postero–anterior accessory movement applied to C2 and a lesser extent C3. Some pain was reproduced over the right C2–C3, and to a lesser extent right C3–C4 zygapophyseal joint. Passive physiological intervertebral movements showed decreased motion between C2 and C3 into extension and right rotation.

Dix-Hallpike manoeuvre

To eliminate dizziness caused by BPPV (the most common cause of dizziness) the Dix-Hallpike manoeuvre was performed. The Dix-Hallpike manoeuvre is a test for positional nystagmus, more specifically for posterior semicircular canal BPPV.[18] The nystagmus is induced by taking the patient rapidly from the erect long-sitting position, into left or right cervical spine rotation (45°) and then to supine head-hanging (30° below the level of the examination table).[7, 19] The test is performed to both sides.

Paroxysmal positional nystagmus is usually geotropic rotary nystagmus, high in frequency with a 3–10 second latency, but dissipates within 30–60 seconds. It has torsional and linear components, and then occurs in the reverse direction when the patient returns to the sitting position. It also exhibits fatigability; that is, with repeated positioning vertigo and nystagmus rapidly disappear.[18, 20] For cervicogenic dizziness, the test may elicit dizziness due to cervical spine movement but would not induce nystagmus. When the test was performed on Howard he complained of mild dizziness when the head was turned to the right, but there was no observable nystagmus.

Balance testing

Balance was assessed by observing Howard in tandem stance (standing with one foot in front of the other), with eyes opened, eyes closed and with his neck in extension. In extension and with his eyes closed Howard felt very unsteady and could not hold tandem stance for 10 seconds.

EVIDENCE-INFORMED CLINICAL REASONING

1 Were the findings from the physical examination consistent with your expectations after the history?

Clinician's answer

Cervicogenic dizziness is generally associated with upper cervical spine (O–C3) mechanical dysfunction. There were a number of findings from the physical examination that supported this hypothesis in Howard's case. Most notably, the marked limitation of active extension and right rotation of the neck, as well as of passive movement predominantly at C2–C3 are

consistent with motion impairment of the upper cervical spine (see Tousignant et al[21] for normative values for cervical spine ROM using the CROM device). In addition, the forward head posture exhibited by Howard may have contributed to this problem by placing the upper cervical spine joints towards end-range extension and the deep neck flexor muscles on stretch, potentially rendering them less effective in controlling cervical spine motion.

The negative Dix-Hallpike manoeuvre also makes it less likely that BPPV is the cause of the dizziness. Collectively, these findings were consistent with expectations following the history and are certainly consistent with cervicogenic dizziness.

2 At this stage of the clinical session, what was your preferred treatment hypothesis and why?

Clinician's answer

At the end of the physical examination, it was decided to treat Howard using Sustained Natural Apophyseal Glides (SNAGs) as described and advocated for cervicogenic dizziness by Brian Mulligan.[22] A randomised controlled trial by Reid et al provides evidence that SNAGs are an effective manual therapy procedure for the treatment of cervicogenic dizziness and related neck pain (Chapter 3).[23] SNAGs were shown in this study to have a clinically and statistically significant immediate and sustained (12 week) effect in reducing dizziness, neck pain and disability caused by cervical spine dysfunction. Given the paucity of research into other interventions for cervicogenic dizziness,[24] and given personal clinical experience of the benefits of SNAGs, this approach seemed most indicated. The other consideration was that SNAGs involve active and passive movement, and therefore may directly improve both joint and muscle receptor dysfunction. In addition, if found effective in the clinic they readily lend themselves to home exercise, potentially enhancing and extending the effects of the therapist's 'hands-on' treatment (see Chapter 2).

TREATMENT AND MANAGEMENT

Howard received SNAG treatment once a week for 4 weeks, as per the treatment regime described in the study by Reid et al.[23]

Treatment 1

A lay explanation was given to Howard about cervicogenic dizziness. It was explained that his neck had become stiff and this was stimulating the receptors in the joints and muscles to send abnormal messages back to the brain. The brain perceives these abnormal messages as dizziness. It was further explained that the SNAG treatment is designed to have an immediate positive effect on the function of both neck joints and muscles, and therefore helps to restore normal signals to the brain and reduce feelings of dizziness.

From the history, cervical spine extension was identified as the offending movement (i.e. the movement that predominantly caused his dizziness in daily activities such as hanging the washing) and was thus used to determine the treatment direction for the SNAG. With Howard in the upright (weight-bearing) sitting position, a sustained passive accessory movement (glide) was applied in an anterior direction to the C2 spinous process while he actively extended his neck through his available physiological range (Table 9.1, Figure 9.3). This was repeated six times. Howard was asked to report any dizziness or other symptoms during the application of the procedure. If he reported any dizziness or neck pain then either the range of active movement was decreased (short of the onset of symptoms), the angle of the glide was slightly altered or the point of application was modified to ensure the treatment was symptom-free. As the extension SNAG was repeatedly performed Howard was able to go further in range with each movement.

After the treatment Howard said his right ear had 'unblocked'. Active cervical spine extension was reassessed and was now 50° and symptom-free.

Treatment 2 (1 week later)

Howard reported he felt better and that he had experienced no headaches over the past week, which was unusual for him. His ear and face felt much clearer. Post-treatment he felt 'magnificent'. He had experienced less dizziness and was able to hang the clothes on the line, looking up at the line, and not lose his balance.

Howard was asked to complete the two VAS self-report measures again. On the VAS for dizziness, he now rated it as 1.5 out of 10. On the VAS for neck pain and headache, he now rated it as 0.6 out of 10.

On examination, cervical spine extension was maintained at 50° and was still symptom-free. Right rotation was 55° with some right-sided neck pain. To progress the treatment at this session, the number of repetitions of the extension SNAG was increased from six to 10. After this treatment, cervical extension increased to 55° and was symptom-free. Howard was also taught how to do a neck retraction exercise while sitting[25] in an effort to reverse the effects of his forward head posture. He was further taught to sit in a neutral upright posture with a normal lumbar lordosis. The use of a lumbar support for prolonged sitting was discussed. Howard

Table 9.1	SNAG for cervicogenic dizziness	
Indication	Dizziness described as imbalance or unsteadiness that is provoked by movements or positions of the neck involving extension	
Positioning	Patient	Sitting in a comfortably erect posture.
	Treated body part	Neutral resting position of the cervical spine.
	Therapist	Standing immediately behind the patient.
	Therapist's hands	Place the palmar aspect of the distal phalanx of one thumb over the spinous process of C2. Reinforce with the other thumb.
Application guidelines	• The therapist pushes in an anterior direction on the spinous process of C2 with both thumbs. • While the therapist sustains the anterior glide of C2 and maintains a constant angle (in relation to the joint plane), the patient slowly extends their neck to end of range. It is critical that the therapist maintains the angle of the glide constant to the neck as it is extended. • Provided there are no symptoms, the patient applies gentle extension overpressure using one hand on their forehead and holds this for a few seconds. • The forward thumb pressure is sustained until the patient returns their neck to the starting position. • Repeat the SNAG six times.	
Comments	• All components of the procedure should be symptom-free. • If symptoms are experienced try slightly altering the direction of the glide or the point of thumb contact.	
Variation	• An extension self-SNAG using a cervical treatment belt (or the selvage of a towel) can be performed by placing the belt over the C2 spinous process and instructing the patient to pull both ends of the belt anteriorly. The patient must maintain the belt in line with the upper jaw as the neck is extended to keep the angle of the glide constant. The procedure must not produce any symptoms and should be repeated 6–10 times. • For dizziness provoked with right rotation, the palmar aspect of the right thumb is placed over the right transverse process of C1, reinforced by the other thumb. Pressure is directed anteriorly and the therapist maintains this as the patient slowly turns their head to the right, so as to keep the angle of the glide constant. The patient applies gentle rotation overpressure using their left hand on their left zygomatic arch and holds this for a few seconds. The procedure is otherwise as described above for an extension problem. If the technique is unsuccessful, try applying the glide to the contralateral transverse process. • A right rotation self-SNAG can be performed using a treatment belt (or towel) by placing the belt over C1 and grasping each end of the belt with the opposite hand. While the left hand remains still (the left elbow can be hooked behind the back of the chair), the right hand pulls the left end of the belt and maintains a constant anterior glide as the neck rotates. The procedure must be symptom-free and should only be repeated two to five times initially as it is a powerful technique.	

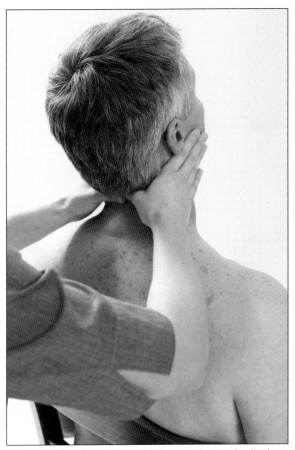

Figure 9.3 Extension SNAG for cervicogenic dizziness produced with neck extension

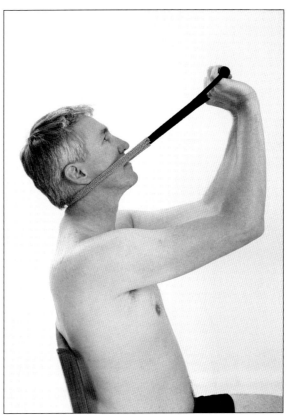

Figure 9.4 Extension self-SNAG for cervicogenic dizziness produced with neck extension

was given written instructions on performing the neck retraction exercise several times throughout the day. To remind him to do this, it was suggested that he might do five repetitions of the exercise each time he sat down.

Treatment 3 (1 week later)
Howard reported feeling much better. He had only experienced one episode of dizziness since the last treatment while working under his caravan, lying on his back with his neck arched in extension. The dizziness settled after 1 hour. He had not had any neck pain, headache, nausea, or feelings of ear or face fullness. He had hung out the washing and did not feel unsteady and had been able to do hedging of high topiary bushes without any problems. On the VAS for dizziness Howard now scored 0.5, and on the VAS for cervical pain and headache he scored 0.

On physical reassessment, active cervical spine extension was measured at 65° and was symptom-free. This represented an improvement of 25° from the initial examination 2 weeks earlier. Right rotation remained unchanged.

Because Howard had reported that sustained cervical spine extension (such as when changing a light bulb or

working under his caravan) produced his dizziness, the SNAG was performed with end-range extension maintained for up to 10 seconds, with gentle overpressure. Howard was also given a cervical spine self-SNAG treatment belt and taught how to undertake self-SNAG extension exercises[22] (Figure 9.4). He was advised to perform the exercise gently and it was stressed that the self-SNAG should be symptom-free. Howard was given written instructions and was asked to do the exercise with 10 repetitions every second day. The cervical retraction exercise was checked and he was advised to continue with this as well.

Treatment 4 (1 week later)
Howard could not recall any episodes of imbalance or dizziness during the last week. He had been able to hang out the washing and go grocery shopping alone, and was feeling much more confident with his driving. He had not experienced any neck pain, headache, or ear or facial symptoms. Howard stated he felt he was able 'to live again' and that he was managing well with the self-SNAG exercise using the treatment belt.

The VASs for dizziness and pain were both rated as 0. The DHI was now scored as 12 which indicates a mild handicap.[2]

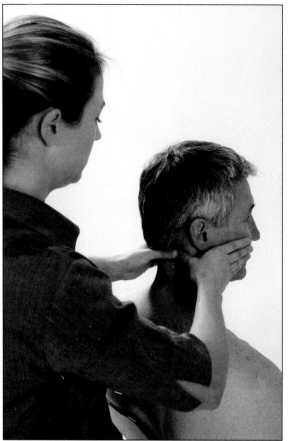

Figure 9.5 Rotation SNAG for cervicogenic dizziness produced with neck rotation

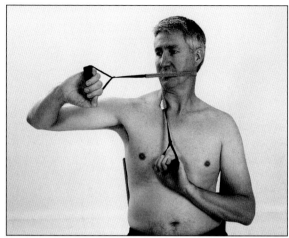

Figure 9.6 Rotation self-SNAG for cervicogenic dizziness produced with neck rotation

Active movements were recorded as:
- flexion: 45°
- extension: 65°
- left rotation: 70°
- right rotation: 55°
- left lateral flexion: 40°
- right lateral flexion: 40°; all movements were symptom-free.

In addition to the extension SNAG applied at the last treatment, a second SNAG into right rotation was added because that direction of movement remained reduced compared to the range to the left. The right rotation SNAG was performed by applying an anteriorly directed force to the right C1 transverse process while Howard slowly rotated his neck as far as possible to the right (Figure 9.5), followed by the application of overpressure. This was repeated 10 times without any symptoms. Anteriorly directed pressure was applied to the right transverse process in this case (as opposed to the left) as this is what enabled Howard to rotate to the right asymptomatically. On reassessment right rotation was now 65°.

Howard was taught a right rotation self-SNAG exercise using the treatment belt (Figure 9.6). He was told he probably only needed to do a session of 10 repetitions of this exercise every second day to regain the final few degrees of right rotation and prevent any recurrence of his symptoms. He was asked to continue the extension SNAG and the retraction exercise as well.

Outcome of intervention

When contacted 6 weeks after completing treatment Howard reported no episodes of dizziness, and rated both his dizziness and pain as 0 on a VAS. On the DHI, Howard scored 6 (mild handicap).

EVIDENCE-INFORMED CLINICAL REASONING

1 Based on the clinical findings and the scientific evidence, why do you think Howard developed cervicogenic dizziness?

Clinician's answer

There is evidence that cervicogenic dizziness is a result of perturbation of the information from sensory afferents in the upper cervical spine.[3, 26] Indeed, it has been shown experimentally that loss of normal input from Type I cervical articular mechanoreceptors leads to dizziness and poor balance.[27] Moreover, studies have shown the presence of mechanoreceptive and nociceptive nerve endings in the cervical zygapophyseal joint capsules, which implies that neural input from these joints is important in proprioception and pain sensation.[10, 27, 28] Not surprisingly therefore, patients experiencing cervicogenic dizziness also frequently experience upper cervical pain and headache.[23]

In Howard's case, the temporal link between the onset of the dizziness (and related pain) and the night job packing grocery shelves and the swimming episode (breathing by turning only to the right), strongly suggests that these activities may have injured joint structures in the upper cervical spine leading to abnormal afferent input from articular mechanoreceptors, and therefore dizziness. The limitations of cervical ROM in extension and right rotation and the abnormal passive accessory movement findings are certainly consistent with this hypothesis.

It is common for people to develop cervicogenic dizziness in the years following a whiplash injury. Some authors[10, 29] propose that trauma to the muscles, ligaments, joint capsules, sensory nerves and other soft tissues of the neck could lead to dizziness in whiplash patients by damaging proprioceptors. Following tearing or significant stretching of upper cervical spine joint capsules and ligaments, firm fibrosis may also develop causing chronic hypomobility in the joints.[30] It has been proposed that joint hypomobility may lead to pain and therefore further reduction in movement,[31, 32] consequently affecting stimulation of the mechanoreceptors and potentially causing dizziness.[32] The history of whiplash could have been a predisposing factor in Howard's case, although the substantial time interval makes this less likely. The immediate and marked response at the first session to just six repetitions of a SNAG, a relatively gentle form of manual therapy, also suggests that it is unlikely that chronic, fibrotic changes related to whiplash trauma were contributing to Howard's symptoms.

The other contributing factor in the development of Howard's dizziness may have been age-related degenerative changes in the upper cervical spine, as evidenced on the radiographic images. Interestingly, Wyke[27] reports that with advancing age there is progressive degenerative loss of mechanoreceptor afferent activity in all tissues in the body.

2 What do you consider is Howard's long-term prognosis? What factors support and refute your hypothesis?

Clinician's answer

Howard's prognosis in the longer term is generally good. He responded quickly and markedly to the SNAG treatment and there was no indication of any regression 6 weeks after the last treatment. Furthermore, he was compliant with his self-management regime and was active and healthy otherwise. On the other hand, there were degenerative changes in the upper cervical spine evident on radiographs and he presented with a long (3-year) history of dizziness and an even longer history of neck pain since sustaining a whiplash injury 40 years ago. His forward head posture was also a possible contributing factor to upper cervical spine dysfunction.

Much would depend on his activities and whether he heeds related advice (e.g. symmetrical rather than one-sided breathing with freestyle). However, Howard now has the capacity to manage his condition himself at the first onset of any dizziness.

AUTHORS' MWM COMMENTARY

If the cause of a patient's dizziness is cervicogenic dizziness then clinical experience and empirical research both indicate there will be a prompt favourable response to manual therapy such as SNAGs applied to the upper cervical spine.[23, 24] A failure to respond after three to four such treatments suggests there is probably another cause for the dizziness.[15, 33] Howard had a marked reduction in his pain and dizziness after the first SNAG treatment. Because Howard had an immediate decrease in his dizziness after manual therapy treatment to the upper cervical spine, it can be inferred that mechanical dysfunction in the upper cervical spine was the likely source of the problem and that the hypothesis of cervicogenic dizziness was probably correct.[8, 26, 34, 35] It also suggests that the SNAG treatment positively addressed this dysfunction.

Several clinical authors including Mulligan contend that once normal joint accessory movement is restored, symptom-free voluntary physiological movement is then facilitated, leading to normal function and resolution of symptoms.[31, 36, 37] This hypothesis is supported by Howard's response to treatment whereby there was parallel improvement in his range of motion, pain and dizziness following the application of SNAGs to the upper cervical spine.

Cervical spine extension was the movement that most notably reproduced Howard's dizziness and was thus the direction of movement initially used in the SNAG treatment. Mulligan[38] reports that extension is the movement most commonly linked to cervicogenic dizziness. This assertion is supported by Reid et al's[23] study in which it was found that cervical spine extension was the provocative movement in 59% of participants. An increase in Howard's range of cervical spine extension was observed post-treatment. Since both his dizziness and extension ROM improved concomitantly this possibly indicates an inverse relationship.

It is proposed that SNAGs, by restoring joint movement in the cervical spine and therefore normalising afferent input of mechanoreceptors and proprioceptors in joints and muscles, will substantially reduce symptoms of cervicogenic dizziness. There is evidence to support the use of SNAGs in this disorder, most notably the randomised controlled trial conducted by Reid et al[23] (see Chapter 3) which demonstrated that such an immediate and profound response to this technique as experienced by Howard is not unusual in chronic cases. A sustained response may, however, require some form of maintenance program.[39] It is also possible that benefits in improving balance may reduce the risk of falls in the elderly, although this remains to be demonstrated.

References

1 Jacobsen GP, Newman CW. The development of the dizziness handicap inventory. Archives Otolaryngology Head Neck Surgery. 1990;116:424–7.
2 Treleaven J. Dizziness Handicap Inventory (DHI). Australian Journal of Physiotherapy. 2006;52(1):67.

3 de Jong PTVM, de Jong JMBV, Bernard C, Jongkees LBW. Ataxia and nystagmus induced by injection of local anaesthetics in the neck. Annals of Neurology. 1977;1:240–6.

4 Furman J, and Cass, S. Balance Disorders: A Case-study Approach. Philadelphia: FA Davis Co 1996.

5 Heikkila H. Cervical vertigo. In: Boyling JD, Jull GA (eds). Grieves' Modern Manual Therapy, the Vertebral Column. Edinburgh, UK: Elsevier Churchill Livingstone 2004.

6 Hain T. Benign Paroxysmal Positional 2004. Online. Available: www.dizziness-and-balance.com/disorders/bpv/bppv.html (accessed 3 November 2009).

7 Wrisley D, Sparto P, Whitney S, Furman J. Cervico-genic dizziness: a review of diagnosis and treatment. Journal of Orthopaedic and Sports Physical Therapy. 2000;30(12):755–66.

8 Oostendorp RAB, van Eupen AAJM, Van Erp J, Elvers H. Dizziness following whiplash injury: a neuro-oto-logical study in manual therapy practice and therapeutic implication. The Journal of Manual and Manipulative Therapy. 1999;7(3):123–30.

9 Heikkila H, Johansson, M, Wenngren B I. Effects of acupuncture, cervical manipulation and NSAID therapy on dizziness and impaired head repositioning of sus-pected cervical origin: a pilot study. Manual Therapy. 2000;5(3):151–7.

10 Hinoki M. Vertigo due to whiplash injury: a neuroto-logical approach. Acta Otolaryngologica (Stockholm) Supplementum. 1985;419:9–29.

11 Humphries B, Bloton J, Peterson C, Wood A. A cross-sectional study of the association between pain and disability in neck pain patients with dizziness of sus-pected cervical origin. Journal of Whiplash and Related Disorders. 2002;1(2):63–73.

12 Ryan GMS, Cope, S. Cervical vertigo. Lancet. 1955;31:1355–8.

13 Wing L, Hargrave-Wilson, W. Cervical vertigo. Austra-lian and New Zealand Journal of Surgery. 1974;44:275–7.

14 Bogduk N. Cervical causes of headache and dizziness. In: Grieve GP (ed.) Modern Manual Therapy of the Vertebral Column. New York: Churchill Livingstone 1986:289–302.

15 Magarey M, Rebbeck T, Coughlan B, Grimmer K, Rivett DA, Refshauge K. Pre-manipulative testing of the cervical spine review, revision and new clinical guide-lines. Manual Therapy. 2004;9:95–108.

16 Rivett DA. The vertebral artery and vertebrobasilar insufficiency. In: Boyling JD, Jull GA (eds). Grieves' Modern Manual Therapy of the Vertebral Column (3rd edn). Edinburgh: Churchill Livingstone 2004:257–73.

17 Rivett DA, Shirley D, Magarey M, Refshauge K. Clini-cal Guidelines for Assessing Vertebrobasilar Insuffi-ciency in the Management of Cervical Spine Disorders. Melbourne: Australian Physiotherapy Association 2006.

18 Baloh R, Honrubia V. Clinical Neurophysiology of the Vestibular System (2nd edn). Philadelphia: FA Davis Company 1990.

19 Bronstein A. Vestibular reflexes and positional manoeu-vres. Journal of Neurology, Neurosurgery and Psychia-try. 2003;74:289–93.

20 Froehling D, Silverstein M, Mohr D, Beatty C. Does this dizzy patient have a serious from of vertigo? Journal of American Medical Association. 1994;271(5):385–9.

21 Tousignant M, Smeesters C, Breton AM, Breton E, Corriveau H. Criterion validity study of the cervical range of motion (CROM) device for rotational range of motion on healthy adults. Journal of Orthopaedic Sports Physical Therapy. 2006;36(4):242–8.

22 Mulligan BR. Manual therapy 'NAGS', 'SNAGS', 'MWMS' etc. (5th edn). Wellington: Plane View Ser-vices 2004.

23 Reid S, Rivett DA, Katekar MG, Callister R. Sustained natural apophyseal glides (SNAGs) are an effective treatment for cervicogenic dizziness. Manual Therapy. 2008;13:357–66.

24 Reid S, Rivett DA. Manual therapy treatment of cervi-cogenic dizziness: a systematic review. Manual Therapy. 2005;10:4–13.

25 McKenzie R, May S. The Lumbar Spine Mechanical Diagnosis and Therapy (2nd edn). New Zealand: Spinal Publications 2003.

26 Brandt T, Bronstein AM. Cervical vertigo. Journal of Neu-rology, Neurosurgery and Psychiatry. 2001;71(1):8–12.

27 Wyke B. Cervical articular contributions to posture and gait: their relation to senile disequilibrium. Age and Ageing. 1979;8:251–8.

28 Hulse M. Disequilibrium caused by a functional distur-bance of the upper cervical spine, clinical aspects and functional diagnosis. Manual Medicine. 1983;1(1):18–23.

29 Fitz-Ritson D. Assessment of cervicogenic vertigo. Journal of Manipulative and Physiological Therapies. 1991;14(3):193–8.

30 Grieve GP. Common Vertebral Joint Problems. Edin-burgh: Churchill Livingstone 1981.

31 Kaltenborn FM, Evjenth O. Manual Mobilization of the Extremity Joints (4th edn). Oslo, Norway: Olaf Noris Bokhandel 1989.

32 Oostendorp R, van Eupen AAJM, Elvers JWH, Bernards J. Effects of restrained cervical mobility on involuntary eye movements. The Journal of Manual and Manipula-tive Therapy. 1993;1(4):148–53.

33 Mulligan BR. Vertigo … Manual therapy may be needed. Manipulative Physiotherapists Association of Australia 7th Biennial Conference, Blue Mountains, Australia, 1991.

34 Karlberg M, Johansson M, Magnussen M, Frannson P. Dizziness of suspected origin distinguished by posturo-graphic assessment of human postural dynamics. Journal of Vestibular Research. 1996;6(1):37–47.

35 Tjell C. Cervicogenic vertigo: with special emphasis on whiplash-associated disorder. In: Vernon H, (ed.) The Cranio-cervical Syndrome. Toronto, Canada: Butter-worth-Heinemann 2001.

36 Maitland G. Vertibral Manipulation (5th edn). London, Butterworth Heineman 1986.

37 Mulligan BR. SNAGS: Mobilisations of the spine with active movement. In: Boyling J, Palastanga N, (eds) Grieves Modern Manual Therapy, the Vertebral Column (2nd edn). Edinburgh: Churchill Livingstone 1994, pp 733–43.

38 Mulligan BR. Manual therapy 'NAGS', ' SNAGS', 'MWMS' etc. (4th edn). Wellington, New Zealand: Plane View Services 1999.

39 Malmström E, Karlberg M, Melander A, Magnusson M, Moritz U. Cervicogenic dizziness-musculoskeletal find-ings before and after treatment and long-term outcome. Disability Rehabilitation. 2007;29(15):1193–205.

Chapter 10
Temporomandibular joint dysfunction: an open and shut case

Mark Oliver

HISTORY

At the time of the initial consultation Catherine was a 33-year-old female production operator in a factory and had one young child. She was sedentary, but had been a ballet dancer until her mid-twenties.

Catherine was referred by an ear, nose and throat (ENT) surgeon who stated in his accompanying letter: 'Her problems are well advanced, but I think the underlying cause needs to be managed before embarking on arthroscopy and surgical treatment'. Her dentist had eliminated the teeth as a source of pain.

Current history

Presenting symptoms were severe left temporomandibular joint (TMJ) pain that was sharp at times, constant but variable left sided pain in the temporal region, maxilla and mandible, bilateral sub-occipital pain with intermittent frontal headaches, and stiffness across the cervical spine (Figure 10.1). Catherine also experienced intermittent clicking in the right TMJ, but this did not concern her and had been present for many years.

Catherine had experienced worsening severe left TMJ pain for the preceding 12 months, but did not know why this was happening. She had been prescribed citalopram hydrobromide, a selective serotonin re-uptake inhibitor commonly used for depression, and took paracetamol intermittently for pain relief.

Past history

Catherine had recently arrived in Australia as an immigrant from Eastern Europe where she had undergone multiple dental procedures. The left and right upper first and third molars were absent, and she had been fitted with multiple dental crowns, necessary because she had fractured teeth by clenching and bruxing.

Catherine had a long history of intermittent left TMJ locking and painful limitation of mouth opening, and was aware that in the past she had clenched and bruxed at night. She had been fitted with an occlusal splint but had stopped using it years earlier. Catherine was of the opinion that she was no longer bruxing at night.

24-hour symptom behaviour

The sharp left TMJ pain occurred when clenching, even very lightly, and consequently Catherine had been forced to adopt a soft food and blended food diet to avoid chewing. She had been doing this for 12 months and was finding it very distressing. Sharp TMJ pain also occurred on mouth opening and the movement was painfully restricted. Consequently, she was not able to place normal sized objects in her mouth and experienced significant pain when yawning.

Pain in the left temporal region, maxilla and mandible was felt to radiate from the left TMJ and was present as a low grade constant ache that became more severe through the day and when the sharp TMJ pain was triggered by clenching or movement. Symptoms in all areas tended to worsen through the day and were less severe in the morning. The bilateral sub-occipital pain and stiffness across the cervical spine were made worse by sustained flexed head and neck positions at work.

Diagnostic imaging

Helical computerised axial tomography (CAT) utilising multi-detector computed tomography was used to produce three-dimensional reconstructions of the TMJs in closed and open mouth positions. These scans gave excellent visualisation of the state of the TMJs and surrounding tissue. The CAT scan of the right TMJ showed moderate anterolateral disc displacement in the closed mouth position with the mandibular condyle being posteriorly situated within the mandibular fossa. With opening, condylar translation was severely restricted, with no disc movement and only mild disc recapture. The supero-lateral joint space was narrowed with early osteoarthritis of the mandibular condyle. The mandibular fossa appeared normal and the articular eminence was pronounced (described by the radiologist as 'a normal variant'). The radiologist commented that it was likely that intra-articular adhesions were present.

The CAT scan of the left TMJ showed moderate to marked anterior disc displacement in the closed mouth position. With opening, there was moderate restriction of condylar translation and the disc was not recaptured.

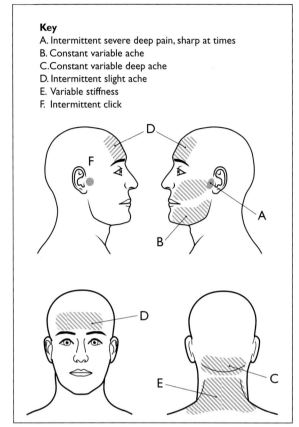

Key

A. Intermittent severe deep pain, sharp at times
B. Constant variable ache
C. Constant variable deep ache
D. Intermittent slight ache
E. Variable stiffness
F. Intermittent click

Figure 10.1 Body chart depicting areas of patient's symptoms

The disc was crumpled and deformed and fluid/synovitis was present in the inferior and to a lesser extent, the superior joint space. There was evidence of prior condylar erosion leaving an irregular articular surface and sub-cortical sclerosis.

EVIDENCE-INFORMED CLINICAL REASONING

1 What factors did you consider had contributed to the maintenance of the present episode of TMJ pain?

Clinician's response

Catherine did not believe that she was clenching and bruxing at night, although she was aware that she had done so in the past. Pain was less in the morning and increased through the day, supporting her contention. If she was still clenching and bruxing it was most likely that this was now occurring during the day. Muscular activity associated with clenching and bruxing often lessens when afferent activity from TMJ ligamentous structures reduces following deterioration of the tissue with concurrent loss of receptors.[1] This may explain why the clenching was not as significant now as it was in the past.

Catherine experienced significant stress, having recently emigrated from Eastern Europe, looking after a young child and employed in a situation that she did not enjoy. She had also lost fitness and was probably not maintaining good nutrition as a result of her altered eating behaviour due to painful mastication.

PHYSICAL EXAMINATION

A comprehensive examination of the spinal column, shoulder girdle and pelvis were performed, but this description is mostly confined to the TMJ component of the presentation and only significant findings are included.

Posture and observation

Spinal posture was poor with head forward position and shoulder girdle protraction.

The left and right upper first and third molars had been extracted 6–7 years ago. There was significant wear on the remaining teeth and crowns. There appeared to be a loss of vertical mouth height, and Catherine confirmed that she thought that her physical appearance around the mouth had changed when compared to that in photographs taken more than 10 years ago.

Active movements

Active jaw opening was painfully restricted to 25 mm with significant left deflection of the mandible in the last one-third of the movement. Pain increased significantly in the left TMJ at end of available range and there was audible and palpable clicking in the right TMJ on jaw opening and closing. Palpation confirmed the marked bilateral restriction of mandibular condylar anterior translation on mouth opening shown in the CAT scans.

Light clench produced sharp pain in the left TMJ. There appeared to be initial tooth contact on the left canines, then a slide of the mandible to the right with poor occlusion (the relationship of the maxillary and mandibular teeth when they are in functional contact).[1] Catherine confirmed that she could feel this movement occurring, and she was aware that her bite had changed significantly. Despite the missing teeth and dental wear, Catherine was certain that the occlusion had been relatively good prior to the onset of the acute left TMJ pain 12 months earlier. Using a tongue depressor in various locations between the teeth reduced clenching pain 20–30%. Pain on occlusion is sometimes reduced significantly by use of a separator that prevents intercuspation of the teeth.[1]

Active left laterotrusion of the mandible moderately increased pain over the lateral pole and posterior portion of the left TMJ, while right laterotrusion produced severe left TMJ pain. Less than 5 mm of lateral movement was possible in each direction before onset of significant pain. Retrusion was not possible actively and passive retrusion was painful in the left TMJ, particularly if the posterior movement was given a left bias. Protrusion was slightly restricted with a slight deviation to the left, increased pain in the left TMJ and a marked click in the right TMJ when returning to the mandibular physiologic rest position (the habitual postural position of the mandible when the patient is resting comfortably in the upright position and the condyles are in a neutral, unstrained position in the glenoid fossae; the mandibular musculature is in a state of minimum tonic contraction to maintain posture and to overcome the force of gravity).[2]

Palpation

The joint capsule, lateral ligament and retrodiscal tissue of the left TMJ were very tender to palpation with significantly less tenderness on palpation of the right joint. In particular, palpation of the left retrodiscal region elicited very sharp pain that radiated into the auricular, mandibular and temporal region.

Although the CAT scans indicated that the right mandibular head was located posteriorly in the mandibular fossa, this was not evident on palpation. Similarly, although the right articular disc was displaced anterolaterally, the mandibular heads were reasonably symmetrically located in the glenoid fossae on palpation.

Passive accessory motion tests

Minimal passive rotation of the mandible to the right decreased left TMJ pain on clenching, but the quality of the bite felt worse. Rotating the mandible minimally to the left resulted in very severe left TMJ pain on light clench. Right transverse translation of the TMJs was slightly restricted but did not produce significant symptoms. Left translation was relatively mobile and pain-free.

Left TMJ posterior translation produced severe sharp pain before a sense of movement or end-feel could be obtained. Left TMJ anterior translation inclined inferiorly to be parallel with the plane of the articular eminence was moderately restricted and produced sharp pain, but pain was not as severe as that occurring on posterior translation. Right TMJ posterior translation was unremarkable while antero-inferior translation was probably slightly–moderately limited compared to normal. Because the discal condylar relationship in both joints had been disturbed in different ways, the comparative movement and end-feel of translation tests was difficult to compare to normal and from left to right.

Muscle function

Orofacial muscle strength and endurance testing was limited by pain, but in view of the long duration of severe symptoms it was anticipated that significant weakness of the masticatory muscles would be present. Swallowing resulted in a slight increase in left TMJ pain occurring as the teeth came together, but the swallowing mechanism appeared normal. Using examination procedures described by Buman et al[3] and von Piekartz,[4] suprahyoid and infrahyoid muscle activity was determined to be relatively normal and symmetrical left to right.

On palpation, tender points were located in the masseter and lateral pterygoid muscles (palpated intra-orally and externally), noticeably worse on the left than the right. The anterior and middle parts of the temporalis muscle were also tender to palpation bilaterally.

Spinal column

Cervical spine left rotation was slightly–moderately restricted producing left mid and upper cervical pain at end of range (EOR), but other cervical movements did not produce remarkable symptoms. On segmental motion testing of C1–C2 using the flexion-rotation method described by Dvorak et al,[5] there was moderate limitation of left rotation with significant tenderness to palpation over the left C1–C2 zygapophyseal joint. There was stiffness in the cervicodorsal junction on palpation and significant local tenderness was elicited on palpation of the anterior tubercles of C4 and C5 on the left and right. The sub-occipital muscles were tender and tight to palpation bilaterally, with tenderness elicited along the superior and inferior nuchal lines bilaterally.

Postural muscle tone was poor in the neck and shoulder girdle region. Studies have demonstrated a clear relationship between head position and occlusion,[6–9] but in this case repositioning of the head, neck and shoulders did not result in significant changes in pain experienced on mouth opening or closing and did not alter occlusion.

EVIDENCE-INFORMED CLINICAL REASONING

1 What was your working diagnostic hypothesis after the physical examination?

Clinician's response

In Catherine's case, the CAT scan of the left TMJ clearly showed that the articular disc was crumpled and deformed, blocking antero-inferior translation of the condyle and constituting a permanent disc displacement. Severe pain was elicited on posterior translation of the mandibular head and the retrodiscal tissue was very painful to palpation with referral of symptoms. The retrodiscal tissue is highly innervated and vascularised.[1] Stress placed on the retrodiscal tissue by a posteriorly displaced mandibular condyle may cause an inflammatory response, with extensive swelling, extravasation of inflammatory fluid into the synovial sacs and pain, especially when the condyle presses against the swollen tissue during maximum intercuspation. The swelling of retrodiscal tissue and intracapsular swelling may also cause acute malocclusion (improper relations of opposing teeth) in the resting occlusal position.[1] It seemed likely that Catherine had an 'acute' malocclusion, even though the severe pain had been present for 12 months. Her CAT scan also showed fluid/synovitis in the left superior and inferior joints, and this swelling may also have been contributing to the malocclusion and restricted jaw movement.

Pain originating from the injured TMJ may also have contributed to the malocclusion and the painful limitation of jaw movement by altering muscle function.[10] This usually takes the form of a protective co-contraction of the masticatory muscles.[11-13] Because the inflammation and pain had been present for a long period, secondary central excitatory effects including referred pain and secondary muscle symptoms such as tenderness and co-contraction of the masticatory muscles[14] had probably also occurred.

Altered orofacial muscular responses and pain may also have been in part due to involvement of the C1–C2 level and the upper cervical spine musculature.[15] Sensory fibres of the upper cervical spinal nerves (C1, C2 and C3) converge on the brainstem and pass into a column of grey matter that is continuous with the trigeminal nucleus. This region of grey matter can legitimately be viewed as either a single or combined nucleus (trigeminocervical nucleus).[16] The trigeminal nucleus receives sensory nerves from the three branches of trigeminal nerve that supplies the face and jaw region. Stimulation of the trigeminocervical nucleus by afferents from tissue damage or stress in the upper cervical spine can result in transmission of nerve

impulses to the thalamus and cortex. Constant afferent nociceptive activity can excite adjacent interneurons from the trigeminal fields giving the patient the perception of pain in the face. If the central excitatory effect involves efferent trigeminal (motor) interneurons, there may also be a resulting alteration in orofacial muscular activity.[14]

2 How did the working diagnostic hypothesis inform your plans for management?

Clinician's response

When treating the TMJ component of longstanding temporomandibular dysfunction (TMD), it is vital to have an accurate diagnosis and appropriate radiological imaging. It is particularly important to differentiate painful movement loss occurring as a result of a reducible disc displacement from painful movement loss occurring as a result of a permanent disc displacement. If a non-reduced disc displacement has not resolved spontaneously, treatment should initially be aimed at reducing the derangement using an appropriate mobilising technique. Application of inappropriate mobilising techniques to a TMJ with a reducible disc displacement may damage the joint sufficiently to result in permanent disc displacement. In particular, using inappropriate stretching techniques may cause permanent elongation of the inferior and superior retrodiscal lamina (Figure 10.2). During full mouth opening the elastic fibres of the superior retrodiscal lamina are fully stretched and produce a slight posterior retractive force on the disc. It is the only structure capable of doing

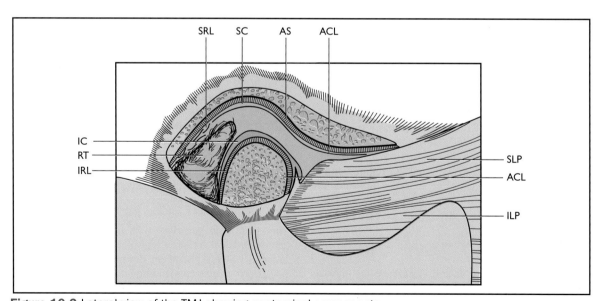

Figure 10.2 Lateral view of the TMJ showing anatomical components
AS, articular surface; IC, inferior joint cavity; ILP, inferior lateral pterygoid; IRL, inferior retrodiscal lamina; RT, retrodiscal tissues; SC, superior joint; SRL, superior retrodiscal lamina. (Source: Okeson 2005, Fig 1.14, p 10, courtesy Dr Julio Turell, University of Montivideo, Uruguay)

so and if damaged it does not regain elasticity, thereby permanently disturbing the relationship between the mandibular condyle and the articular disc.[1]

The pain that Catherine was experiencing was very severe, so initial treatment needed to be directed at eliminating or controlling external factors contributing to painful loading of the TMJs, and also at pain generators in the TMJs, orofacial musculature and cervical spine. Attention also needed to be directed at the mechanical disturbance of TMJ movement and occlusion, with TMJ Mobilisation with Movement (MWM) techniques indicated. In Catherine's case, there was no chance of restoring the normal anatomical relationship between the disc and the mandibular condyle, so there was no need to be concerned about causing irreversible damage to the joint with stretching techniques.

Other factors that needed to be addressed were stress, nutrition, and exercise levels.

The referring ENT surgeon did not expect the severe symptoms to settle with conservative treatment and had considered surgical options, but it was hoped that if symptoms and signs could be controlled referral to a prosthodontist for assessment of the teeth was a possibility. If pain could not be controlled, referral to a clinical psychologist or pain specialist may have been appropriate. As financial constraints were a factor, where possible self-treatment techniques needed to be used. Catherine was very keen to do whatever she could and had excellent motor skills, comprehension and motivation.

TREATMENT AND MANAGEMENT

To apply TMJ MWM techniques effectively, the therapist must have a sound knowledge of TMJ and orofacial anatomy. There is significant variation in the slope of the articular eminence between individuals. On jaw opening, the steeper the slope, the more the condyle is forced to move inferiorly as it moves anteriorly.[1] In a person with a flat eminence, there is a minimum amount of posterior rotation of the disc on the condyle during opening. As the steepness increases, more rotational movement is required between the disc and the condyle during forward translation of the condyle.[17]

The treatment plane of the superior joint of the TMJ is parallel to the slope of the articular eminence (Figure 10.3). To determine the slope of the articular eminence, the angle of application of an antero-inferior glide is varied to produce the maximal amount of translation. The angle that produces the greatest range of translation is parallel to the slope of the articular eminence and forms the treatment plane of the superior joint. Refer to Chapter 2 for more detail on the treatment plane concept, movement and force applied.

Treatment 1

The first treatment included instruction on the optimal rest position of tongue and jaw integrated with simple spinal postural correction exercises. Because the TMJ

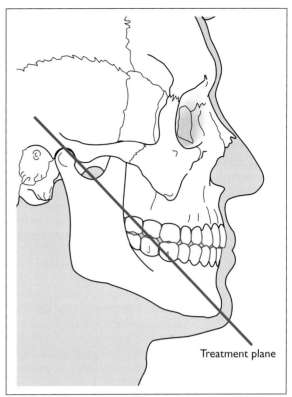

Figure 10.3 Treatment plane of the superior joint of the TMJ parallel to the slope of the articular eminence The treatment plane of the inferior joint lies across the concave inferior surface of the articular disc

pain was worse through the day, it was considered important to control daytime clenching. The significance of prolonged upper and lower teeth contact was explained to Catherine, and she was instructed that if she became aware of the upper and lower teeth making contact to adopt the corrected jaw rest position (combined with spinal postural correction) and maintain it for three normal breaths. She was also instructed to make this correction five times every hour from day 2 post-treatment.

Catherine was further instructed to practise opening the mouth with the anterior half of the tongue gently resting on the hard palate in order to re-establish symmetrical roll in the first stage of jaw opening, and to repeat this six times on six occasions during the day. She was instructed to combine this exercise with the posture correction exercises.

Trigger point release techniques[18] were used for the masseter and lateral pterygoid muscles, but stretching techniques were not used to avoid aggravation of the TMJs. Gentle reverse natural apophyseal glides (NAGs) were performed from C7–T3.

Catherine did not seem to be clenching or bruxing at night and although the symptoms were improved in the mornings, correction of pillow height, sleeping position and avoiding hand contact with the jaw was discussed.

Treatment 2 (1 week later)

Catherine was unsure of her habitual tongue and teeth position, and was asked to evaluate this between the current and the previous appointment. She reported that the tongue was pushing forwards behind the mandibular anterior teeth and that the top and bottom teeth were frequently in contact, even though the contact produced pain. She was gradually establishing the protective rest position for the tongue and teeth as instructed in Treatment 1.

Catherine was experiencing bilateral frontal headaches that were probably worse than those she had experienced prior to treatment. The jaw symptoms were unchanged.

The left C1–C2 joint restriction into left rotation was still evident on segmental movement testing.

A trial sustained natural apophyseal glide (SNAG) for the left C1–C2 joint was performed into left rotation. When the SNAG was performed, Catherine could rotate her neck to the left without pain and with full range. As described in Chapter 2, when there is a substantial improvement with the MWM glide in place, further repetitions are warranted. Two sets of six movements with EOR overpressure were subsequently applied and restored pain-free full range left cervical rotation.

Strengthening exercises were provided for the interscapular muscles and the deep cervical flexors.

Lateral pterygoid and masseter muscle trigger point release techniques (without stretching) were repeated.

Treatment 3 (2 weeks later)

Catherine had experienced significant emotional stress in the period between the second and third treatment sessions, and this made her aware that increased stress worsened her clenching and was associated with headaches and increased jaw pain when eating. She had also become aware that adopting the corrected jaw and spinal posture markedly eased her headaches and neck stiffness. Despite the stress-related provocation of symptoms, generally neck pain and stiffness and the headaches were much less severe and occurred less frequently. Catherine was managing well with the strengthening exercises.

On physical examination, the pain-free range of active physiological cervical left rotation had been sustained, and on segmental motion testing C1–C2 movement was equal to the left and right. The C4 and C5 levels were less tender to palpation over the anterior tubercles, but were still slightly stiff. Mouth opening ROM and pain was unchanged, and jaw clenching was still painful. There was less resistance to antero-inferior translation of the left TMJ mandibular condyle, but posterior translation still increased left TMJ pain. There

was significantly less tenderness on palpation of the lateral pterygoid and masseter muscles. High abnormal masticatory muscle tone can make TMJ MWM techniques difficult to perform, but with lessening of the protective co-contraction tone in the masticatory muscles this was thought to be an ideal time to use a MWM.

A TMJ MWM for jaw closing to maximal tooth contact was chosen (Table 10.1 and Figure 10.4). To avoid painful compression of the retrodiscal tissue, the mandible was repositioned slightly antero-inferior. Sufficient force was used to stop the left mandibular head from moving posterior in the mandibular fossa when clenching. If the corrected position of the mandibular head was maintained, there was no pain on clenching. Catherine was then asked to actively open the mouth approximately 10 mm, then to close again to produce a light clench. Throughout the movement, the therapist maintained sufficient anteroinferior pressure on the left mandible to keep left and right condylar movement symmetrical. On retesting after two sets of three movements, closing to clench was significantly less painful and there was slight lessening of pain on jaw opening.

The patient was then shown how to perform the technique as a self-MWM (Figure 10.5). When first trying the technique, Catherine released the antero-inferior force during the technique and experienced sharp left TMJ pain, but when she maintained the correct amount of force throughout the manoeuvre she could close and clench repeatedly without pain. Catherine was instructed to repeat this technique up to six times on six occasions per day. She was able to perform the technique successfully in either supine lying or sitting.

Small amplitude end-range antero-posterior unilateral mobilisation techniques were also applied to the C4 and C5 anterior tubercles[19] with the cervical spine in the neutral position.

Catherine telephoned seven days later and reported that there had been a significant improvement in jaw ROM and marked lessening of pain on opening and closing the jaw. She was instructed to continue with the exercises.

Treatment 4 (5 weeks later)

The next appointment was 5 weeks later as the therapist had been away from practice. Catherine had repeated the self-MWM regularly since the last consultation. She could now eat and clench without much pain but mouth opening was still painfully restricted. She had not used medication since the last visit.

On examination, jaw closure and clenching was pain-free and Catherine reported that the teeth felt like they were meeting normally. Jaw opening was limited to 30 mm with a slight left deviation and slight-moderate pain around the left TMJ at EOR, increased with application of overpressure. Left laterotrusion

Table 10.1	TMJ MWM for pain on jaw closure (see Figure 10.4)	
Indication	Pain on closure of mouth with or without acute malocclusion. This technique is used for acute malocclusion caused by muscular dysfunction or by acute TMJ derangement, but not for malocclusion caused by dental mal-alignment.	
Positioning	Patient	Supine lying or sitting facing mirror.
	Treated body part	TMJ in rest position.
	Therapist	Standing at the head of the plinth if the patient is lying supine or behind the chair of a seated patient.
	Therapist's hands	The hands rest with the palms on either side of the head and the fingers over the jaw so that the fingertips point inferiorly with the fourth fingers resting just behind the mandibular ramus.
Application guidelines	• The guidelines provided are specifically for the presentation in this case study. • The therapist's palms are used to stabilise the head while the proximal parts of the fingers are used to position the mandible to restore comfortable jaw closure when the patient clenches. • Mobilisation directions are performed with respect to the treatment planes of the superior and inferior TMJ. • The left fingers are used to move the left mandibular head slightly anterior in the mandibular fossa (less than 1 mm). Sufficient pressure is used to prevent the mandibular head from moving posteriorly into the painful retrodiscal tissue as the patient slowly closes the jaw. • Subtle changes in the position of the mandibular head in any direction can be made until a position that renders the movement painless is found. • When the mobilisation forces have been applied and maintained, the patient is asked to close the jaw more firmly. • If normal occlusion is possible and pain-free, end of range overpressure is effectively applied by asking the patient to clench lightly. • As a trial treatment, two sets of three movements are performed, and jaw closure is then reassessed. • If the trial treatment is successful, a further 2–3 sets of six movements are performed.	
Comments	• If painful jaw closure has occurred in association with an acute malocclusion, the pain-easing position should coincide with restoration of a comfortable normal 'bite'. • Minimal pressure is required for this technique. • If the occlusion is poor or the teeth are painful, the patient can close against a tongue depressor or a bite plate, but it is important to note that on occasion using the bite plate or the depressor alone (without the MWM) will render the movement pain-free. • If the opposite joint is symptomatic, it may be necessary to apply gentle anterior force to prevent the mandibular head from moving into the painful posterior part of that joint.	
Variation	• The mandibular head of the painful joint may be moved in any direction that renders jaw closure pain-free and restores comfortable occlusion. This may include medial or lateral translation, anterior or posterior translation, and medial or lateral rotation. • The technique can be performed as a self-treatment (Figure 10.5). The patient's hands are positioned over each mandible so that the distal phalanx of the thumb is resting behind the mandibular ramus with the inter-phalangeal joint at the angle of the jaw and the lower border of the mandible resting between the thenar and hypothenar eminences. The fingers will then be pointing in a postero–superior direction so that the index fingers pass over the TMJs. The patient uses the left hand to move the jaw slightly forwards and inferior on the left, while using the right hand to prevent the right mandibular condyle from moving backwards in the right glenoid fossa. The patient is then instructed to follow the guidelines used for the therapist administered technique to render jaw closure painless. If the trial treatment is successful, the patient can perform the self-MWM as a home exercise. If symptoms are acute, initially the self-MWM may be performed up to six times per day with 6 movements each time, progressively reducing frequency as the condition improves. The self-MWM may be used as a maintenance technique 3–4 times per week in chronic conditions. If pain is experienced on jaw closure when eating, one set of 6 self-MWMs should be performed just before each meal. If pain is experienced when eating, the patient can also apply and maintain gentle forward pressure or lateral pressure on the mandibular ramus while chewing.	

was not painful, but application of gentle EOR overpressure elicited mild pain in the left TMJ. Right laterotrusion was slightly limited and produced slight pain in the left TMJ region with application of EOR overpressure.

A TMJ MWM for mouth opening was trialled (Table 10.2 and Figure 10.6). The left deviation was easily controlled and a significant range of pain-free opening was possible. One set of six repetitions with EOR

overpressure was performed resulting in 35 mm range of opening with minimal left deviation at EOR and significantly less left TMJ pain.

Catherine then attempted a TMJ self-MWM for mouth opening (Figure 10.7). The particular technique chosen was 'the scream stretch' as it is most suitable to achieve maximum EOR stretch, and is easy for the patient to perform. Using the self-MWM, Catherine was able to obtain more range than was possible using

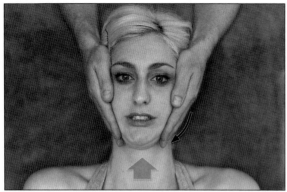

Figure 10.4 TMJ MWM for acute malocclusion and pain on jaw closure

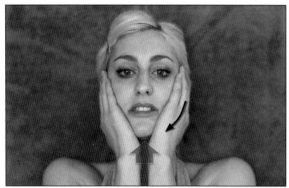

Figure 10.5 TMJ self-MWM for acute malocclusion and pain on jaw closure

the therapist technique. Six TMJ self-MWM scream stretches were performed under supervision and resulted in a further increase in range of mouth opening with minimal deviation to the left from the midline. Maximal tooth contact remained pain-free.

Catherine had demonstrated that she could learn and perform exercises and self-MWM procedures easily and had been diligent in performing these. As the self-treatment technique could be performed at home, it made it possible to perform it more frequently and also reduced financial stress on the patient. Catherine was instructed to perform a set of five TMJ self-MWM scream stretches 1–2 times per day for the next week, reducing to once every second day if the improvement in ROM and pain was sustained. She was also to continue to perform the other exercises. Finally, NAGs were again performed at the cervicodorsal junction and anterior mobilisation techniques at the C4 and C5 levels.

Treatment 5 (4 weeks later)

Catherine was now experiencing only very occasional shooting pain in the left TMJ. She could chew comfortably, but continued to avoid hard food.

On examination, there was only a slight left deviation on opening and much better ROM (40 mm). There was no pain on clenching, and occlusion was probably as good as could be expected with the condition of the teeth. C1–C2 segmental rotation left and right remained symmetrical and asymptomatic.

Catherine was performing the TMJ self-MWM opening and closing techniques well and no modification was required. The cervical mobilisation techniques were repeated as for treatment 4.

Final outcome (12 weeks later)

A 3-month follow-up check was conducted. Catherine had not experienced significant pain, and eating was now very comfortable with a wider range of food options possible. She was instructed to continue a softer food diet and to avoid tearing food in view of the pathological state of the joints.

Jaw movements were of adequate range. The quality of TMJ movement had improved with a reasonable range of translation available in both joints. There was a 'sandy' sensation in the right TMJ on palpation, but no significant clicking.

At one point Catherine had stopped the TMJ self-MWM exercises for 3 weeks and noticed that the pain started to return. When she recommenced the exercises the pain lessened again. In view of this experience and the severity of the joint pathology, it was agreed to continue the exercises on an ongoing basis at least 3–4 days per week.

Considering the radiological examination findings and the severity and duration of symptoms on initial presentation, the outcome to this point was considered satisfactory.

Catherine now had adequate range of jaw opening, relatively pain-free jaw function, no facial pain, minimal neck discomfort and no headaches that could be attributed to the jaw or cervical spine.

The exercises for the neck and jaw were now structured as a maintenance program. The jaw exercises were to be performed 3–4 times per week, with ongoing attention to posture, mouth position, general cardiovascular fitness and strength. Isometric jaw strengthening exercises were given with an emphasis on directions that were weak.

Catherine was reviewed by the ENT surgeon who was now of the opinion that surgical and arthroscopic procedures were not indicated. Plans were made for a prosthodontic opinion on restoration of teeth, but this was dependent on financial considerations.

AUTHOR'S MWM COMMENTARY

Patterns of mandibular movement are entirely different between the upright and the supine lying rest positions,[20] so it is important that, as with MWM techniques for other joints, TMJ MWMs are performed in the upright position where possible.

Table 10.2	TMJ MWM for painful limitation of mandibular depression (see Figure 10.6)	
Indication	**Painful or non-painful limitation of mandibular depression with or without lateral deviation**	
Comment	The limitation may: • be caused by a mild TMJ internal derangement without reduction • remain after spontaneous or therapist reduction of a moderate to severe internal derangement • be due to capsular and/or intra-articular adhesions, or masticatory muscle dysfunction. If the movement limitation Is caused by a modcrate to severe reducible internal derangement, this should be treated using an appropriate MWM technique or another reduction technique such as that described by Okeson.[1] If the cause of the limitation is unknown, a full dental and radiological examination may first be necessary. The technique described is for a more complex presentation than that of the case study: • deflection of the mandible to the left when opening the jaw with restricted range of motion and pain in the left TMJ • limited anterior gliding of the left mandibular head and excessive anterior gliding of the right mandibular head on jaw opening and on accessory movement testing • left mandibular head positioned slightly posteriorly in the mandibular fossa • displacement of the mandibular heads transversely to the left so that on palpation the left head is prominent laterally in the mandibular fossa, and the right mandibular head is recessed medially into the right mandibular fossa.	
Positioning	Patient	Sitting facing mirror.
	Treated body part	TMJ in relaxed rest position.
	Therapist:	Standing behind patient.
	Therapist's hands	The hands lie over the temporalis muscles with the fingers pointing down so that the thumbs lie over the zygomatic arches. The hands and thumbs are used to stabilise the head. The left index finger lies parallel to and just in front of the posterior border of the mandible passing over the TMJ. The left third and fourth fingers are placed behind the posterior border of the ramus of the mandible just above the angle. The right fingers can be located the same as the left, or the index and middle fingers can be placed on the lateral aspect of the body of the mandible just in front of the anterior border of the masseter muscle.
Application guidelines	• The purpose of the technique is to maintain a midline position and maintain correct (or 'best possible' in the case of a permanently deranged joint) anatomical relationships of the TMJ components as the patient fully opens the mouth. • This is achieved by moving the mandible sideways to correct any transverse displacement of the mandibular heads, applying a forward gliding force on the side of the limited anterior glide, and controlling the unrestricted side so that excessive forward gliding is not permitted. • If there is no problem with mouth closure, the patient is then asked to gently clench and relax the jaw several times to lessen muscle tension. • The palmar aspect of the left index finger gently glides the mandible to the right to correct the transverse displacement of the mandibular heads. • While this position is maintained, the patient is instructed to open the jaw while the third and fourth fingers of the left hand apply an anterior translation force (directed anteroinferiorly along the treatment plane of the superior joint) to the left TMJ and the fingers of the right hand prevent excessive anterior gliding of the right TMJ. The combined forces keep the mandible in the midline as it opens. • At end of range, the patient applies overpressure into depression with the fingers of one hand on the chin. No lateral excursion is permitted. The midline position is maintained as the patient releases the overpressure and closes the jaw. • Using the hand located over the chin, the patient can assist by helping to control deflection or deviation from the midline as well as applying overpressure. • The mobilisation is initially performed 3 times then reassessed. Two to three sets of 6 repetitions will often produce a significant change in unassisted movement.	
Comments	• If a reducible derangement is not recognised, application of an inappropriate technique may cause permanent damage to the joint. • A stretching sensation may be reported in the hypomobile joint, but as with all MWMs, no pain should be produced during the technique. • The MWM technique protects the normal or hypermobile joint while allowing fairly strong mobilisation of the limited joint. • It is important to use just enough force to control movement of the opposite normal or hypermobile TMJ, because if excessive posterior force is applied the technique may be painful, particularly if the retrodiscal tissue is sensitive. • If clicking is present in the hypermobile or hypomobile joint, it will often be significantly lessened or eliminated when the technique is being performed and there may be long-term lessening of the clicking. • If muscular forces exerted by the masticatory muscles are too great to be controlled, techniques directed at lessening muscle overactivity may need to be used before applying the MWM technique. • A mirror is very useful for the therapist and patient to monitor the movement of the mandible. It also prepares the patient for home exercises using a mirror. • If the correct movement pathway cannot be maintained, the range of motion during the MWM must be limited to that which can be controlled.	

(Continued)

Table 10.2	TMJ MWM for painful limitation of mandibular depression (see Figure 10.6)—cont'd
Indication	**Painful or non-painful limitation of mandibular depression with or without lateral deviation**
Variation	• An alternative therapist hand position is cradling the mandible between the two hands to control movement. • The technique can be used for painful limitation of movement in other directions, particularly laterotrusive movements. • Once good range and symmetry have been achieved, the patient may be able to perform the technique using their own hands in front of a mirror, as only minimal pressure is required. • If indicated, the technique can be integrated into jaw muscle re-education and resisted isometric exercises, reducing any associated pain. • If full range of mandibular depression cannot be restored using this technique, a self-MWM termed 'the scream stretch' can be used (Figure 10.7). The patient sits facing a mirror with one hand over the mandible so that the deepest part of the first web space is in the midline of the mandible just above the chin, with the lateral border of the index finger running just above the edge of the mandible on one side and the medial aspect of the thumb running just above the edge on the other side. The other hand is placed horizontally over the forehead. The mouth is opened actively as far as possible with the anterior half of the tongue maintaining contact with the roof of the mouth. This should allow no more than 20 mm of opening. When this point is reached, the tongue is lowered and the jaw is opened to comfortable end of range. The hand around the chin is used to correct any deflection or deviation from the midline. If movement cannot be maintained in the midline, do not proceed to the next stage of the MWM. When end-range mandibular depression has been reached, the mandible is held in position by the hand over the jaw. The patient then looks up and actively extends the upper cervical spine so that the jaw opens further. If no pain is experienced and the movement can be maintained in the midline, the hand on the forehead is used to apply gentle overpressure into cervical extension. This stretch is maintained for 2–3 seconds, then the patient looks down and lowers the head to close the jaw. When the head has been lowered to the starting position, the patient releases the hold on the chin and closes the mouth fully. The stretch is repeated 3–4 times. If intraarticular adhesions are limiting jaw opening, the stretch can be repeated 2–3 times per day with 3–6 repetitions each time. If cervical problems are present, they must be treated before this technique can be used.

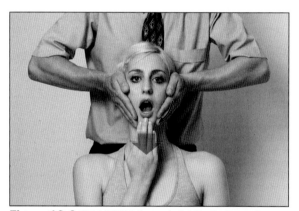

Figure 10.6 TMJ MWM for painful limitation of mandibular depression

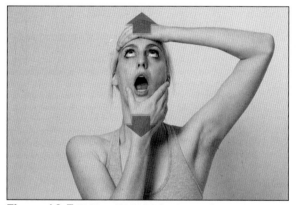

Figure 10.7 TMJ self-MWM for loss of mandibular depression (the scream stretch)

A clear link between neck movement and movement of the jaw has been shown,[21–24] but to date TMJ mobility exercises have not included the cervical spine contribution to TMJ movement. It has been hypothesised that a possible functional significance for the coupling between neck and jaw movements is to extend jaw gape. Cervical spine extension could contribute to a wider jaw gape by reducing tension in the jaw opening muscles and reorientating these muscles so that they obtain a more favourable position for jaw opening.[25] The MWM scream stretch is the only way to achieve full range jaw opening. It also utilises the oculocervical reflex by making the patient look up,

thereby facilitating appropriate activity of the upper cervical extensors and flexors.

The use of the MWM principles to render movement painless can be readily integrated into existing TMJ exercise programs described elsewhere.[26–28] The addition of the MWM component to render the movement painless likely removes masticatory muscle neuromuscular inhibitory mechanisms (see Chapter 7). Once any derangement has been reduced, MWM techniques may also help to maintain correct anatomical relationships between the condylar head and the disc while normal movement patterns are re-established.

References

1 Okeson JP. Management of Temporomandibular Disorders and Occlusion (5th edn). St Louis: Mosby 2003.

2 Mosby's Dental Dictionary (2nd edn). Sydney:Elsevier 2008.

3 Buman A, Lotzmann U, Mah J. TMJ Disorders and Orofacial Pain: the Role of Dentistry in a Multidisciplinary Diagnostic Approach. Sydney:Elsevier 2002.

4 von Piekartz H. Craniofacial Pain: Neuromusculoskeletal Assessment, Treatment and Management. Edinburgh: Butterworth-Heinemann 2007.

5 Dvorak J, Antinnes JA, Panjabi M, et al. Age and gender related normal motion of the cervical spine. Spine. 1992;17(10 Suppl):S393–8.

6 Ishii M, Koide K, Ueki M, et al. Influence of body and head posture on deviation of the incisal point undergoing dental treatment. Prosthodontic Research & Practice. 2007;6(4):217–24.

7 Makofsky HW, Sexton TR, Diamond DZ, et al. The effect of head posture on muscle contact position using the T-Scan system of occlusal analysis. Cranio. 1991;9(4):316–21.

8 Visscher CM, Huddleston Slater JJ, Lobbezoo F, et al. Kinematics of the human mandible for different head postures. Journal of Oral Rehabilitation. 2000;27(4):299–305.

9 Yamada R, Ogawa T, Koyano K. The effect of head posture on direction and stability of mandibular closing movement. Journal of Oral Rehabilitation. 1999;26(6):511–20.

10 Broton JG, Sessle BJ. Reflex excitation of masticatory muscles induced by algesic chemicals applied to the temporomandibular joint of the cat. Archives of Oral Biology. 1988;33(10):741–7.

11 Lund JP, Olsen KA. The importance of reflexes and their control during jaw movement. Trends in Neurosciences. 1983;6:458–63.

12 Smith AM. The coactivation of antagonist muscles. Canadian Journal of Physiology and Pharmacology 1981;59:733–47.

13 Stohler C, Yamada Y, Ash MM, Jr. Antagonistic muscle stiffness and associated reflex behaviour in the pain-dysfunctional state. Schweiz Monatsschr Zahnmed. 1985;95(8):719–26.

14 Okeson JP. Bell's Orofacial Pains (5th edn). Chicago: Quintessence Publishing 1995.

15 Hu JW, Yu XM, Vernon H, et al. Excitatory effects on neck and jaw muscle activity of inflammatory irritant applied to cervical paraspinal tissues. Pain. 1993;55(2):243–50.

16 Bogduk N. Headache and the neck. In: Goadsby PJ, Silberstein SD (eds) Headache. Boston: Butterworth-Heinemann 1997:369–81.

17 Bell WE. Temporomandibular Disorders (3rd edn). Chicago: Year Book Medical Publishers 1993.

18 Simons DG, Travell JG, Simons LS. Travell & Simons' Myofascial Pain and Dysfunction: the Trigger Point Manual (vol 1): Upper Half of the Body (2nd edn). Philadelphia: Lippincott Williams and Wilkins 1999.

19 Snodgrass SJ, Rivett DA, Robertson VJ. Manual forces applied during cervical mobilization. Journal of Manipulative and Physiological Therapeutics. 2007;30(1): 17–25.

20 Tingey EM, Buschang PH, Throckmorton GS. Mandibular rest position: a reliable position influenced by head support and body posture. American Journal of Orthodontics and Dentofacial Orthopedics. 2001;120(6): 614–22.

21 Eriksson PO, Haggman-Henrikson B, Nordh E, Zafar H. Co-ordinated mandibular and head-neck movements during rhythmic jaw activities in man. Journal of Dental Research. 2000;79(6):1378–84.

22 Eriksson PO, Zafar H, Nordh E. Concomitant mandibular and head-neck movements during jaw opening-closing in man. Journal of Oral Rehabilitation. 1998;25(11):859–70.

23 Haggman-Henrikson B, Nordh E, Zafar H, Eriksson PO. Head immobilization can impair jaw function. Journal of Dental Research. 2006;85(11):1001–5.

24 Yamabe Y, Yamashita R, Fujii H. Head, neck and trunk movements accompanying jaw tapping. Journal of Oral Rehabilitation. 1999;26(11):900–5.

25 Koolstra JH, van Eijden TM. Functional significance of the coupling between head and jaw movements. Journal of Biomechanics. 2004;37(9):1387–92.

26 Kraus SL. Physical therapy management of TMD. In: Kraus SL (ed.) Clinics in Physical Therapy: Temporomandibular Disorders (2nd edn). New York: Churchill Livingstone 1994.

27 Morrone L, Makofsky HW. TMJ home exercise program. Clinical Management in Physical Therapy 1991;11(2):20–6.

28 Rocabado M, Iglarsh ZA. Musculoskeletal Approach to Maxillofacial Pain. New York: Lippincott 1991.

Chapter 11
Golfer's back: resolution of chronic thoracic spine pain

Stephen Edmondston

HISTORY

David was referred by a sports medicine physician who he had consulted in relation to chronic, unilateral mid-thoracic pain. He was aged 42 years at the time of referral, was married with two young children and worked full-time as an administrator. He was a keen recreational runner who had completed five marathons, and played golf socially about twice a month.

Previous history

Nine months prior to his referral, he had been playing golf. On the eighth tee he hit a drive (right-handed golfer) and felt a sudden onset of sharp pain in the mid-thoracic spine during the follow-through phase of the swing. The pain initially felt centrally located but by the end of the day was predominantly right-sided. David was unable to continue playing due to the sharp pain associated with any attempt to swing the club. David described the pain during the first week after his injury as a moderate, constant ache, with bursts of more severe pain with activities which required reaching across the body or overhead, or rotation of his neck to the symptomatic side (such as reversing the car). He did not require any time off work.

After 2 weeks the constant ache had eased but was still present, as was the pain with movement. At that time he attempted to return to golf and running but found his thoracic pain was immediately aggravated to the extent that he could not continue. David was prescribed oral anti-inflammatory medication by his general practitioner, which he took for the first 2 months after the injury. After 4 months he had eight chiropractic treatments but did not notice any significant change in his symptoms and did not continue. David did not seek any further medical opinion or physical treatment prior to his consultation with the sports physician.

Current presentation

At the initial physiotherapy consultation, David described a constant low-grade ache in the right mid-thoracic region (Figure 11.1). The ache was generally less intense in the morning but increased during the day, especially when sitting at work (5/10 maximum on a verbal pain scale). He had no pain at night and described a feeling of 'stiffness' in the symptomatic region, which was slightly worse on waking in the morning. David indicated that he could perform most activities of daily living without much pain provocation, although he tended to move cautiously and avoid quick movements.

Symptom behaviour

Sustained sitting would increase the ache to a moderate level but did not limit David's capacity to sit or perform his work activities. Although David had no respiratory pain or pain with walking, he was still unable to run due to the immediate onset of his thoracic pain, which would get worse if he continued and he was also unable to play golf due to the pain associated with his attempts to swing the club. His pain would ease to the baseline intensity within 5 minutes if provoked by these activities. His ache was eased by moving into thoracic flexion and was completely relieved by lying down for 15 minutes. David described feeling that his back needed movement or 'stretching', but he had been unable to do this in a way that had made any long-term change to his disorder.

Medical history and investigations

David was currently not taking any medication for this thoracic pain, or any other prescribed medication. His plain X-rays showed diffuse early degenerative changes, specifically anterior vertebral body lipping which was most prominent between T3 and T7. He had not had any other medical or radiological investigations of his current symptoms. David had no previous history of thoracic pain but had experienced an episode of acute low back pain (LBP) playing soccer 2 years ago. That episode had ultimately settled but had taken a number of months to fully resolve. Screening in relation to thoracic pain 'red flags' was negative.

David indicated that his motivation for seeking further treatment was to determine whether there was anything which could be done to help improve his back

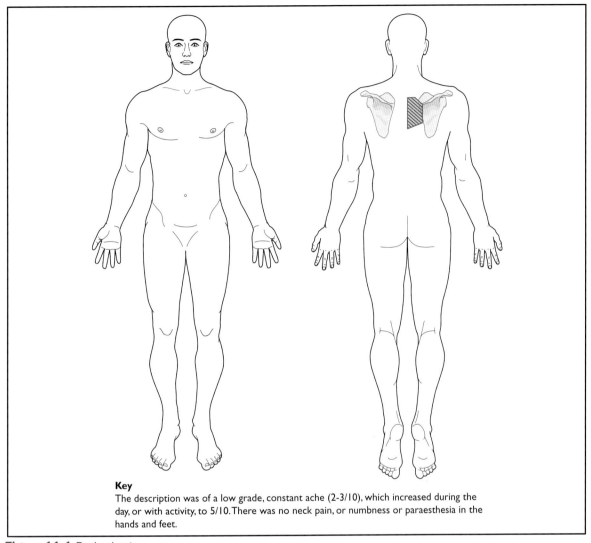

Key
The description was of a low grade, constant ache (2-3/10), which increased during the day, or with activity, to 5/10. There was no neck pain, or numbness or paraesthesia in the hands and feet.

Figure 11.1 Body chart

problem. In particular, his goals were to return to running and golf.

EVIDENCE-INFORMED CLINICAL REASONING

1 What were the key diagnostic case features at this stage with respect to recognising any clinical pattern?

Clinician's response
The key diagnostic features from the history include:

- Mechanism of injury — suggests a tissue 'sprain' due to mechanical overload (golf swing). The mechanics of the golf swing may have been a factor in the development of the injury, and could also be important in relation to recurrence.

- Symptom history — suggests recovery from acute pain, but non-resolution of abnormal tissue physiology; that is, inflammation causing ongoing pain and incomplete recovery of thoracic mechanics.
- Unilateral pain location with good localisation — indicative (but not definitive) of a posterior element pain source.[1]
- Symptom behaviour linked to mechanical function — some pain provoked by static loading (sitting), but more readily by dynamic loading (running) and movement (golf).
- X-ray findings — mild disc degeneration is common in people this age and poorly correlated with the presence of symptoms.[2] However, disc degeneration is likely to influence segmental mobility and tolerance of the motion segment to high rates or magnitudes of loading (single or repetitive).[3, 4]

2 Did you consider any additional non-diagnostic thoughts? Did you hypothesise beyond diagnosis?

Clinician's response

Additional thoughts not directly related to diagnosis included:

- David requires a logical explanation as to the reason for his ongoing pain and functional limitation. He seems motivated to assist his recovery.
- Treatment goals have been clearly defined by David and seem appropriate based on the history provided.
- Poor response of this injury to physical treatment (chiropractic) may be important in relation to prognosis. Full details of that treatment were not available, but it appears that David was not provided with any clear plan in relation to exercise and related self-management.
- Slow resolution of the previous LBP episode may have prognostic significance for this injury.

PHYSICAL EXAMINATION

Posture

In standing, there was no obvious frontal plane deformity (antalgic or structural) or asymmetry of extensor muscle activity or bulk. In the sagittal plane, the mid-thoracic spine appeared mildly hyper-kyphotic but this was not due to pain avoidance. In sitting, David had an habitual relaxed posture which promoted end-range thoracolumbar flexion. He found this posture comfortable, and his pain was mildly provoked when asked to sit more upright. The pain with sitting in a more upright posture may have been due to a limitation of motion in the symptomatic segments of the spine, or the increase in load associated with the extensor muscle contraction. His thoracolumbar posture correction was a global movement, driven by his long erector spinae muscles.

Active movements

All active movements were examined in sitting. Thoracic flexion was full range and pain-free (easing). Extension was pain-limited and associated with significant reproduction of the right thoracic spine pain. Right rotation was similarly pain-limited to about 25° (observational measurement), with a flattening of the characteristic 'S' curve in the mid-thoracic region.[3] This movement was more limited and painful when performed with the arms fully elevated. Left rotation was about 45° and did not produce pain, although David described a feeling of tightness in the area of pain at the end of range. Right lateral flexion reproduced mild local pain, and was mildly restricted with an observed decrease in the mid-thoracic contribution to the range. Left lateral flexion was not obviously restricted but was associated with right-sided 'tightness' with overpressure. Inspiration at the end of the available ranges of extension and right rotation caused a further (mild) increase in the thoracic pain.

Isometric muscle tests

When tested in the neutral spine position, isometric testing of rotation in both directions produced minimal discomfort. When tested at the end of the available pain-free range of right rotation there was moderate reproduction of the right thoracic pain, but not when tested in left rotation. Isometric testing of extension in the neutral position also reproduced the right-sided thoracic pain at a moderate intensity.

Palpation and passive accessory motion tests

There was significant tenderness and reactivity to palpation in the paravertebral musculature in the area of pain. There was increased tenderness of the T3 to T5 spinous processes compared to adjacent levels. The corresponding right costo-transverse junctions (ribs 3 to 5) were very sensitive to palpation, as were ribs 3 to 5 on the right when palpated over the postero-medial aspect. Rib 4 on the right and the related costo-transverse junction were more sensitive than the adjacent levels.

Tests of postero–anterior (PA) 'accessory' intervertebral motion could not be performed for the T3 to T5 spinal segments due to the tenderness provoked with palpation through the paravertebral muscles. Similarly, PA force could not be applied to the right ribs 3 to 5 due to local tenderness. With care, gliding movements of these ribs could be tested in the cephalad-lateral and caudad-medial directions. The key finding was a significant restriction of caudad-medial gliding of ribs 4 and 5 compared to that of the comparable left ribs.

Passive physiological motion tests

Testing was performed only in those directions identified as restricted in the active movement examination. Segmental rotation (assessed in side-lying) was moderately restricted to the right at T3–T4 and T4–T5. In sitting, right lateral flexion was mildly restricted, while the movement into extension was very limited at all segments from T3–T4 to T5–T6. Posterior rotation of the right ribs 4 and 5 was also restricted when tested passively with right thoracic spine rotation in sitting. Examination of rib rotation is performed by palpation of the posterior aspect of the rib during passive rotation of the thorax while seated.

Neural tissue provocation tests

There was no pain reproduction with full neck and thoracic flexion in sitting. Similarly, there was no symptom reproduction in the full slump position with either unilateral or bilateral knee extension.

EVIDENCE-INFORMED CLINICAL REASONING

1 What were the key findings from the physical examination and how did they assist your diagnostic reasoning?

Clinician's response

The key findings from physical testing included:

- Movement impairment to the symptomatic side with pain provocation, especially right rotation and extension. Pain relief in flexion is probably due to 'unloading' of painful structures (if sustained the altered patterns of load transfer within the symptomatic segment are likely to provoke pain as pain was provoked with sustained sitting). The localised pain location and consistent pain/movement pattern may be indicative of an articular pain source, most likely involving the posterior joints (e.g. facet or costo-transverse). Examination of combined movements was not performed initially due to the irritability of David's symptoms, and that consistent movement impairments related to the symptoms had been identified with the uni-directional movements.
- Seated trunk rotation in shoulder elevation isolates movement more in the mid-thoracic segments. This test may assist in the identification of pain-related movement impairment in this region of the thoracic spine, as the associated spinal extension will constrain movement in the low thoracic region.
- Tightness associated with left rotation and lateral flexion may represent decreased soft tissue extensibility in the symptomatic region of the thorax.
- Where muscle is a significant pain source it would be expected that pain would be reproduced with isometric tests in the neutral position. The pain provocation associated with isometric testing towards the end of range in the painful directions is likely to be due to increased spinal loading. The vertical orientation of the thoracic extensor muscles produces compressive loading of the related vertebral segments.

2 What were your primary hypotheses at the end of the physical examination? How did these relate to your plans for management?

Clinician's response

Identification of a specific pain (structural) source is difficult for spinal pain disorders.[5] In the thoracic spine, identification is even more difficult as it is not possible to directly palpate either the costo-vertebral or the costo-transverse joints as they are located anterior to the transverse process. Furthermore, passive accessory motion tests which apply force to the rib will influence both joints so it is not possible to determine which joint is the pain source on the basis of these tests. Dif-ferentiation may be assisted through correlation with nuclear medicine imaging such as a bone scan.

Despite this, it would be reasonable to hypothesise that David has a chronic sprain injury, most likely involving structures associated with the T3–T4 to T5–T6 spinal segments and/or related rib joints. This is based on the history of a specific injury event, localisation of symptoms and physical examination findings. The dominant impairment of spinal function is that of mobility in which pain is associated with three mechanically linked directions of movement and relieved by movement in the opposite direction. The postural loading component of David's pain would be considered secondary in the interpretation of the disorder but is an important consideration in the overall management plan.

The ongoing symptoms could be due to the non-resolution of abnormal tissue physiology which was a response to the initial injury. Since tissue physiology is strongly influenced by mechanical factors,[6] the inability of the patient to independently restore normal spinal mechanics may be the stimulus for the ongoing abnormal tissue physiology and associated pain.

Physical treatment is indicated based on this interpretation of the disorder and the absence of features which would contraindicate treatment of this nature (red flags). Passive or assisted mobilisation of the thorax in directions which David cannot achieve independently could be considered a positive stimulus to assist the recovery of active movement, and consequently the resolution of abnormal tissue physiology. While the abnormal thoracic mechanics may be a key factor contributing to the ongoing symptoms, it is also important that David's limited understanding of the disorder and strategies for self-management are addressed. These later elements of the management plan may not have been addressed adequately in David's previous chiropractic treatment.

TREATMENT AND MANAGEMENT

Treatment 1

The first priority was to provide David with an explanation of the diagnosis and some thoughts as to why his injury had not resolved. This formed the basis for an explanation of the treatment plan and how this would help him. In particular, the importance of David's active participation in management was stressed, additional to treatment in the clinic. It was also indicated that while it was likely that the treatment would have a favourable outcome, it was not possible to be certain of that given the symptom duration, plateau in recovery and poor response to previous physical treatment.

The primary objective of the physical treatment was to improve the impairments of thoracic spine mobility. A key consideration was the high level of sensitivity of the soft tissues overlying the hypomobile segments. The initial approach was to use longitudinal and transverse soft tissue massage to the paravertebral muscles in the symptomatic region. During this part of the treatment David reported a gradual decrease in the local tenderness and there was a palpable associated relaxation of the paravertebral muscles in response to this technique. On reassessment, the tightness felt with active left rotation had improved but there was no change in right rotation.

The initial approach to treating the right rotation restriction was to use a Mobilisation with Movement (MWM) with hand contact over the 4th rib (Figure 11.2 and Table 11.1). It was felt that this would be a more comfortable technique than one which required a direct oscillatory force or application of direct pressure to the symptomatic structures. It was also considered useful to see how readily the movement restriction could be changed with the spine loaded in sitting. The biomechanical rationale for selecting this technique is that the force applied to the rib will modify the starting position prior to the movement. This would assist the restoration of the normal pattern of posterior rib rotation and related caudad glide at the costo-transverse joint.

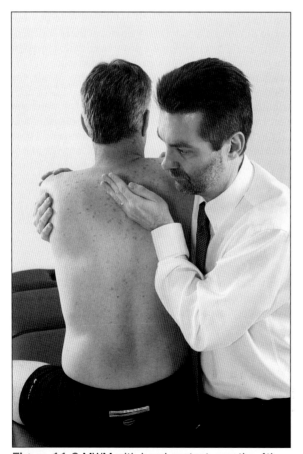

Figure 11.2 MWM with hand contact over the 4th rib

During application of the MWM David was able to achieve about 40° of right rotation range prior to the onset of pain. The technique was repeated six times (up to the point of pain) and on reassessment the rotation range achieved during the MWM was maintained on active movement. However the range of active thoracic spine extension was unchanged on reassessment. David reported an increase in the resting ache at this point so no further mobilisation was performed in this treatment session. To help maintain the improvement in right rotation, David was shown a rotation mobility exercise in four-point kneeling to perform twice per day at home with six repetitions on each occasion (Figure 11.3). This exercise position was chosen as the compressive load on the spine is reduced during the movement, and the patient is able to stretch more passively into the movement restriction. David was also encouraged to continue with his usual level of activity and to take note of any changes in his symptoms.

Treatment 2

Four days later David reported experiencing a slight increase in his thoracic ache following the previous treatment, but this had recovered to the usual level by the next day. He had performed the rotation exercise as instructed and had felt generally less stiffness and pain with movement. The pain associated with sitting was about the same.

On examination, thoracic right rotation was now 40° with the onset of mild pain at end-range, but the extension range of motion (ROM) and pain response were unchanged. Left thoracic rotation was now full range with no 'tightness' felt at end of range. The tenderness over the paravertebral muscles had decreased and it was possible to apply a unilateral PA force over the right T4 and T5 transverse processes. Movement in response to this PA force (applied via the ulnar border of the hand) was markedly less than that achieved with the same test on the left side.

Given the evident improvement in the thoracic movement impairment disorder, the initial treatment in this session was to repeat the right rotation MWM to rib 4. During this application it was possible for David to achieve full range of right rotation without pain. Two sets of six repetitions of this technique were applied, after which active right rotation had improved to full range without pain, although there was still mild pain with overpressure. Thoracic extension had not improved compared to the initial examination so an extension MWM to rib 4 was applied. This did not produce any change in the range of extension and a similar response occurred with an MWM applied to rib 5. As the paravertebral tissue tenderness had improved, a thoracic spine Sustained Natural Apophyseal Glide (SNAG) was attempted for extension with contact under the right transverse process of T4 (Figure 11.4). With this technique, David was able to extend fully with pain only

Table 11.1	Thoracic SNAG	
Indication	**Pain and/or loss of movement during thoracic spine movement**	
Positioning	Patient	Patient sitting astride the treatment table facing away from the therapist.
	Treated body part	Thoracic spine in neutral.
	Therapist	Standing behind the patient on the symptomatic side.
	Therapist's hands	*Stabilising hand*: forearm placed anteriorly over the chest, at approximately the vertical position of the symptomatic level. This arm assists the vertical force from the gliding hand. *Gliding hand*: the hypothenar eminence is placed between the ribs contacting the transverse process on the symptomatic side.
Application guidelines	• Force generated through the gliding and stabilising hands must be directed up along the vertically orientated facet joint plane. • Hand contact tenderness can be minimised by the use of sponge rubber. • Ask the patient to perform the painful or restricted movement but stop at the onset of pain, to avoid forcing a painful movement. A positive treatment outcome is to significantly improve the restricted range without pain. • As a precaution, apply gentle gliding force initially, particularly if the disorder is acute. Stronger gliding force is usually required when the thoracic movement is limited by stiffness more than pain. If the patient's movement is not completely pain-free, stronger gliding force can be employed. • Try altering the angle of force if pain-free rotation cannot be obtained. Variations in normal anatomy may dictate a change in direction of gliding force. • Change the thoracic vertebral level at which the SNAG is applied if the movement is either unchanged or if it is made worse on the first application. • Attempt no more than four trials to obtain pain-free movement, as failure to relieve pain over this number of trials will prove counterproductive. • Repeat the movement 6–10 times once pain-free movement is achieved. • Subsequent reassessment should reveal a significant improvement in pain-free range of thoracic movement. • Three to five sets of further repetitions can be performed depending on the severity, irritability and nature of the disorder.	
Comments	• Maintain the glide force throughout the movement until the patient returns to the starting position. • It is important to encourage the patient to achieve the maximum end-range position where overpressure may be applied if necessary.	
Variations	• The contact point of the gliding hand for application of the thoracic SNAG can be the transverse process, spinous process or rib (Figures 11.2 and 11.4). • Once full range active movement is achieved with overpressure, the thoracic SNAG technique can be performed in a combined or out of neutral position. An example of this would be extension in a starting position of rotation. • Self-treatment techniques (Figure 11.5) are very important to reinforce the effectiveness of the SNAGs used in the clinic. A thoracic self-SNAG requires the use of a self-treatment strap or narrow cloth strip. The purpose of the strap is to replicate the gliding force provided by the therapist's hand at the spinous process of the involved level. The patient pulls upward and forward on the strap, following the facet joint plane, with the strap positioned beneath the symptomatic level. The thoracic self-SNAG is best performed in sitting (Figure 11.5). The exercise must be repeated 10 times at least three times per day.	

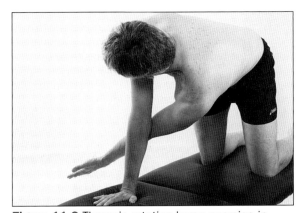

Figure 11.3 Thoracic rotation home exercise in four-point kneeling position

at the extreme of range. The T4 unilateral SNAG was repeated six times, and the range of extension achieved during treatment was maintained on reassessment of active extension. The treatment did not produce any increase in the pain at rest. David was shown a localised thoracic extension stretch in supine lying, and asked to perform this six times twice per day, in addition to the rotation exercise prescribed in Treatment 1. It was also suggested that David try a short run to see if there was any change in the pain response to this activity.

Treatment 3

One week later, David reported he had not experienced any exacerbation of his symptoms following the previous treatment, and that the pain associated

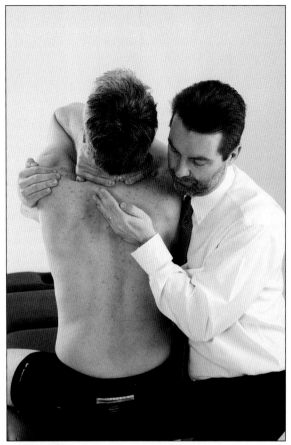

Figure 11.4 Thoracic extension SNAG with contact under the right transverse process of T4

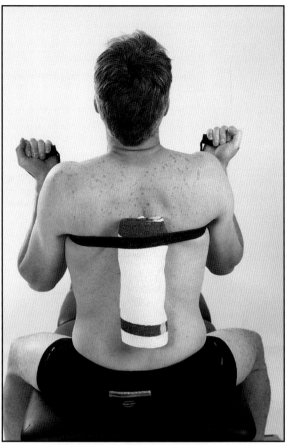

Figure 11.5 Thoracic extension SNAG as a home exercise using a mobilisation strap

with sitting had decreased. He also considered there was some improvement in the feeling of thoracic stiffness described in his initial history. David had completed two runs of about 5 minutes duration and experienced no pain during or after each run. He had attempted the extension mobility exercise but found it was too uncomfortable to perform and had stopped doing it. The rotation exercise had been continued without any problems. On examination David had mild end-range pain with active right thoracic rotation and no pain with left rotation. Thoracic extension was still limited by pain of moderate severity, but the range achieved at the end of the previous treatment had been retained.

The extension SNAG to the right T4 transverse process was repeated and David was able to extend fully with mild pain at the extreme of range. The technique was repeated six times after which the active extension range was improved to the same extent as that achieved during the application of the technique. A further set of six repetitions resolved the end-range pain during the application of the SNAG, but the pain persisted on active reassessment of extension. At this

stage, David was taught a self-SNAG with the force applied to the T4 spinous process[7] (Figure 11.5). Using this technique David was able to extend to end-range with no pain, but the response was still not retained on active movement testing after five repetitions of the technique.

On passive accessory movement examination, the movement response to a PA force over the right T4 transverse process was still limited compared to that on the left side. Given the positive response to mobilisation and the regular pattern of movement impairment, the indications were present for the application of a manipulative thrust technique.[8] It is proposed that the manipulative thrust technique might cause a transient increase in joint volume, and an associated increase in ROM.[9] After an explanation of the technique, a high-velocity thrust was applied in supine lying to the T4–T5 motion segment.[10] On reassessment, the end-range pain was still present with extension, but at a reduced intensity to that reported prior to the manipulation. David was advised to continue the self-SNAG at home using six repetitions, three times per day. Since his main activity limitations now were his sporting activities, it was suggested he increase his running frequency and duration, as his fitness allowed, in order to determine the symptom response. He was advised not to play golf until after the next review.

Treatment 4

David had followed the self-SNAG treatment advice since the last treatment session 2 weeks previously and noticed a gradual decrease in the pain with end-range extension. His pain in sitting and at the end of the day had resolved, as had the feeling of stiffness in his thoracic spine. He had run on alternate days for up to 30 minutes and had not experienced any pain at all.

On examination, David had full range rotation in both directions with no pain. He still had mild pain at the extreme of active extension. The movement response to PA pressure over the right T4 transverse process was still slightly restricted with a firm end-feel, but minimal pain. The extension SNAG was modified by positioning David's thoracic spine into slight right rotation prior to asking him to move into extension (Figure 11.6). The extension SNAG, which relieved the end-range pain, was repeated six times in slight

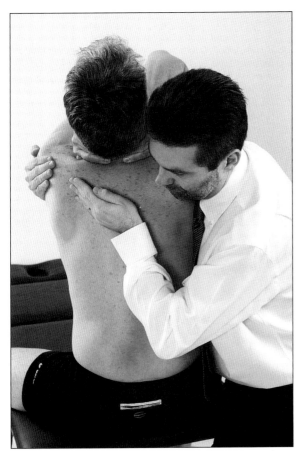

Figure 11.6 Thoracic extension SNAG commencing from slight right rotation

right rotation. On reassessment, active extension was now full range and without pain. The technique was repeated and on the final reassessment extension was still full range and without pain, as were active movements into rotation. The high velocity thrust technique applied in supine lying to T4–T5 was repeated at the end of this treatment session.

David was shown how to modify his extension self-SNAG to include the rotation component and asked to continue this exercise at home using six repetitions, once per day. He was also advised to continue to progress the duration of his running and note any pain response. As David was keen to play golf it was suggested he try some slow practice swings at home, initially without a ball. If this did not cause any pain, he was to hit a few balls at the practice range to determine the response during and after this exercise. On the basis that this could be achieved, it was agreed that he could return to play nine holes of social golf.

Final outcome

David was reviewed 3 weeks later and had played golf twice since his last treatment. He reported no pain when playing but some soreness in the area of his injury after the first game, but this was less obvious after his second game. David had continued with the extension self-SNAG with decreasing frequency, and found this exercise useful in maintaining his pain-free range. He had continued running without pain and had no pain at the end of his workday.

On physical examination, David now had full range of active movement in all directions with no pain during or at the end of ROM. There was still some tenderness to palpation over the right costo-transverse junctions at T4 and T5, but the movement response to PA force applied over the transverse processes and ribs was now similar to that identified on the left side.

David returned to the clinic 2 months later with acute LBP which had developed when pushing a wheelbarrow full of sand. While he was in considerable discomfort in his lumbar spine, he indicated that he had experienced no problems with his thoracic spine.

AUTHORS' MWM COMMENTARY

The sprain injury which David sustained while playing golf, would have resulted in physiological responses (inflammation) both within the joint and in the related extra-articular tissues.[11, 12] While this is a normal response to injury, it would be expected that resolution of such a response would occur within 2–3 weeks.[13] The mechanical environment within which healing tissues function is likely to be an important factor in the resolution of the abnormal tissue physiology and associated symptoms.[14, 15] The inability of the patient to independently restore normal mechanical function, due to pain or changes in tissue mechanics, may be a contributing factor in the non-resolution of the abnormal tissue physiology and associated pain (see Chapters 6 and 7 for related information).

The initial selection of the MWM technique was based on two key issues in David's clinical presentation. Firstly, the pain-related functional limitations (i.e. running and golf) require thoracic movement under load-bearing conditions. Secondly, the high level of local tenderness in the region of the symptomatic segments made the application of effective passive mobilisation techniques very difficult. The MWM techniques address both of these issues as they are applied under physiological loading conditions, and with a sustained mobilisation force, which can be applied to minimise contact discomfort. Experience in the application of MWMs in the thorax suggests that impairments of rib mobility should be addressed before treating the related spinal segment. However, consideration should also be given to the relative degree of restriction of spinal and rib mobility.

It is hypothesised that the MWM and SNAG techniques included in David's treatment were the stimulus for the recovery of normal mechanical function of the injured structures, and consequently the resolution of the abnormal tissue physiology and associated pain (see Chapters 5–7 for further information). While this hypothesis is based on current knowledge of tissue biology, it requires considerable further evaluation in laboratory and clinical studies.

References

1 Dreyfuss P, Tibiletti C, Dreyer S. Thoracic zygapophyseal joint pain patterns. A study in normal volunteers. Spine. 1994;19(7):807–11.

2 Girard C, Schweitzer M, Morrison W, et al. Thoracic spine disc-related abnormalities: longitudinal MR imaging assessment. Skeletal Radiology 2004;33(4):216–22.

3 Edmondston S. Clinical biomechanics of the thoracic spine including the ribcage. In: Boyling J, Jull G (eds) Grieve's Modern Manual Therapy (3rd edn). Edinburgh: Churchill Livingstone 2004:55–65.

4 Lotz J, Hsieh A, Walsh A, et al. Mechanobiology of the intervertebral disc. Biochemical Society Transactions 2002;30(6): 853–8.

5 Chou R, Qaseem A, Snow V, et al. Diagnosis and treatment of low back pain: a joint clinical practice guideline from the American College of Physicians and the American Pain Society. Annals Internal Medicine. 2007;147(7):478–91.

6 Adams M, Dolan P. Spine biomechanics. Journal of Biomechanics. 2005;38(10):1972–193.

7 Austin G, Benesky W. Thoracic pain in a collegiate runner. Manual Therapy 2002;7(3):168–72.

8 Hing W, Reid D, Monaghan M. Manipulation of the cervical spine. Manual Therapy 2003;8(1):2–9.

9 Gibbons P, Tehan P. Manipulation of the spine, thorax and pelvis — an osteopathic perspective (2nd edn). Edinburgh: Churchill-Livingstone. 2005.

10 Monaghan M. Spinal Manipulation: a Manual for Physiotherapists. Nelson: Aesculapius 2001.

11 Muto T, Shigeo K, Kanazawa M, et al. Ultrastructural study of synovitis induced by trauma to the rat temporomandibular joint (TMJ). Journal of Oral Pathology and Medicine. 2003;32(1):25–33.

12 Woo S-Y, Abramowitch S, Kilger RL, et al. Biomechanics of knee ligaments: injury, healing, and repair. Journal of Biomechanics. 2006;39(1):1–20.

13 Kannus P, Parkkari J, Jarvinen T, et al. Basic science and clinical studies coincide: active treatment approach is needed after sports injury. Scandinavian Journal of Medicine and Science in Sports. 2003;13:(3)50–4.

14 Buckwalter J, Grodzinsky A. Loading of healing bone, fibrous tissue, and muscle: implications for orthopaedic practice. Journal of the American Acadamy of Orthopaedic Surgeons. 1999;7(5):291–9.

15 Pitsillides A, Skerry T, Edwards J. Joint immobilization reduces synovial fluid hyaluronan concentration and is accompanied by changes in the synovial intimal cell populations. Rheumatology. 1999;38(11):1108–12.

Chapter 12
Mobilisation with Movement in the management of swimmer's shoulder

Pamela Teys and Bill Vicenzino

HISTORY

Janet was a 26-year-old female who presented with a 6 week history of unresolved right-sided anterolateral shoulder pain following a return to swimming of 1500 metres a day for 1 week. Freestyle stroke and associated drills predominated in these sessions. She had previously not been swimming for 2 years. Janet undertook no treatment apart from cessation from swimming during those 6 weeks.

Her swim practise and competition history revealed that she had been an elite national level Canadian swimmer from the age of 16 years. She had been swimming competitively since she was 10 years old and first noticed the onset of shoulder pain when she was moved to senior squad at 13 years of age. This move included a significant increase in training to two daily sessions covering 10–12 kilometres per day. She increased the number of training days and her primary stroke was freestyle.

Symptom behaviour

On initial presentation to our clinic, the patient reported a constant deep ache over the anterolateral aspect of her right shoulder that she rated as 3/10 on a visual analogue scale (VAS) (Figure 12.1). This increased to a sharp pain rated 9/10 on a VAS when she attempted any overhead activities. She also reported intermittent numbness and pins and needles down her right arm if she slept on her right side, which subsided in 5 minutes upon changing position.

EVIDENCE-INFORMED CLINICAL REASONING

1 At the end of the interview, what were your thoughts or hypotheses regarding Janet's shoulder pain?

Clinician's response

The presenting symptoms and their behaviour are consistent with an unaccustomed overuse injury of the shoulder, with impingement of the structures within the subacromial space, especially the supraspinatus tendon. There is very little space for the rotator cuff muscles and subacromial bursa, especially when the arm is in the overhead position, as in swimming, where they can be compromised with repetitive movement. Pins and needles are not uncommon symptoms and are thought to occur in the presence of anterior capsule laxity whereby the humeral head shifts forward and compromises the neural structures from the brachial plexus.

2 Given the information from the history did you have any treatment and prognosis hypotheses under consideration at this early stage? If so, what factors in the patient's history, based on your experience and scientific evidence, support your treatment hypothesis?

Clinician's response

Swim training involves highly repetitive loading of the muscles of the upper limb, specifically the rotator cuff muscles. A commonly accepted notion in sports medicine is that a previous injury predisposes the athlete to another injury. The exact mechanism for this is not known but changes to motor control and to soft tissues about a joint are frequent sequelae following pain and injury. These may be the mediators for further problems down the track.

In our experience it is not uncommon for people who have performed at an elite or a high level in sport to overestimate (or to not think about) their capacity to recommence the sport after a long time away from that sport. Janet is characteristic of this in that she resumed swimming 1500 metres per day without any build up. While this distance is much less than she was used to doing when she last practised swimming, it transpired to be sufficiently excessive to create issues. It is likely that going from no swimming to this distance per day, without a day off to allow for the body to recover and adapt to the imposed physical demands, was in part responsible for her shoulder problem.

PHYSICAL EXAMINATION

On observation, the right humeral head appeared slightly anterior compared to the left humeral head on a base of bilaterally protracted, abducted and internally rotated scapulae. There was a mild flattening of the mid thoracic spine region; that is, she presented

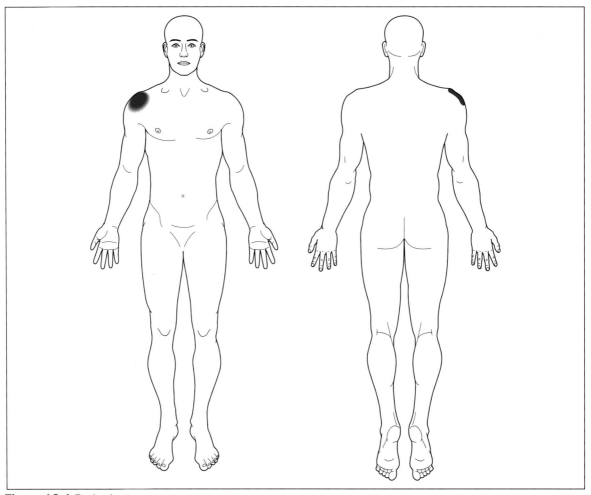

Figure 12.1 Body chart

with a relatively typical swimmer's shoulder-thorax region posture. Active range of motion (ROM) testing revealed limited external rotation (performed in neutral elevation) on the right with 25° to pain onset compared to 65° on the left. Shoulder abduction was 85° to pain onset and limited to 110° (3/10 pain), but there was full range of flexion with some minimal pain at end of range. Hand behind back as measured by the spinal level the wrist could reach was T6 on the right and T2 on the left. Palpation of the supraspinatus tendon and soft tissues of the anterior and anterolateral glenohumeral joint elicited the patient's pain (~6/10). Muscle contraction tests in abduction and internal rotation reproduced pain (5/10) as did the empty can test. The reverse can test was negative. Muscle length tests revealed a tight pectoralis minor bilaterally and some tightness of the right latissimus dorsi. There was 30° of isolated internal rotation available when performed in 90° of abduction, compared to 60° on the left side.

Pain was also reproduced with impingement tests of Neer and Hawkins-Kennedy. Accessory glide testing in the plane of the glenoid (load and shift test of Hawkins[1, 2]) revealed excessive anterior translation and increased resistance to posterior translation on the right compared to the left, which seemed consistent with the humeral head observation initially on examination. Horizontal flexion was limited to neutral when the scapula was stabilised onto the rib cage, indicative of tightness in the posterior shoulder capsule.

Repeating abduction while the therapist manually positioned the scapula in a more ideal posture resulted in pain onset at 125°, which was also the point at which the patient experienced pain at a 3/10 level. To place the scapula in this position, the therapist placed her hand over the dorsum of the scapula and applied a slight adduction force, posterior rotation and external rotation before the patient commenced elevation. While the patient performed the shoulder abduction movement, the therapist applied an upward rotation

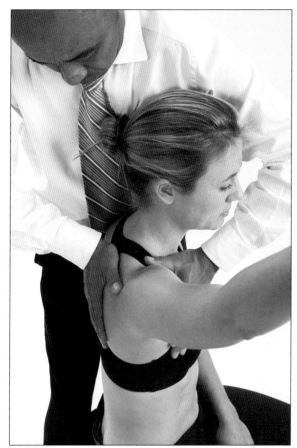

Figure 12.2 Scapulothoracic joint MWM for elevation

glide of the scapula as well as encouraging posterior rotation and external rotation (aiming to replicate/facilitate normal scapulothoracic motion relationships as the patient moved through elevation). This is essentially a scapulothoracic Mobilisation with Movement (MWM) (see Figure12.2 and Table 12.1).

Two other attempts at normalising scapula position by varying the therapist's manual contact and applied force direction were undertaken with little improvement in gained abduction ROM in the scapular plane. In order to test if this was the best possible outcome, the therapist then moved to the glenohumeral joint and exerted a posterolateral glide of the humeral head on the glenoid (Figure 12.3, Table 12.2). This resulted in a marked increase in range of abduction to 180° pain-free with overpressure. This was also the case when the same glide was applied in external rotation; that is, full pain-free ROM occurred with the glide maintained.

There was full range of cervical spine motion and some local tenderness to palpation centrally at C3–4 (postero–anterior glide). Neurological testing revealed no deficits in power, sensation or reflexes. Neurodynamic tests of the upper limb were not provocative.

Muscle tests revealed a side-to-side difference in strength of the scapular stabilisers on the right with resisted internal rotation of the arm in neutral abduction. The medial border of the scapula started to internally and downwardly rotate. Decreased strength was noted in the external rotators on the right (Grade 4). Janet found it difficult to maintain humeral head centring while performing internal and external rotation at 90° abduction. This was exaggerated with increased speed of the movement.

EVIDENCE-INFORMED CLINICAL REASONING

1 After the physical examination, was your hypothesis following the interview confirmed? What clinical findings were most relevant in coming to this decision?

Clinician's response

Janet's physical examination supported a working hypothesis of impingement secondary to an abnormal humero-scapula relationship, likely secondary to anterior capsule laxity, posterior structure tightness and rotator cuff muscle fatigue. There is also an element of practise error in that Janet selected a workload in the water for which she was not yet prepared (e.g. too much too soon). However, once established, the pain did not settle with rest alone, which is not that uncommon for such overuse injuries. According to Magarey and Jones,[3] there is some evidence (albeit indirect) that pain and injury are associated with disruption of rotator cuff function, especially its function as a deep (close to joint) stabiliser. If there is injury to or fatigue of these muscles, the humeral head may not remain centred. It is known that the subscapularis is prone to fatigue in swimmers because of its continual activity throughout the freestyle stroke. This can lead to pain and limitation of range of elevation.[4] The sensory symptoms may be triggered by the lack of rotator cuff control maintaining centring of the humeral head with subsequent forward shift of the humeral head irritating the pain sensitive structures that traverse the anterior aspect of the humeral head.

Interestingly, in a systematic review of clinical tests of rotator cuff pathology, Hughes et al[5] reported that a positive Hawkins-Kennedy test did not increase the likelihood of the presence of rotator cuff pathology (impingement syndrome), but rather a negative test increased the likelihood of no such pathology being present. They recommend the focus move away from a pathological based system to one in which the signs and symptoms are emphasised along with a triage system to exclude serious pathology. In the 'Shoulder Symptom Modification Procedure', described by Lewis,[6] physical manoeuvres of the scapula and shoulder (e.g. scapular positioning, humeral head translations) are trialled during the physical examination in an effort to best direct and structurally target the

Table 12.1	Scapulothoracic joint MWM for shoulder elevation (see Figure 12.2)	
Indication	**Pain and/or limitation of movement of shoulder elevation through abduction or flexion**	
Positioning	Patient	The patient sits in a good relaxed posture.
	Treated body part	The patient's arm rests by their side with the forearm supinated, fingers and thumb extended and the thumb pointing laterally in the direction of the movement.
	Therapist	The therapist stands facing the patient, on the opposite side of the painful shoulder.
	Therapist's hands	The therapist reaches across the patient's trunk. To affect the right shoulder the therapist places the palm of the left hand over the clavicle with the right hand on the medial aspect of the scapula with the fingers spread across the dorsal aspect of the scapula controlling the scapula position.
Application guidelines	• Both hands will apply corrective force to reposition the scapula to the optimal position. In this case an adduction force, with posterior rotation and external rotation was employed. In other cases different corrections may be chosen based on evaluation of the patient's resting posture. Ultimately a positive response to MWM is the most important factor for determining scapula repositioning. • While maintaining optimal scapula position the patient is asked to actively elevate their arm through abduction to the point of pain onset and return to the starting point. • While the patient performs abduction, the therapist allows upward rotation of the scapula as well as encouraging posterior rotation and external rotation (aiming to replicate/facilitate normal scapulohumeral rhythm). • If the technique is indicated, the patient will be able to achieve considerably greater elevation range without pain. • If pain persists, even after modifications are considered, the technique should not be used. • Possible modifications if pain persists include subtle alteration in the direction of force that repositions the scapula. Further modifications include repositioning the scapula together with repositioning the humerus at the glenohumeral joint. • Repeat the movement 6–10 times before reassessing the active movement independent of scapula repositioning. Subsequent reassessment should reveal a significant improvement in pain-free range of movement. Further sets of 6–10 repetitions may be employed.	
Comments	• Ensure that gentle and not excessive force is applied to reposition the scapula. Excessive force may cause discomfort or pain preventing application of the technique. This is particularly true for an acute injury where there may be significant local tenderness over the area. It is advisable to use a thick piece of sponge rubber to soften the contact in cases of local tenderness. • The patient must experience no pain or other symptoms at any stage of the mobilisation or active movement. Should pain occur, the technique should be modified by altering the scapula position.	

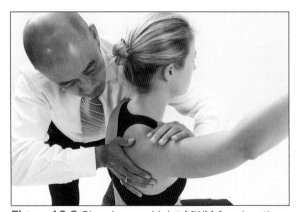

Figure 12.3 Glenohumeral joint MWM for elevation

treatment approach. This aligns well with the Mulligan MWM approach in which a joint glide is sustained while a previously painful movement is repeated pain-free (see Chapter 2).

2 What were your primary hypotheses with respect to management? Was the Mulligan Concept indicated and, if so, why?

Clinician's response

In terms of management, there was evidence from the clinical examination that pointed to soft tissue imbalance about the glenohumeral joint, which would reasonably be expected to be amenable to exercise therapy. Manual therapy is often used as an adjunct to exercise therapy to hasten pain-free motion and muscle contraction, which then facilitates pain-free exercise.[7, 8]

On the basis of the resistance to posterior glide, the forward sitting humeral head and the marked improvement in ROM with the application of a posterior glide to the humeral head, it is tempting to speculate that a positional fault existed in this case. However, as discussed in the positional fault hypothesis chapter (Chapter 4) improvement in shoulder elevation with the application of a MWM does not constitute sufficient evidence of a positional fault existing. Notwithstanding the consideration of positional faults, in particularly their existence at the shoulder joint, it is salient to the decision-making process that this patient responded in such a way to provide a high degree of confidence that MWM would be helpful in the management of the shoulder problem.[6]

Table 12.2	Glenohumeral joint MWM for shoulder elevation (see Figure 12.3)	
Indication	Pain and/or limitation of movement of shoulder elevation through abduction or flexion and/or external rotation	
Positioning	Patient	The patient sits in a good relaxed posture.
	Treated body part	The patient's arm rests by their side with the forearm supinated, fingers and thumb extended and the thumb pointing laterally in the direction of the movement.
	Therapist	The therapist stands facing the patient, on the opposite side of the painful shoulder.
	Therapist's hands	The therapist reaches across the patient's trunk. To affect the right shoulder the therapist stabilises the scapula with the thenar eminence of the right hand placed above the spine of the scapula and the fingers below. The gliding hand is placed such that the palm of the hand cups the anterior aspect of the humeral head, ensuring comfort for the patient. This hand should be immediately lateral to the coracoid process.
Application guidelines	• Posterolateral force is directed as a glide of the humeral head along the plane of the glenoid. Ensure adequate stabilisation of the scapula when applying the glide. • While maintaining this posterolateral glide the patient is asked to actively elevate their arm through abduction to the point of pain onset and return to the starting point. • Ensure that the scapula is allowed to move normally through lateral rotation. Simply blocking the scapula will disrupt normal shoulder biomechanics and limit the range of abduction achievable. • If the technique is indicated, the patient will be able to achieve considerably greater abduction range without pain. • If pain persists, even after modifications are considered, the technique should not be used. • Possible modifications if pain persists include varying the glide force and glide angle. Further modifications include repositioning the scapula together with repositioning the humerus. • Repeat the movement 6–10 times before reassessing the active movement independent of the glide. Subsequent reassessment should reveal a significant improvement in pain-free range of movement. Further sets of 6–10 repetitions may be employed.	
Comments	• Ensure that gentle and not excessive force is applied to the anterior humeral head. Excessive force may cause discomfort or pain preventing application of the technique. This is particularly true for an acute injury where there may be significant local tenderness over the area. It is advisable to use a thick piece of sponge rubber to soften the contact in cases of local tenderness. • The patient must experience no pain or other symptoms at any stage of the mobilisation or active movement. Should pain occur modify the technique by altering the amount and direction of the mobilisation force on the humeral head.	
Variation	• Two strips of sports tape, one stretch (hypoallergenic) and the other non-stretch, may be applied on top of each other to enhance the effect of the mobilisation (Figure 12.4). A manual therapy belt may be used in place of the therapist's hands. A home exercise replicating this MWM has also been described. The reader is directed to Mulligan's books for more details of this exercise and other technique variations.	

There is preliminary evidence from one randomised controlled trial of the initial effects of an MWM technique[9] that supports the use of MWM for improving shoulder elevation initially on application. In a double-blind randomised controlled trial, 24 subjects with pain-limited shoulder elevation showed a statistically significant improvement in both ROM in the plane of the scapula and pressure pain threshold (PPT) after just one application of shoulder MWM treatment.[9] In another report, by DeSantis and Hasson,[10] a patient responded to 12 treatment sessions of the same shoulder MWM plus other manual therapy techniques to the extent that he recovered full shoulder ROM, improving from 95° to 180°, and the numerical pain rating scale (NPRS) reduced from 7/10 to 0/10 with abduction. Notwithstanding these two papers, it is important to remember that the conclusion of our systematic review (Chapter 3) indicates that there is, on the whole, a low level of research quality in this area and the evidence that exists remains equivocal on balance.

During normal shoulder movement the humeral head is considered to remain relatively centred (in an anterior-posterior direction), predominantly through small translatory glides along the glenoid.[11] This allows the upper extremity to function with precision and force. According to Magarey and Jones,[3] the rotator cuff functions as a stabiliser of the glenohumeral joint, with some evidence of its disruption leading to pain. If there is injury to or fatigue of these muscles, the humeral head may not remain centred. Likewise, if there is tightness of the rotator cuff or parts of the capsule,[12] there may be an interference to the centring of the humeral head. It is conceivable that with this set of circumstances when the swimmer subjects the shoulder to repeated loading, glenohumeral function is compromised and may then lead to some degree of laxity in the glenohumeral joint,[13] which in turn contributes to the pain and impairment reported by Janet.

During freestyle swimming, the hand enters the water forward of and lateral to the head and medial to the shoulder, a position not unlike those devised and described as impingement tests (e.g. Neer and Hawkins-Kennedy tests). A number of authors have demonstrated that patients with shoulder impingement had greater proximal translation of the humeral head and a reduced subacromial space, which likely compromises its contents (e.g. supraspinatus and bursa).[14, 15]

TREATMENT AND MANAGEMENT

The patient was managed by a combination of MWM, taping and exercise over 7 weeks involving six face to face physiotherapy consultations.

Treatment 1

In the first instance the therapist applied the posterior MWM glide that improved ROM in the physical examination (see Table 12.1 for full description). This was applied six times for shoulder abduction, during which there was full ROM achieved, including overpressure of abduction at end of range. Following the application of the MWM, re-assessment of abduction revealed some mild pain in the last 30° of abduction. Shoulder external rotation was approximately 45° to pain onset. The patient was not asked to do any self-treatment between sessions, but asked to monitor shoulder pain and to continue to refrain from aggravating the shoulder with swimming.

Treatment 2

Three days later the patient returned reporting less constant ache (~1/10) since the previous session, but overhead activities were still problematic (~8/10). On examination the ROM was much the same as on the first session before MWM was applied. The same MWM (with overpressure) was applied and improvements in range were again noted. As there was no exacerbation of the condition following the first session and no sustained improvement, repetitions were increased to 10 in the first set. Reassessment revealed that abduction was still somewhat painful in the last 30° (~2/10). A second set of 10 repetitions was then performed with pain reducing to approximately 1/10 within the last 10° of shoulder abduction on reassessment. External rotation was now 55° to pain onset. This was accepted as a sufficient gain in this session and a decision to augment the effect of the therapist-applied MWM with tape was made. The tape consisted of a posterior glide on the humeral head and continued down to the right upper thorax to about the level of T10. Abduction with this tape in place was now pain-free and full range.

Treatment 3

The patient attended a week after the first session reporting a marked reduction in the constant ache (0/10) and improving use of the arm with overhead activities being less concerning (~3/10). Janet also indicated that she no longer had been feeling the pins and needles or

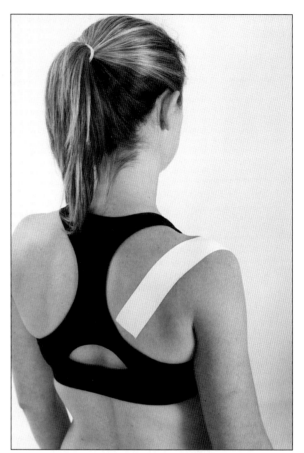

Figure 12.4 Shoulder taping to replicate MWM of the glenohumeral joint

numbness she had described at the first session. The tape was still in place and so was removed prior to assessment and the skin cleaned. Physical examination revealed an arc of pain from approximately 120–140° through abduction but no pain at end of range. External rotation was 45° to onset of pain and hand behind back was much the same as at first assessment in session one. Palpation of the anterior and anterolateral glenohumeral joint soft tissues was still reasonably pain provocative (~4/10) but muscle contraction tests into abduction and internal rotation were eliciting less pain (2/10). Internal rotation isolated to the glenohumeral joint was still 30° when performed in 90° of abduction and there was a tendency to allow the scapula to move off the treatment table earlier on the affected side during this test.

The focus of this session was to ascertain if Janet was capable of controlling her humeral head position in much the same way as the MWM. This was accomplished by applying the MWM in sitting with the upper limb fully supported and asking Janet to sense the humeral head change. Once she felt she had a reasonable sense of the displacement and the direction, Janet was asked to attempt the same motion underneath the therapist's hands. Janet exhibited a sound kinaesthetic awareness and was able to draw back the humeral head to a more central position within the glenoid in reasonably short time. After practising this 10 times, she then held the humeral head position and superimposed some active inner range external rotation followed by some assisted active anti-gravity elevation in the scapula plane (to 60°) both for six repetitions. The last three abduction movements were conducted actively without assistance. Following this, reassessment of abduction revealed that the painful arc was easier but still present. The therapist then applied three sets of 10 repetitions of MWM with abduction, after which there was full abduction ROM without any pain. External rotation exhibited some pain in the last 5°.

The tape was re-applied and reassessment revealed full pain-free abduction. Janet was then asked to practise the humeral head re-positioning exercise in three sets of six, with no more than 60 seconds set-rest intervals. She was asked to do this as frequently as possible (at least two times per day, but with at least an hour between practise sessions) over the next 3 days.

As a precursor to future exercises, Janet was counselled about the bilateral scapulae positioning, how it was less then optimal and how she could move and practise a more optimal position of the scapulae. This was performed in supine first, using the treatment bench (floor at home) for tactile input, and then when she had the idea of the required scapular movement she was asked to perform it in a standing position without tactile input. These scapular posture exercises were to be performed at least twice a day separated by at least several hours (2–4 hours). The supine lying position was also used as a stretch for the pectoralis minor muscle, asking Janet to increasingly sustain the holds of exaggerated scapulae retraction, posterior rotation and external rotation for periods starting at 15 seconds to 60 seconds by 8–12 repetitions once a day.

Treatment 4

Janet returned 3 days later reporting that she had not experienced any constant ache and was only having mild pain with overhead activities (~1/10). As instructed she had removed the tape prior to attending physiotherapy. There was full and pain-free range of abduction and some mild pain on the last 10° of external rotation. She reported having practised the humeral head repositioning exercises a minimum of four times per day, which was borne out on examination as she demonstrated good execution. The scapular postural exercises were also going well, indicating that Janet was able to replicate these well. The quality of motion and control of humeral head position during internal rotation with the shoulder at 90° abduction (performed in supine) had changed little from the first session, but there was now easily 50° of internal rotation.

The MWM technique was applied, but this time with external rotation being the target motion. One set of 10 repetitions achieved full pain-free range of external rotation motion. Reassessment showed full ROM into abduction and external rotation. Humeral positioning exercises were then progressed to full range, which Janet was able to do well. Taping was not re-applied at this session.

Focus then progressed to the control of humeral head and scapular posture during internal rotation at 90° of abduction. A similar tactile approach to the humeral head re-positioning manoeuvre described above was followed with good effect.

Janet was then instructed to perform a series of simple rotator cuff strengthening exercises using three sets of eight repetitions structure at a starting load of 10RM (using elastic band resistance) but emphasising that no pain was to be felt during or after the exercise. The exercises were essentially external rotation and internal rotation through the entire range available, but on a base of a soundly positioned scapula and humeral head (i.e. humeral head centred within glenoid). These exercises were commenced with the arm by the side (i.e. 0° elevation) and when control of the scapula and humeral head was attained, the position of the glenohumeral joint was progressed from 0° to 45° and then 90°. This occurred over the next 2 weeks.

Treatment 5

Ten days after treatment 4 Janet reported that she was happy with progress, not having any pain with day-to-day activities including those involving overhead movement. Swimming had not been recommenced yet. Physical examination focused on the exercises. Janet had a good command over all exercises and none were painful to perform. She now could better control humeral head position during internal rotation of the shoulder at 90° of abduction (without elastic band resistance — she had not graduated to 90° abduction on the resisted rotation exercises yet).

Impingement tests were still slightly provocative, but muscle contraction and empty can tests were normal. Palpation revealed tenderness over the region of the supraspinatus tendon, but this was much improved from the initial session.

Janet was performing her rotator cuff strengthening exercises well and was instructed in progression of these exercises (higher resistance elastic bands). Having experienced elite level weight training, Janet was confident of being able to progress her shoulder exercise positions and loads in 2 to 3 weeks time.

She was counselled about her return to swimming approach. A discussion was undertaken regarding the need to gradually resume swimming with adequate recovery and adaptation/recovery periods in between the swimming sessions while progressively increasing distance and intensity within each swim session. Janet had not included swimming drills within her return to swimming (e.g. kicking drills and use of other swimming strokes) and was encouraged to break up her swim session into a series of different drills, many of which she could recall from her earlier swimming days. The need to include other exercise sessions in her overall fitness program was also canvassed; for example, the use of bike ergometer and elliptical trainers as well as gym-based weight sessions were considered.

Treatment 6

Janet attended a physiotherapy consultation a month later reporting that she was now swimming 3 days a week without any shoulder problems. She was also now including three sessions at a gym, during which she mixed some cardiovascular exercises on an elliptical trainer with endurance-based weight training. Physical examination revealed that she had retained her capacity to control her humeral head position at rest and during shoulder rotation and elevation. There was no pain or impairment noted with active movement and muscle contraction. Impingement tests were now non-provocative but there was still some tenderness on palpation over the anterolateral glenohumeral region.

When contacted by phone two months later, Janet reported that her shoulder and return to physical fitness was progressing well without any problems.

AUTHORS' MWM COMMENTARY

Tate et al[16] have shown that repositioning the scapula immediately reduces pain during impingement tests in 46 of 98 athletes they studied with impingement syndrome. They concluded that using scapular repositioning might be useful in an impairment-based classification in managing shoulder conditions.[16] Interestingly, the scapulothoracic MWM that we included in our physical examination of Janet has many similarities to that of the scapular repositioning manoeuvre described by Tate et al. Even with finessing the scapulothoracic MWM we were unable to achieve a substantial change in impairment (ROM) in our patient and so progressed to applying a MWM to the glenohumeral joint. This is not unlike the Shoulder Symptom Modification Procedure described by Lewis.[6] He proposed that the practitioner may test the effect of scapular, glenohumeral, cervical or thoracic spine manoeuvres on symptoms in order to assist the clinical decisions regarding the treatment to be undertaken.

Our initial application of the scapulothoracic MWM was based partly on our knowledge of the study of Tate et al,[16] but also on our observations of scapulothoracic mal-posture. In retrospect, if we weighed the observation of bilaterally poor posture of the scapulothoracic regions against unilateral humeral head forward positioning, we may have selected to apply the MWM to the glenohumeral joint in the first instance. It seems a sensible approach for practitioners to use their perceived observations of bony and joint mal-alignment, albeit usually subtle, to guide their initial application of MWM. In this case the direction of the applied MWM glide would be one that opposes the observed poor posture. It is salient to remember that a positive response on a MWM provides clinical guidance to both the clinician and client in treatment selection and overall management of the shoulder condition. It should not be used to validate positional faults (see Chapter 4).

The role of the MWM in overall management is most likely an adjunctive but not lesser one to exercise therapy in cases like Janet. For a MWM to be included in a management program there has to be, on physical examination, a substantial improvement in impairment immediately on application with at least some carry over (see Chapter 2). Thus, by this operational definition of MWM, it is compelling to include MWM in the management program as a means by which to reduce pain-impaired motion and muscle contraction in order to optimise exercise performance (and its compliance). In our case, the glenohumeral MWM helped the patient regain ROM and symptom-free function, which helped her to strengthen her rotator cuff muscles.

The imbalance of soft tissues about the glenohumeral joint and in particular the tightness of the posterior capsule would also need to be considered when using MWM. If on applying the glenohumeral MWM the response was not of the magnitude observed in this case, we would have considered using techniques (both manual therapy and active exercise) to improve posterior translation of the humeral head and possibly extensibility of the posterior capsular structures. Cadaveric studies have demonstrated a positive response to a caudally directed glide on the humeral head and have also demonstrated stretching of the posterior capsule as being the reason for this.[17]

References

1 Krishnan SG, Hawkins RJ, Warren RF. The Shoulder and the Overhead Athlete. Philadelphia: Lippincott, Williams & Wilkins 2004.
2 Ellenbecker T. Clinical Examination of the Shoulder. St Louis: Elsevier 2004.
3 Magarey M, Jones M. Dynamic evaluation and early management of altered motor control around the shoulder complex. Manual Therapy. 2003;8(4):195–206.
4 Zachazewski J, Magee D, Quillen W. Athletic Injuries and Rehabilitation. Philadelphia: WB Saunders 1996.
5 Hughes PC, Taylor NF, Green RA. Most clinical tests cannot accurately diagnose rotator cuff pathology: a systematic review. The Australian Journal of Physiotherapy. 2008;54(3):159–70.
6 Lewis J. Rotator cuff tendinopathy: a model for the continuum of pathology and related management. British Journal of Sports Medicine. 2010;44(13):918–23.
7 Conroy D E, Hayes K W. The effect of joint mobilization as a component of comprehensive treatment for primary shoulder impingement syndrome. Journal of Orthopaedics and Sports Physical Therapy. 1998;28(1):3–14.

8 Bang MD, Deyle GD. Comparison of supervised exercise with and without manual physical therapy for patients with shoulder impingement syndrome. Journal of Orthopaedics and Sports Physical Therapy. 2000;30(3):126–37

9 Teys P, Bisset L, Vicenzino B. The initial effects of a Mulligan's mobilization with movement technique on range of movement and pressure pain threshold in pain-limited shoulders. Manual Therapy. 2008;13(1):37–42.

10 DeSantis L, Hasson S. Use of a mobilisation with movement in the treatment of a patient with sub-acromial impingement: a case study. Journal of Manual and Manipulative Therapy. 2006;14(2):77–87.

11 Graichen H, Stammberger T, Bonel H, et al. Glenohumeral translation during active and passive elevation of the shoulder — a 3D open-MRI study. Journal of Biomechanics. 2000 2000;33(5):609–13.

12 Lin J, Lim H, Yang J. Effect of shoulder tightness on glenohueral translation, scapular kinematics, and scapulohumeral rhythm in subjects with stiff shoulders. Journal of Orthopaedic Research. 2006;24(5):1044–51.

13 Malicky D, Kuhn J, Frisancho J, et al. Nonrecoverable strain fields of the anteroinferior glenohumeral capsule under subluxation. Journal of Shoulder and Elbow Surgery. 2002;11(6):529–40.

14 Ludewig P, Cook T. Translations of the humerus in persons with shoulder impingement symptoms. Journal of Orthopaedic and Sports Physical Therapy. 2002 June 2002;32(6):248–59.

15 Hallstrom E, Karrholm J. Shoulder kinematics in 25 patients with impingement and 12 controls. Clinical Orthopaedics and Related Research. 2006;448:22–7.

16 Tate AR, McClure PW, Kareha S, et al. Effect of the scapular reposition test on shoulder impingement symptoms in overhead athletes. Journal of Orthopaedics and Sports Physical Therapy. 2008 38(1):4–11.

17 Hsu AT, Ho L, Ho S, et al. Immediate response of a caudally directed translational mobilization: a frech cadaveric study. Archives of Physical Medicine and Rehabilitation 2000;81(11):1511–6.

Chapter 13
A recalcitrant case of aircraft engineer's elbow

Leanne Bisset and Bill Vicenzino

HISTORY

Allan is a 50-year-old male who presented in June 2003 with right lateral elbow pain of 12 years' duration. The pain had begun during his former job as an aircraft maintenance engineer, a job that requires a reasonably heavy manual workload, often with long bouts of repetitive manual tasks. The elbow pain was recalcitrant, as it did not respond to a range of treatments including surgery and eventually led to Allan ceasing his aircraft maintenance work to take up deskwork. He was unable to enjoy recreational sporting activities with his sons (e.g. playing cricket, throwing a ball) and his family life was affected. He was a scout guide in his leisure time, but was unable to go away on camping weekends, due to the pain and poor level of function in his dominant affected arm. When asked about his condition, Allan was unsure of the underlying problem, because he had had surgery to remove the offending tendon and the condition had not responded. He presented to our unit after hearing about our research into tennis elbow and expressed a desire to be entered into one of our trials. Allan's presentation made him ineligible for the trials that we were conducting at that time, but he was offered a consultation with a view to instituting treatment if warranted.

Past history

The pain in his right (dominant) elbow (Figure 13.1) developed while working as an aircraft maintenance engineer in 1991. His job involved repetitive arm movements under load as he was working on large aircraft engines at the time. The elbow pain started after a particularly busy time at work, it came on gradually and worsened over a week until he felt that it was a severe pain that was limiting his upper limb function. This pain was easily aggravated by activities such as a light throwing action (e.g. a paper plane), computer keyboard typing, driving a car and any combination of gripping with supination or pronation (e.g. using a screwdriver). Allan lodged a workers compensation claim in 1991 and was managed with a range of treatments, including three corticosteroid injections, a brace, non-steroidal anti-inflammatory medications, physiotherapy and acupuncture. The physiotherapy treatment he received included deep friction massage, stretching of the forearm extensor muscles and ultrasound. Still suffering severe pain and functional loss, he underwent surgery in 1993, which failed to relieve his chronic elbow pain. Unable to continue in his occupation, he changed jobs and started as an aircraft inspection officer in 1995. His workers compensation claim was ceased in 1995. The new job took him into predominantly office work and away from the tools of his trade. Despite this change in work activity levels, his pain did not abate.

Symptom behaviour

On initial examination he reported lateral elbow pain in the region of his lateral humeral epicondyle (Figure 13.1), which was still being aggravated by the activities he recalled in his history.

There were no neurological symptoms, such as paraesthesia or anaesthesia, reported. Nor did Allan experience any pain or stiffness in his neck, shoulder, wrist or hand. At the time of presentation, the worst pain he had experienced in the past week was 2/10 on a numerical pain rating scale. However, the relatively low level of pain was due to drastic modification of all upper limb activities in order to avoid any exacerbation of his symptoms. He reported that, should he attempt any aggravating activities, the pain would quickly rise to 8/10 and pain would remain for the rest of the day, reflecting an irritable nature to his condition. There was occasional soreness in the elbow on rising in the morning and he reported often waking early with pain in the elbow, which then settled quickly with gentle active movement. He generally slept well and was not woken by the pain at night unless he lay on the affected arm, but it would settle quickly if he changed positions.

Medical history and investigations

There were no other co-morbidities, including no previous history of fractures and Allan was not taking any medication for his elbow pain. There were no 'red flags' on detailed questioning.

Baseline measures of pain and function

In order to improve the internal validity of the case report, we determined the stability of the condition by measuring pain and function on eight different

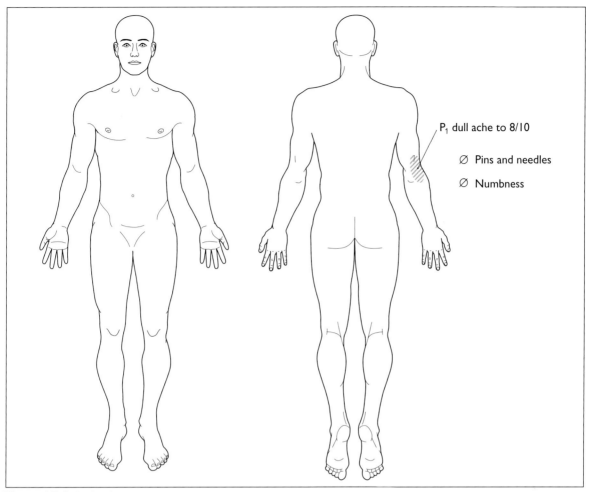

P₁ dull ache to 8/10

Ø Pins and needles

Ø Numbness

Figure 13.1 Body chart

occasions over a 3-week baseline period in which no treatment was implemented. Over this period, the patient rated his condition at a mean 69 points (standard deviation 11) on the Patient Rated Elbow Evaluation questionnaire,[1] 69 (14) mm on a 100 mm pain visual analogue scale for worst pain experienced in the past week (VAS, where 100 mm represents worst pain imaginable) and 54 (15) mm on function VAS (100 equates to full function and 0 to arm in a sling).

EVIDENCE-INFORMED CLINICAL REASONING

1 At the end of the history, what were your thoughts or hypotheses regarding Allan's elbow pain?

Clinician's response

Allan presented with the classic symptoms and history of lateral epicondylalgia (otherwise termed tennis elbow or lateral elbow tendinopathy), which is characterised by a pain at the lateral elbow (focalised to the lateral epicondyle) that is brought on by repetitive manual work.[2] Though the prevalence of this condition within the general community is approximately 3%,[3] there is a higher prevalence (~15%) in jobs that require repetitive hand tasks such as food processing, construction, assembly, manufacturing and forestry.[4–6] Not only was Allan's presentation typical in terms of mechanism of onset, location and behaviour of symptoms, he also was within the classic age range (35–55 years) and had injured his dominant upper limb.[3, 7–10] Allan was atypical in that he had a persistent problem that was resistant to previous treatments and even surgery, whereas the majority of patients with this condition tend to recover within 6–24 months.[11–14]

Chronic or recurrent cases, which have become recalcitrant to conservative treatments, may eventually undergo surgery.[4] While various surgical approaches have been described in the literature, there is very little evidence of the efficacy of surgery for lateral epicondylalgia. Interestingly, in a Cochrane systematic review of surgical interventions for lateral epicondylalgia,[15] the authors reported that there were no published randomised controlled trials of surgery for lateral elbow pain and that the efficacy of such an intervention is as yet unknown.

Pain that is irritable and severe after such a prolonged period of time and remains present despite a range of treatment interventions is suggestive of dysfunction of the nociceptive system (Chapter 6). There is evidence that the nociceptive system is impaired in patients with lateral epicondylalgia, with higher levels of glutamate reported[16, 17] and signs commensurate with secondary hyperalgesia.[18–20] For quite some time researchers have reported a distinct lack of inflammatory mediators in lateral epicondylalgia, suggesting it is not an inflammatory condition.[21–23] Thus, treatments such as non-steroidal anti-inflammatory medication and corticosteroid injections are not likely to provide lasting improvements in this condition.[24]

2 Given that Allan's condition was long lasting and recalcitrant, did you have any treatment and prognosis hypotheses under consideration at this early stage? If so, what factors in the patient's history, based on your experience and the scientific evidence, support your treatment hypothesis?

Clinician's response

After the interview it was apparent that Allan had a chronic lateral elbow pain that appeared to be related to physical activity in its inception and since then in its provocation, thus it was likely mechanically induced and musculoskeletal in origin. This type of pain is usually amenable to manual therapy and exercise. Allan did not recollect strengthening exercises or joint manipulations as part of his previous physiotherapy treatment. His presentation, apart from the surgery, is not that dissimilar to previously reported cases of chronic upper limb pain (including lateral epicondylalgia) that responded to Mobilisation with Movement (MWM).[25–28] Vicenzino and Wright[28] reported a case of lateral epicondylalgia in a 39-year-old patient that had originated after a bout of heavy repetitive manual work and had failed to respond to physical therapy (involving deep massage and electrotherapy). They showed that a lateral glide MWM of the elbow produced immediate pain-relieving effects within a session and that this effect became long lasting after several sessions of MWM plus patient self-treatment with the MWM and exercises to strengthen the forearm muscles (Figures 2.1 and 2.8). The immediate effect of this MWM technique has been previously demonstrated in laboratory studies that employed examiner blinded and placebo control methodology (Chapter 3).[29–31]

A progressive and graduated program of exercise should not be overlooked for Allan because studies by Pienimaki et al[32, 33] showed that this is superior to ultrasound in both the short and long term. Pienimaki et al[32, 33] studied patients that were similar to Allan in that they had all failed conservative management (including injections, medication, physical therapies) and were chronic (most had the condition for more than 3 months). They demonstrated that an 8-week graduated progressive exercise program, performed in a pain-free manner, was effective in relieving pain and lessening sick leave and the use of other treatments, including surgery.[32, 33] There will no doubt be a substantial de-conditioning of the forearm muscles through the initial injury (and the subsequent injections and surgery perhaps), pain inhibition and possibly disuse (protective behaviours of avoiding use of the injured limb, moving from high to low load manual work). This is predictable as there are a number of studies that have shown muscle and motor deterioration with this condition.[34–37] Pienimaki et al also showed that the exercise program improved grip and extensor strength when compared to ultrasound.[33]

The foregoing favourable perspective of Allan's condition in terms of prognosis and treatment needs to be counter-balanced with the knowledge that his condition has not responded to previous treatments. Of these previous treatments, corticosteroid injections have been shown to provide highly effective short-term relief, though recurrence rates are higher when compared to a wait-and-see policy.[38] Other factors that may signal a poor prognosis are Allan's level of pain severity and duration of symptoms. Smidt et al[39] showed that prognosis is worse in those with worse pain and longer duration of symptoms. Over the baseline period Allan's pain was 69 mm (SD 14), which was significantly ($t_7 = 2.689$; $p = 0.03$) in excess of the mean of 55.3 (SD 23.6) reported by Smidt et al. Allan's 12-year duration of pain is also in excess of the average 15 weeks (SD 22) in the prognosis study.[39]

PHYSICAL EXAMINATION

Screening and range of motion tests

On observation there was some muscle wasting around the forearm muscles, particularly the forearm extensor group on the affected side. Otherwise normal resting sitting posture of the trunk and neck was observed. The elbow pain was reproduced by palpation over the lateral humeral epicondyle. Physical testing revealed that isometric contraction against minimal resistance for wrist, 2nd and 3rd finger extension reproduced lateral elbow pain, the latter being most severe (8/10). Table 13.1 shows the range of motion (ROM) data for the affected and unaffected elbow, shoulder and cervical spine.

Table 13.1 Summary of the findings from the physical examination. Cervical, shoulder and elbow movements not stated were normal full range of motion and pain-free

Joint motion	Dominant (affected) side	Non-dominant (unaffected) side
Elbow extension	–5° end of range stiffness limited	√√
Elbow pronation	Full ROM, lateral elbow pain provoked EOR	√√
Neural provocation test 2b (radial nerve bias)[26]	Full available elbow extension, shoulder abduction to 30° lateral elbow pain provoked	Full elbow extension, shoulder abduction to 45°
Shoulder internal rotation (hand behind back)	Wrist to L1, no pain EOR	√√Wrist to T10
Shoulder external rotation	3/4 ROM, shoulder pain provoked EOR	√√

ROM, range of motion; √√, full pain-free ROM; EOR, end of range; T10, spinal segment

Pain-free grip force

A series of physical outcome measures were used to assess the severity of the condition and assist in evaluating the effectiveness of the treatment program. Pain-free grip (PFG) force was measured using an electronic grip dynamometer (MIE Medical Research Ltd) with the patient in the supine lying position, upper limb by side and in a standardised position of elbow extension and forearm pronation with a grip size allowing the index finger to touch the thumb.[7, 40] Allan was asked to grip the dynamometer until the first onset of pain at which point he was to stop gripping. The amount of force reached was then recorded and three measures were taken for both the unaffected and affected sides, the former tested first. At least 30-seconds rest was given in between measures to limit any residual soreness or exacerbation of pain with the testing. As the unaffected side was completely pain-free, maximal grip strength was recorded. The PFG force on the affected side was 290N and on the unaffected side 344N. Application of a static, sustained lateral glide to the ulna resulted in an increase in force of 24% (from 290N to 360N) on repeat PFG force testing.

Pressure pain threshold

Apart from pain with gripping being a key indicator of lateral epicondylalgia ('tennis elbow') patients will report tenderness and sensitivity to pressure over the lateral humeral epicondyle. This may be measured to some extent using a pressure pain algometer. We used an electronic digital algometer (Somedic AB) to measure the pressure pain threshold (PPT) over the most sensitive area of the elbow. The test probe, which consists of a force transducer and a $1\ cm^2$ probe tip, was applied at a constant rate.[41] The mean (standard deviation) of a series of five repeated measures was 324 (49) on the affected side compared to 427 (85) on the unaffected side, a deficit of 24%.

A neurological assessment demonstrated normal deep tendon reflexes and normal light touch sensation in both upper limbs. Passive physiological intervertebral movement assessment of the cervical spine revealed minor reactivity (resistance to movement) at C5–6 on right lateral flexion and rotation, however elbow symptoms were not reproduced. Otherwise, all cervical spine palpation was unremarkable for his age group.

EVIDENCE-INFORMED CLINICAL REASONING

1 After the physical examination, was your hypothesis of lateral epicondylalgia and the condition's prognosis confirmed? What clinical findings were most relevant in coming to this decision?

Clinician's response

The primary clinical feature of lateral epicondylalgia is pain that is aggravated by palpation, gripping and/or resisted wrist or finger extension.[7] Lateral epicondylalgia is commonly understood to involve the extensor carpi radialis brevis and common extensor muscles and tendons at their proximal insertion.[3, 7–10] Diagnosis is made on clinical presentation and further investigations are not overly helpful unless to exclude alternative diagnoses. Allan presented with the classic signs and symptoms of lateral epicondylalgia. He also has signs that are found in many chronic cases, such as limitation to elbow extension and shoulder rotation[42] as well as positive signs of mechanical neural provocation tests.[43, 44]

After the interview we hypothesised that based on previous research indicating poor prognosis with greater duration and severity of pain Allan had a poor prognosis. However, the two key characteristics of lateral epicondylalgia measured by PFG and PPT on physical examination showed relatively small deficits (~16%) compared to the unaffected side when considered in light of published deficits (e.g. ~50%). [29, 31, 45] These relatively lower deficits of Allan's when compared to the literature is suggestive of a less severe condition than that portrayed in the interview, which conceivably modifies in a favourable direction our initial hypothesis of a poor prognosis. The disparity between the interview and the physical examination may also signal to the practitioner that proactively managing the pain is a priority as opposed to allowing the patient to adopt a wait-and-see approach or even an exercise program that elicits his pain.

2 What were your primary hypotheses with respect to management? Was the Mulligan Concept indicated and, if so, why?

Clinician's response

A recent randomised controlled trial demonstrated the efficacy of a treatment approach that coupled MWM with exercise in patients with chronic lateral epicondylalgia (Chapter 3).[38] However, the effectiveness of this combined MWM and exercise treatment approach in patients with long-term persistent pain that is recalcitrant to other treatments (including surgery) has not been investigated within a clinical trial.

To be confident in the anticipated positive outcomes associated with the application of a MWM technique, it is necessary to establish a quantifiable client-specific outcome measure prior to treatment and to quantify the effects of the MWM technique during and immediately after its application. For patients with lateral epicondylalgia, the cardinal sign is often pain reproduction and force deficits during a gripping task.[37, 46–48] Therefore, it is appropriate to use PFG as a means of quantifying the immediate effects of the MWM technique (Chapter 2). A lateral glide of the ulna MWM is applied and sustained and the patient is asked to repeat the PFG test. The extent to which the PFG should improve in order for the practitioner to have a high level of confidence in applying the MWM has not been studied sufficiently. One post-hoc analysis of a clinical trial showed that the probability of success following treatment with MWM and exercise is 85% if the initial effect in PFG is > 25% of pre-application PFG levels.[49] Our patient exhibited 24% improvement on a trial application of an MWM in the physical assessment, which appears to be close to supporting the successful application of the MWM and exercise program in this patient.

The afore cited post-hoc analysis also derived a preliminary clinical prediction rule for MWM and exercise in the management of lateral epicondylalgia.[49] The derived clinical prediction rule indicated that the success of improvement would range from 87–100% if one, two or all three of the following baseline characteristics were present: younger than 49 years, a PFG force on the affected side greater than 112N and a maximum grip strength of less than 336N on the unaffected side (LR: 1.8, 37 and infinity, respectively). At 50, Allan is just over 49 years of age, has a PFG on the affected side of 290N (which is clearly > 112N) and a maximum grip on the unaffected side that is marginally larger than 336N. Thus it would be reasonable to suggest that treatment with MWM and exercise would

increase the probability of his condition improving considerably, given the condition had been stagnant in this regard for over a decade.

Although in the above we have focussed on a lateral glide applied at the elbow, because lateral glides appear to be the direction of first choice at most joints (see Chapter 4), there are other MWM techniques that can be applied at the elbow (e.g. postero–anterior glide of the radial head) or at the neck (see Mulligan[50] and Vicenzino[51] for examples). With respect to the neck, the minor reactivity on palpatory motion assessment of the cervical spine is not that uncommon.[52]

TREATMENT AND MANAGEMENT

A multi-modal treatment approach of this condition utilising elbow MWM, taping and an exercise program that has been shown to be efficacious[38] was undertaken. The treatment protocol consisted of ten 30-minute treatment sessions over 8 weeks, of Mulligan's MWM manual therapy technique to the elbow[29, 31, 52] (Figure 13.2 and Table 13.2), a taping technique that mimicked the MWM technique (Figure 13.3)[51] and a graded therapeutic exercise program.[51, 53]

Treatment 1

Five repetitions of an MWM were applied to the elbow, which consisted of a lateral glide to the ulna with pain-free grip as the movement task (Table 13.2). This was followed immediately by two sets of 10 repetitions of lateral glide MWM to the ulna with active elbow flexion/extension through ROM (Table 13.3). This was performed to reduce the possibility of a flare up in pain immediately after the application of the MWM with PFG (see Chapter 2) but also had the effect of improving extension range at the elbow. The MWM improved the PFG on the affected side by 29.5% (86N) of baseline measurement (290N) at this session (which represents a 159% reduction in the deficit between the affected and unaffected sides (344N)). Allan was then taught to

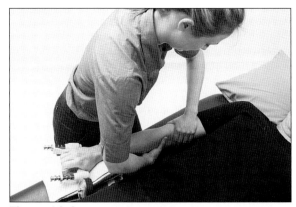

Figure 13.2 Lateral glide MWM of the elbow with PFG

Table 13.2	Instructions for application of lateral glide MWM of the elbow for PFG (see Figure 13.2)	
Indication	Pain over lateral elbow on gripping that is worse than tenderness to direct palpation over the lateral epicondyle	
Positioning	Patient	Supine with upper limb fully supported on treatment table.
	Treated body part	Relaxed extension of the elbow with pronation of the forearm.
	Therapist	Adjacent to the affected elbow facing across the body of the client.
	Therapist's hands	Stabilising hand: heel and first web space placed on the lateral surface of the distal humerus. Gliding hand: index finger and first metacarpal placed on the medial surface of the ulna just distal to the joint line.
Application guidelines	• First ensure that the client has a reproducible aggravating action prior to applying glide (i.e. pain-free grip in this case). • A grip dynamometer is used to quantify the outcome measure, allowing for accurate assessment of treatment effects. • Apply a laterally directed glide across the elbow joint. • While sustaining the glide have the client repeat the isometric gripping action until the onset of pain and no more. • Note the grip strength obtained before relaxing the grip and then release the glide. • Repeat several times (e.g. 6–10X) in a session, BUT ONLY IF there is a substantial relief of pain with gripping during the application of the technique and there is no latent pain immediately following the treatment technique (see Chapter 2 for guidelines in regards to volume of MWM).	
Comments	• Ensure that the stabilising hand does not compress the lateral epicondyle in such a way as to cause pressure pain that reproduces the client's symptoms. • Directing the glide in a purely lateral or slightly posterior of lateral (approximately 5°) direction will be effective in most cases.[45] If pain relief is not achieved then inclining the glide anterior to lateral some 5° or slightly caudad should be trialled before discarding the technique. Attempt no more than four trials to elicit a positive response in any one treatment session, as failure to relieve pain over this number of trials will prove counterproductive. • Do not release the sustained lateral glide before grip has been relaxed. • We have evaluated in a pilot study the amount of force that should be applied during this treatment technique and found it to be approximately two-thirds that of the therapist's maximal force application across the joint.[54]	
Variations	• An alternate position may be used in which the upper limb is not resting on the bed, now supported, instead, by the therapist. The therapist's right hand is stabilising the distal humerus while the left hand performs the lateral glide.[51] • A treatment belt may be used to lessen the manual work load on the therapist but care should be taken not to be overly vigorous.	

apply the lateral glide MWM himself and given a home exercise of two sets of five repetitions with a 6-second hold of isometric wrist flexion/extension.

Treatment 2

Allan reported a significant reduction in pain during light activities after the first treatment, but there was some minor exacerbation of elbow pain during the isometric wrist flexion/extension exercises. This pain quickly settled with the application of self-glides. The self-glide technique and the isometric wrist flexion/extension exercises were checked for correctness of performance and to facilitate compliance. The lateral glide MWM to the ulna was repeated, this time using the Mulligan treatment belt (Figure 13.4). As the patient responded well to the first treatment in which the MWM with gripping was applied, three sets of four repetitions of the lateral glide MWM to the ulna with gripping was applied in the second treatment session,

followed by one set of 10 repetitions of MWM. In addition, taping was applied to the elbow to supplement the pain-relieving effects of the treatment (Figure 13.3). The taping was also effective at changing PFG. The patient was advised about the potential for skin reactions from the tape and instructed on how to remove the tape should a skin reaction occur. If there was no reaction from the tape, then Allan was instructed to wear the tape for as long as he felt it was being effective. In order to normalise muscle performance function of the forearm muscles,[33, 51] one set of five repetitions of 6-second holds of isometric forearm supination/pronation was added to the home program.[51]

The exercise program was implemented as part of the home program. The aim of the home program was to address PFG force deficits (possibly of neuromotor[34, 55] and local morphological origin[36]), and altered wrist posture (which was not optimal when the patient performed PFG testing, the wrist assuming some flexion[35]

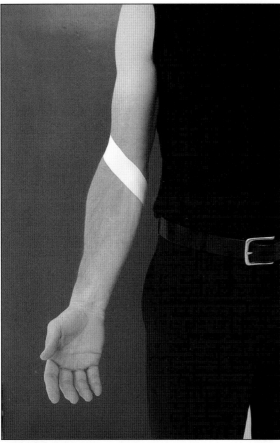

Figure 13.3 Taping of the elbow to mimic the MWM

and ulnar deviation). It is essential to the success of this program that all exercises are pain-free.

Treatments 3–10

Allan reported a continuing and significant reduction in his elbow pain, placing particular emphasis on the effectiveness and comfort of the tape. An improvement in PFG was also evident on reassessment (affected side PFG was now 450N). Treatment was continued and the home program was expanded to include general upper limb exercises (i.e. bench press, shoulder press, bent over rowing, biceps curls, triceps extensions) and local forearm exercises for the flexor/extensors and supinator/pronators. The general upper limb exercises were added to encourage integration of the gains expected from the local forearm exercises, as well as to condition all upper limb exercises in order to allow re-institution of a higher level of activity that generally uses the upper limbs. This is based on the findings of global weakness in the upper limb in chronic and recovered tennis elbow.[34] The lateral glide MWM to the ulna with gripping was continued at two to three sets of three repetitions per set. The lesser volume of MWM was chosen because PFG had improved substantially over the first few sessions and to compensate for the increased load of exercise generally in the home treatment program. In addition, the lateral glide MWM to the ulna with resisted wrist extension (Figure 13.5) was included from treatment session number 5 onwards. Rubber tubing that provided light to moderate resistance was

Table 13.3	Instructions for the lateral glide MWM during elbow flexion/extension	
Indications	• Pain over the lateral elbow that is worse with movements of the elbow	
	• After the MWM lateral glide to the ulna with gripping when there may be pain on first moving out of the extended position	
Positioning	Patient	Supine with upper limb fully supported on treatment table.
	Treated body part	Arm positioned by side with sufficient abduction to allow therapist access to medial side of the upper limb.
	Therapist	Facing across the client's head.
	Therapist's hands for flexion	Stabilising hand: heel on the lateral surface of the distal humerus. Gliding hand: lateral border of second metacarpal placed on the medial surface of the ulna just distal to the joint line.
	Therapist hands for extension	Stabilising hand: first web space and lateral border of second metacarpal placed over the lateral surface of the distal humerus. Gliding hand: first web space placed on the medial surface of the ulna just distal to the joint line.
Application guidelines	• Determine which motion (flexion, extension or both) are painful and or limited.	
	• Apply a laterally directed glide across the elbow joint in a non-painful part of the range (i.e. start in extension if flexion is the problem and vice versa).	
	• While sustaining the glide have the client repeat the painful movement and if pain-free at end of range then with overpressure (see Chapter 4).	
	• Only release the sustained glide when the movement has returned to the start position.	
	• Repeat several times (6–10X) in a session.	

(Continued)

Table 13.3	Instructions for the lateral glide MWM during elbow flexion/extension—cont'd
Comments	• In addition to comments in Table 13.2. • Therapist should foresee any restriction to flexion movement that may be due to the placement of digits over the anterior part of the joint and avoid this scenario.
Variation	• A treatment belt may also be used with care being taken to place the stabilising hand in such a way that does not interfere with elbow movement and the belt placement such as to be close to the joint line and orientated such that when end of range is reached the lateral glide through the belt is effective. • Self-treatments as per lateral glide as in Table 13.2 with the exception that instead of gripping, the patient moves the elbow through ranges of flexion and extension. • This technique can be used when pain on pain-free grip strength test occurs in a position other than extension but without movement (i.e. grip in the provocative position).

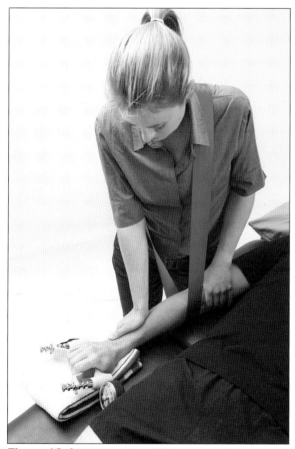

Figure 13.4 Lateral glide MWM of the elbow applied with a treatment belt

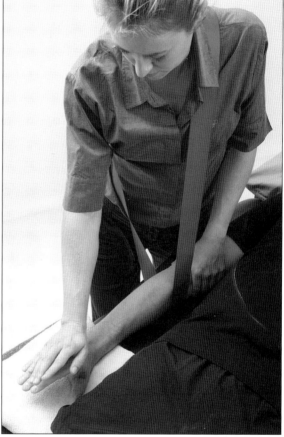

Figure 13.5 Lateral glide MWM of the elbow with wrist extensor exercises

used during this technique and also as part of the home program.

OUTCOME OF INTERVENTION

After the 3-week baseline period, the 8-week treatment plan was implemented and outcome measured at 3, 6, 12, 18, 24 and 52 weeks from the start of treatment.

All measures were stable over the 3-week baseline period, with no significant trend for either a worsening or improvement in symptoms (Figure 13.6). After the 8-week treatment intervention, significant improvements were noted across all outcome variables. There was a positive change across all outcome measures over the treatment phase, that was maintained even at 52 weeks (Figure 13.6).

Allan's self-rated general improvement was assessed on a 6-point Likert scale, with categories of 'Much Worse, Worse, No Change, Improved, Much

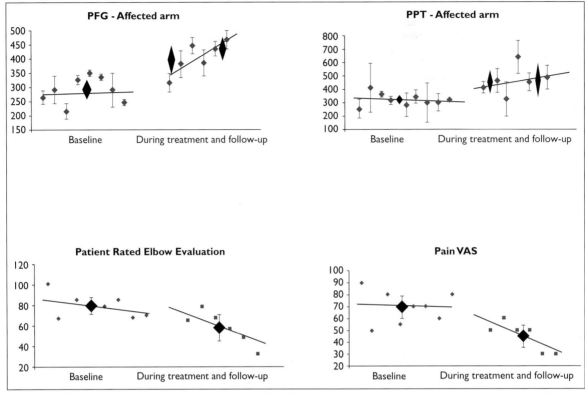

Figure 13.6 Primary outcome measures at baseline (8 measures in 3 weeks), during treatment and 3, 6, 12, 18, 24 and 52 week follow up

The higher the score represents poorer function and more severe pain.

Average of three repeated measures and 95% confidence intervals for each assessment session at baseline, each treatment session and during follow up. The large black diamonds represent the mean and 95% confidence intervals for the baseline and the treatment and follow-up periods.

Improved and Completely Recovered'. He rated himself 'Much Improved' by 3-weeks follow-up and this was maintained over the 52-week follow-up period. At 52-weeks follow-up, he reported 90% function (on function VAS) and was able to grip maximally without pain to 465N, which was stronger than his maximal grip force on his unaffected arm (412N). The lateral elbow pain had also subsided with a PPT of 490 kPa on the affected arm and 548 kPa on the unaffected arm. Moreover, he had resumed recreational activities he had not been able to participate in for several years, including canoeing, throwing a football and playing tennis.

In summary, lateral epicondylalgia can be a difficult condition to manage effectively and there is little evidence of the long-term effectiveness of any treatment. We found that the application of a lateral ulna glide MWM in conjunction with taping to reduce pain and a graded exercise program to restore function was effective in reducing pain and improving grip strength in the long term (1 year) in a patient who had a 12-year history of the condition with many failed previous treatments, including surgery.

AUTHORS' MULLIGAN CONCEPT COMMENTARY

This case demonstrated the utility of MWM on an individual basis in managing a patient who had a chronic tendinopathy that was resistant to a range of treatments including surgery. In doing so, this case provided an example of how to implement the findings of a recently published clinical trial of MWM and exercise for the management of lateral epicondylalgia.[38]

In a systematic review we found that there was good efficacy in the short term for exercise, and in the immediate term for taping and elbow MWM.[56] MWM has been shown to provide substantial improvement in PFG in chronic lateral epicondylalgia but not in the unaffected elbow[31, 45] indicating that MWM likely affects clinical outcomes through some pain–motor system interaction rather than being solely a direct mechanical stimulus to enhancing motor system function (see Chapter 7). Coupling the pain-relieving effect of MWM on gripping with a graduated exercise program intuitively addresses the presenting impairments of this condition. Rapidly resolving pain allows exercise to progress at a greater rate, instils patient confidence in the therapist and facilitates adherence to the rehabilitation program. Thus, the aim of rehabilitation is to resolve symptoms expeditiously with MWM and then to restore motor system function through graduated pain-free exercises. Interestingly, ensuring a pain-free exercise program is perhaps the most clinically significant difference between lateral epicondylalgia and other chronic tendinopathies such as Achilles or patella tendinopathy, where some exacerbation of pain (but not disabling) is considered essential in determining the correct exercise load.[57]

Allan's grip strength of 344N on his unaffected side (as well as 290N on affected side) was at the lower end of normative data for his age (mean: 500N; range: 284–774N).[58] There is some evidence that those with chronic lateral epicondylalgia who have not restored full and normal grip strength are more prone to recurrences,[32] underscoring the importance of a progressive graduated exercise program for Allan. At 12 months after starting treatment Allan's grip strength was close to the average for his age group, which is likely to serve a protective role in prevention of recurrence.

Exercises that are typically prescribed in the management of musculoskeletal disorders may result in an aggravation of pain, which inevitably creates an environment from which there arises a negative motivation for the patient to continue with the program. The advantage of performing the MWM and taping in conjunction with the exercise program is their immediate effect on reducing pain and allowing pain-free exercise to occur. Teaching the patient to perform the MWM and taping as part of self-management assists in maintaining compliance with the exercise program at home.

An effective and consistently applied home program of MWM self-glides and exercises is a key component to the overall success of this management approach in patients with lateral epicondylalgia. The approach described in this case requires the patient to be motivated in adhering and complying with a program of self-treatment for a period of time. Clinically, we find a good way in which to emphasise the importance of the home program is to ask the patient to demonstrate the self-treatment before doing any physical examination or treatment at follow-up sessions. This inherently demonstrates to the patient the importance of their participation in their management. A number of things we are particularly interested in observing is the ability of the patient to improve the PFG with the self-applied MWM and also their ability to perform the self-applied MWM technique and exercises correctly. Another indicator of patient compliance is the improvement in PFG and exercise load after the third week of the program. This approach can be used as feedback on good performance or to identify poor performance and guide correction of the technique as required. It also identifies

lack of compliance and possibly the need to address issues other than solely the elbow condition.

The underlying mechanisms by which the MWM produces a rapid change in a previously painful motor activity is not fully understood, but is thought to involve activation of endogenous pain control mechanisms. It has been postulated that the afferent input that is provided by the application of the MWM is sufficient to trigger these innate mechanisms. Chapters 5, 6 and 7 provide more detail regarding these possible mechanisms.

References

1 MacDermid JC. Outcome evaluation in patients with elbow pathology: issues in instrument development and evaluation. Journal of Hand Therapy. 2001;14(2):105–14.

2 Mani L, Gerr F. Work-related upper extremity musculoskeletal disorders. Primary Care. 2000;27(4):845–64.

3 Allander E. Prevalence, incidence and remission rates of some common rheumatic diseases or syndromes. Scandinavian Journal of Rheumatology. 1974;3(3):145–53.

4 Chiang HC, Ko YC, Chen SS, et al. Prevalence of shoulder and upper limb disorders among workers in the fish-processing industry. Scandinavian Journal of Work Environment and Health. 1993;19(2):126–31.

5 Kurppa K, Viikari-Juntura E, Kuosma E, et al. Incidence of tenosynovitis or peritendinitis and epicondylitis in a meat-processing factory. Scandinavian Journal of Work, Environment and Health. 1991;17(1):32–7.

6 Ranney D, Wells R, Moore A. Upper limb musculoskeletal disorders in highly repetitive industries: precise anatomical physical findings. Ergonomics. 1995;38(7):1408–23.

7 Haker E. Lateral epicondylalgia: Diagnosis, treatment and evaluation. Critical Reviews in Physical and Rehabilitative Medicine. 1993;5(2):129–54.

8 Binder A, Hazleman B. Lateral humeral epicondylitis — a study of natural history and the effect of conservative therapy. British Journal of Rheumatology. 1983;22(2):73–6.

9 Hamilton PG. The prevalence of humeral epicondylitis: a survey in general practice. Journal of the Royal College of General Practitioners. 1986;36(291):464–5.

10 Shiri R, Viikari-Juntura E, Varonen H, et al. Prevalence and determinants of lateral and medial epicondylitis: a population study. American Journal of Epidemiology. 2006;164(11):1065–74.

11 Murtagh J. Tennis elbow. Australian Family Physician. 1988;17(2):90, 91, 94–5.

12 Hay E, Paterson S, Lewis M, et al. Pragmatic randomised controlled trial of local corticosteroid injection and naproxen for treatment of lateral epicondylitis of elbow in primary care. British Medical Journal. 1999;319(7215):964–8.

13 Smidt N, van der Windt DAWM, Assendelft WJJ, et al. Corticosteroid injections, physiotherapy, or a wait-and-see policy for lateral epicondylitis: a randomised controlled trial. Lancet. 2002;359(9307):657–62.

14 Hudak PL, Cole DC, Haines AT. Understanding prognosis to improve rehabilitation: the example of lateral elbow pain. Archives of Physical Medicine and Rehabilitation. 1996;77(6):586–93.

15 Buchbinder R, Green S, Bell S, et al. Surgery for lateral elbow pain. The Cochrane Database of Systematic Reviews: DOI: 10.1002/14651858.CD003525 2002(1).

16 Alfredson H, Ljung B, Thorsen K, et al. In vivo investigation of ECRB tendons with microdialysis technique — no signs of inflammation but high amounts of glutamate in tennis elbow. Acta Orthopaedica Scandinavica. 2000;71(5):475–9.

17 Alfredson H, Lorentzon R. Chronic tendon pain: no signs of chemical inflammation but high concentrations of the neurotransmitter glutamate. Implications for treatment? Current Drug Targets. 2002;3(1):43–54.

18 Vicenzino B, Souvlis T, Wright A. Musculoskeletal pain. In: Strong J, Unruh AM, Wright A, Baxter GD (eds) Pain: a Textbook for Therapists. Edinburgh: Churchill Livingstone 2002, pp 327–49.

19 Wright A, Thurnwald P, O'Callagan J, et al. Hyperalgesia in tennis elbow patients. Journal of Musculoskeletal Pain. 1994;2(4):83–97.

20 Wright A, Thurnwald P, Smith J. An evaluation of mechanical and thermal hyperalgesia in patients with lateral epicondylalgia. The Pain Clinic. 1992;5(4): 221–7.

21 Khan KM, Cook JL, Kannus P, et al. Time to abandon the 'tendinitis' myth. British Medical Journal Clinical Research Edition. 2002;324(7338):626–7.

22 Kraushaar BS, Nirschl RP. Tendinosis of the elbow (tennis elbow) — Clinical features and findings of histological, immunohistochemical, and electron microscopy studies. Journal of Bone and Joint Surgery — American Volume. 1999;81-A(2):259–78.

23 Nirschl R, Pettrone F. Tennis Elbow: The surgical treatment of lateral epicondylitis. Journal of Bone and Surgery — Amercian Volume. 1979;61-A(6): 832–9.

24 Green S, Buchbinder R, Barnsley L, et al. Non-steroidal anti-inflammatory drugs (NSAIDs) for treating lateral elbow pain in adults. Cochrane Database of Systematic Reviews 2001;Issue 4. Art. No.: CD003686. DOI: 10.1002/14651858.

25 Backstrom K. Mobilization with movement as an adjunct intervention in a patient with complicated de Quervain's tenosynovitis: a case report. Journal of Orthopaedic and Sports Physical Therapy. 2002;32(3):86–97.

26 Folk B. Traumatic thumb injury management using mobilization with movement. Manual Therapy. 2001;6(3):178–82.

27 Scaringe J, Kawaoka C, Studt T. Improved shoulder function after using spinal mobilisation with arm movement in a 50 year old golfer with shoulder, arm and neck pain. Topics in Clinical Chiropractic. 2002;9:44–53.

28 Vicenzino B, Wright A. Effects of a novel manipulative physiotherapy technique on tennis elbow: a single case study. Manual Therapy. 1995;1(1):30–5.

29 Paungmali A, O'Leary S, Souvlis T, Vicenzino B. Hypoalgesic and sympathoexcitatory effects of mobilization with movement for lateral epicondylalgia. Physical Therapy. 2003;83(4):374–83.

30 Paungmali A, O'Leary S, Souvlis T, et al. Naloxone fails to antagonize initial hypoalgesic effect of a manual therapy treatment for lateral epicondylalgia. Journal of Manipulative and Physiological Therapeutics. 2004;27(3):180–185.

31 Vicenzino B, Paungmali A, Buratowski S, et al. Specific manipulative therapy treatment for chronic lateral epicondylagia produces uniquely characteristic hypoalgesia. Manual Therapy. 2001;6(4):205–12.

32 Pienimaki T, Karinen P, Kemila T, et al. Long-term follow-up of conservatively treated chronic tennis elbow patients. A prospective and retrospective analysis. Scandinavian Journal of Rehabilitation Medicine. 1998;30(3):159–66.

33 Pienimaki TT, Tarvainen TK, Siira PT, et al. Progressive strengthening and stretching exercises and ultrasound for chronic lateral epicondylitis. Physiotherapy. 1996;82(9):522–530.

34 Alizadehkhaiyat O, Fisher AC, Kemp GJ, et al. Upper limb muscle imbalance in tennis elbow: a functional and electromyographic assessment. Journal of Orthopaedic Research. 2007;25(12):1651–7.

35 Bisset LM, Russell T, Bradley S, et al. Bilateral sensorimotor abnormalities in unilateral lateral epicondylalgia. Archives of Physical Medicine and Rehabilitation. 2006;87(4):490–5.

36 Ljung BO, Lieber RL, Friden J. Wrist extensor muscle pathology in lateral epicondylitis. Journal of Hand Surgery (Br). 1999;24(2):177–83.

37 Pienimaki T, Sura P, Vanharanta H. Muscle function of the hand, wrist and forearm in chronic lateral epicondylitis. European Journal of Physical Medicine and Rehabilitation. 1997;7(6):171–178.

38 Bisset L, Beller E, Jull G, et al. Mobilisation with movement and exercise, corticosteroid injection, or wait and see for tennis elbow: randomised trial. British Medical Journal. 2006;333(7575):939–41.

39 Smidt N, Lewis M, van der windt D. Lateral epicondylitis in general ractice: course and prognostic indicators of outcome. Journal of Rheumatology. 2006;33(10): 2053–9.

40 Stratford PW, Levy DR, Gowland C. Evaluative properties of measures used to assess patients with lateral epicondylitis at the elbow. Physiotherapy Canada. 1993;45(3):160–4.

41 Brennum J, Kjeldsen M, Jensen K, Jensen T. Measurements of human pain pressure thresholds on fingers and toes. Pain. 1989;38(2):211–17.

42 Abbott JH. Mobilization with movement applied to the elbow affects shoulder range of movement in subjects with lateral epicondylalgia. Manual Therapy 2001;6(3):170–7.

43 Vicenzino B, Collins D, Wright A. The initial effects of a cervical spine manipulative physiotherapy treatment on the pain and dysfunction of lateral epicondylalgia. Pain. 1996;68(1):69–74.

44 Yaxley G, Jull G. Adverse tension in the neural system. A preliminary study in patients with tennis elbow. Australian Journal of Physiotherapy. 1993;39(1): 15–22.

45 Abbott JH, Patla CE, Jensen RH. The initial effects of an elbow mobilization with movement technique on grip strength in subjects with lateral epicondylalgia. Manual Therapy. 2001;6(3):163–9.

46 Pienimaki TT, Siira PT, Vanharanta H. Chronic medial and lateral epicondylitis: a comparison of pain, disability, and function. Archives of Physical Medicine and Rehabilitation. 2002;83(3):317–321.

47 Stratford PW, Levy DR. Assessing valid change over time in patients with lateral epicondylitis at the elbow. Clinical Journal of Sport Medicine. 1994;4(2): 88–91.

48 Stratford P, Levy DR, Gauldie S, Levy K, Miseferi D. Extensor carpi radialis tendonitis: a validation of selected outcome measures. Physiotherapy Canada. 1987;39(4):250–255.

49 Vicenzino B, Smith D, Cleland J, et al. Development of a clinical prediction rule to identify initial responders to mobilisation with movement and exercise for lateral epicondylalgia. Manual Therapy. 2009;14(5):550–4.

50 Mulligan B. Manual therapy — 'NAGS', 'SNAGS', MWMS' etc (4th edn). Wellington: Plane View Services 1999.

51 Vicenzino B. Lateral epicondylalgia: A musculoskeletal physiotherapy perspective. Manual Therapy. 2003;8(2):66–79.

52 Vicenzino B, Cleland JA, Bisset L. Joint manipulation in the management of lateral epicondylalgia: A clinical commentary. The Journal of Manual and Manipulative Therapy. 2007;15(1):50–56.

53 Vicenzino B, Bisset L. Physiotherapy for tennis elbow. Evidence-Based Medicine. 2007;12(2):37–38.

54 McLean S, Naish R, Reed L, et al. A pilot study of the manual force levels required to produce manipulation induced hypoalgesia. Clinical Biomechanics. 2002;17(4):304–8.

55 Coombes BK, Bisset L, Vicenzino B. A new integrative model of lateral epicondylalgia. British Journal of Sports Medicine. 2009;43(4):252–8.

56 Bisset L, Paungmali A, Vicenzino B, et al. A systematic review and meta-analysis of clinical trials on physical interventions for lateral epicondylalgia. British Journal of Sports Medicine. 2005;39(7):411–22.

57 Silbernagel K, Thomee R, Thomee P, et al. Eccentric overload training for patients with chronic Achilles tendon pain — a randomised controlled study with reliability testing of the evaluation methods. Scandinavian Journal of Medicine and Science in Sports. 2001;11(4):197–206.

58 Gunther CM, Burger A, Rickert M, et al. Grip strength in healthy Caucasian adults: reference values. Journal of Hand Surgery (Am). 2008;33(4):558–65.

Chapter 14

A chronic case of thumb pain and disability with MRI identified positional fault

Chang-Yu J Hsieh, Bill Vicenzino, Chich-Haung Yang, Ming-Hsia Hu and Calvin Yang

Note: This study is revised and adapted from Hsieh, Vicenzino, Yang, Hu and Yang[1]

HISTORY

Joan is a 79-year-old female who presented with right thumb pain of 7 months duration following a fall on her hand. Although the problem was less severe initially, it had become more significant and she now had difficulty with activities of daily living, causing her significant disability.

Current and past history

The pain in her right thumb (Figure 14.1) began after a fall that occurred while alighting from a bus. The right thumb was stressed into hyperabduction as Joan held onto her umbrella during the fall. In the fall she landed on her knees and right cheek, sustaining abrasions of these areas. She also noticed some swelling of her right thumb soon thereafter. Later in the evening Joan noticed some bruising over the dorsum of her right thumb and the web space, and also some local thumb pain. Because it was not initially disabling, she did not consult a health professional. One month prior to attending the first physiotherapy consultation, the pain worsened during a visit to her daughter, who lived in a cold climate.

Symptom behaviour

At the time of consultation, Joan reported right thumb pain that was still being aggravated by activities, such as opening the cap of a jar, sewing and picking up tiles in Mah-Jong. She experienced moderate to severe pain when using a can opener (pain intensity rated 6 out of 10 on an analogue scale with 10 being the worst pain imaginable), and slight pain when wringing a washcloth.

Medical history and diagnostic imaging

Joan reported she suffered from osteopenia, diabetes mellitus and osteoarthritis, all of which were controlled by medication. Radiographic examinations of the right thumb showed marginal erosion of about 6.4 mm of the

right first metacarpal head on the radial side. A healed fracture of the metacarpal head was suspected. A hyperabduction stress view of the metacarpophalangeal joint (MPJ) of the right thumb was also performed.[2] The findings were an approximation of the base of the first proximal phalanx into the bony erosion, and no excessive joint space separation on either the radial or ulnar side of the MPJ. The patient reported moderate pain (6 out of 10) on the radial aspect of the MPJ of her thumb during the stress test. No apparent positional fault was observed when the right thumb was maximally flexed. MRI examination confirmed the X-ray findings and showed no abnormal fluid accumulation inside the interphalangeal joint (IPJ) and no significant capsule or tendon injury.

EVIDENCE-INFORMED CLINICAL REASONING

1 At the end of the interview, what were your thoughts or hypotheses regarding Joan's thumb pain? How do the diagnostic imaging findings fit with the history?

Clinician's response

Falling onto an abducted thumb may result in fracture, dislocation and/or rupture of the supporting capsular and ligamentous structures of the MPJ. A Bennett's fracture-dislocation of the first MPJ joint may occur following this type of injury,[3] though it would be expected that this will be associated with substantial pain and disability. Joan did not recount such symptoms, but did mention noticing bruising and swelling later in the evening after the fall. Hyperabduction of the thumb may also lead to ruptures of the soft tissue supporting structures of the MPJ joint, not unlike what is commonly referred to as 'skier's thumb'. On balance, this historical recollection of her condition indicates a likely soft tissue injury of the MPJ joint. However, the X-rays and MRI tend to indicate a different clinical picture with evidence of a previously healed fracture of the metacarpal head, an intact capsule and no excessive joint space separation with hyperabduction of the MPJ of the thumb.

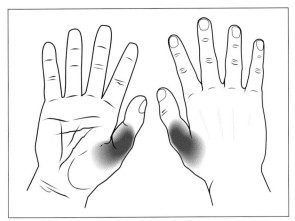

Figure 14.1 Body chart

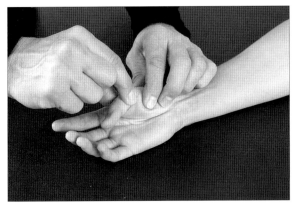

Figure 14.2 Supination MWM during thumb flexion

2 Given the information from the history and the MRI, did you have any treatment or prognosis hypotheses under consideration at this early stage? If so, what factors in the patient's history, based on your experience and the scientific evidence, support your hypotheses?

Clinician's response

Given the apparent mismatch between the recalled history of events surrounding the injury and the diagnostic imaging, some care needed to be exercised in conducting the physical examination, as well as in planning treatment and prognostication. However, this could be balanced against an elapsed period of 7 months following the injury during which the patient had not sought medical care, indicating a lower level of injury severity.

From a manual therapy perspective, the reported functional restrictions with tasks such as opening a jar, using a can opener and wringing a washcloth, along with the absence of resting pain, suggest a condition that is mechanical in nature and one which should be amenable to Mobilisation with Movement (MWM) intervention. On the other hand, there is little in the way of evidence from clinical trials of MWM for the thumb (or wrist and fingers) that can be used in informing a clinical decision regarding a treatment hypothesis.

In terms of prognosis, there are some underlying medical conditions that should be factored into any clinical decisions. For example, Joan reports diabetes mellitus that, although under control with medication, would likely be associated with delayed healing and as such may indicate a longer period for resolution of her problem. Osteopenia may also complicate matters considering the diagnostic imaging findings of a previously healed fracture and bony irregularity just proximal to the distal phalanx of the right thumb.

PHYSICAL EXAMINATION

Physiological movements

On initial examination, goniometric measurement revealed a reduced range of flexion of the IPJ and the MPJ of the right thumb, that is, 45° and 46° respectively, as compared to 72° and 53° for the uninjured left thumb. There was pain both at the IPJ and MPJ at the end of the motion and Joan rated the intensity as 5 out of 10. There was a slight discomfort reported with abduction of her right thumb. However, when passively hyperabducted, there was a rather sharp pain at the radial aspect of the MPJ of the right thumb. These were the most remarkable findings on examination of motion.

Grip strength

Over three trials using a Jaymar hand dynamometer (Therapeutic Equipment Corporation, Clifton, USA), there was a reduction of the grip strength in her right hand (mean 13.9 kg (SD 1.9)) compared to her left hand (mean 16.1 kg (SD 0.7)).[4] Pain during gripping with her right hand was 4–6 out of 10.

MWM trial

In an attempt to see the effect of a MWM, a medial glide and a lateral glide of the base of the proximal phalanx was attempted but did not reduce the patient's pain with flexion. However, a MWM that supinated the proximal phalanx totally relieved her MPJ pain during the movement (Figure 14.2 and Table 14.1).

As suggested by the positional fault hypothesis (see Chapter 4), a possible explanation for the rapid change in pain and range of motion (ROM) may be the reduction of a positional fault of the proximal phalanx. In order to evaluate this hypothesis, a number of MRI scans were taken before and during the application of a MWM, and then after a course of MWM treatment.

Table 14.1 Directions for applying a supination MWM during thumb flexion (see Figure 14.2)

Indication	Pain and/or limitation of movement of the MPJ or IPJs of the thumb or fingers. The following example is for a flexion limitation of the first MPJ	
Positioning	Patient	Patient lays supine or sits with the elbow flexed and forearm resting on a table.
	Treated body part	The patient's forearm is supinated with the wrist in the neutral position. The dorsal aspect of the hand rests on the supporting surface, allowing free movement of the thumb in any direction.
	Therapist	The therapist stands facing the patient.
	Therapist's hands	The therapist stabilises the distal end of the first metacarpal using the thumb and index finger of one hand while the thumb and index finger of the other hand grips the proximal end of the proximal phalanx on the ulnar and radial aspects to allow free movement of the MPJ into flexion.
Application guidelines	• The supination force is applied as a spin rotation. • While maintaining the supination force the patient is instructed to actively flex the thumb (Figure 14.2). • If the technique is indicated, the patient will be able to achieve considerably greater flexion range without pain. • If pain persists, even after modifications are considered, the technique should not be used. • Repeat the movement several times before reassessing the active movement independent of the glide. Subsequent reassessment should reveal a significant improvement in pain-free range of movement. • If full range and pain-free active flexion can be achieved with the supination glide, the therapist then applies gentle, passive flexion overpressure for 1–2 seconds. It is important that this movement is also pain-free.	
Comments	• Ensure that gentle and not excessive supination force is applied to the proximal phalanx. Excessive force may cause discomfort or pain preventing application of the technique. This is particularly true for an acute injury where there may be significant local tenderness and swelling. It is advisable to use a thick piece of sponge rubber to soften the contact in cases of local tenderness. • The patient must experience no pain or other symptoms at any stage of the mobilisation or active movement. Should pain occur the technique should be modified by altering the direction of the mobilisation force on the proximal phalanx or the amount of force applied.	
Variation	• Two thin strips of non-stretch sports tape may be applied one on top of the other to reproduce the effect of the supination mobilisation. • With careful instruction the patient may be able to reproduce the MWM as a home exercise (Figure 14.3).	

MRI scans before treatment

MRI examination of both thumbs with a GE 1.5 Tesla Signa short bore magnet was performed in knee surface coils. Imaging was conducted first while both thumbs were fully flexed (in a painful position on the injured side), and then with the right thumb with the MWM in situ. The scanning for the first position took approximately 40 minutes, and for the second approximately 20 minutes. The patient tolerated the procedures well with a rest interval of about 5 minutes between positions in which the patient walked and stretched. The axial sections of the MRI were examined to determine rotational positions of the phalanx and adjacent metacarpal. On visual inspection, it was noted that the right first proximal phalanx and the first metacarpal were both more pronated than their left counterparts.[1]

When comparing the relative position of the proximal phalanx to the first metacarpal in the axial plane using the MRI digitizer, the right proximal phalanx was found to be 9° relatively pronated to the right first metacarpal. In comparison, the left proximal phalanx was 5° relatively pronated to its adjacent metacarpal. Thus, the proximal phalanx of the right thumb had a relative 4° pronation 'positional fault' compared to the left thumb. The MRI image of the thumb during MWM showed a 'correction' of this positional fault, with a more supinated position of the right proximal phalanx compared to the pre-MWM condition.[1]

EVIDENCE-INFORMED CLINICAL REASONING

1 After the physical examination, was your hypothesis of a positional fault confirmed? What clinical findings were most relevant in coming to this decision?

Clinician's response

It may be tempting to infer that the physical examination alone, which included the application of a trial of MWM, confirms a positional fault. However, it is not currently possible to clinically determine the existence of a positional fault at the first MPJ and IPJ, so clinicians should not assume the amelioration of impairment and pain with a specific MWM confirms the existence of a positional fault. In this case, in addition to the clinical examination, an MRI examination was conducted in order to specifically assess the positional fault hypothesis. The MRI examination arguably found a positional fault (in relation to the opposite asymptomatic side), which was in the opposite direction to that of the pain relieving and ROM improving MWM. It is important to note that the physical examination and the MRI measurements were conducted by health professionals who were blind to each other's assessment findings, which strengthens the validity of the reported results.

2 What were your primary hypotheses with respect to management? Was the Mulligan Concept indicated and, if so, why?

Clinician's response

The primary hypothesis regarding management was that the application of passive supination to the right MPJ, which ameliorated pain with the patient's primary problem (i.e. flexion) on initial application, would likely produce longer-term improvements in impairment if applied frequently enough. That is, the initial marked effect observed on application of the MWM could be viewed as sufficient evidence to include it in the management of this patient's thumb condition.

TREATMENT AND MANAGEMENT

Treatment 1

Based on the clinical findings and without the benefit of the MRI findings, Joan was instructed to perform self-MWM by supinating the right proximal phalanx with her left index finger and thumb while actively flexing her right thumb (Figure 14.3). This self-MWM alleviated the thumb pain. She was instructed to carry out six repetitions every 2 hours, with the emphasis strongly on pain-free performance.

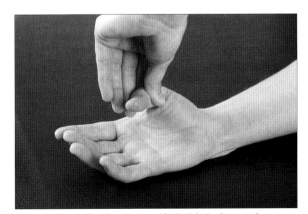

Figure 14.3 Supination self-MWM during active thumb flexion

Treatment 2

After 1 week, Joan reported that she continued to experience pain in her thumb when performing the aggravating activities noted in the first session, which involve flexion of the thumb (e.g. opening a jar or can, picking up Mah-Jong tiles). Upon reassessment, there was 47° of MPJ flexion and 50° of active IPJ flexion with only some 'tight' sensation reported along the MPJ and the IPJ. There was no pain at all with this movement but the patient reported a 'click' sound at the MPJ. Indeed when adding flexion overpressure to the supination MWM a clicking sound at the MPJ of the flexed thumb was noted two out of four times. Additional examination of the right MPJ showed that distraction was painful but compression was painless. Abduction and adduction (i.e. valgus and varus) stress tests produced pain in the lateral and medial aspects of the MPJ respectively. The patient was instructed to continue self-MWM treatment of her thumb as previously instructed, provided there was no pain during the application of the technique.

Treatment 3

After the second week of MWM, Joan reported an overall improvement but continuing discomfort (1–2/10) of her right thumb with sewing and lifting. The 'click' sound was still intermittently noticed by Joan. Upon reassessment, there was 50° of MPJ flexion and 53° of IPJ flexion with no pain elicited. Passive valgus, varus, supination and pronation tests of the MPJ of the right thumb were also painless. Only distraction elicited slight pain deep in the centre of the MPJ, which was 50% less than the previous week.

OUTCOME OF INTERVENTION

After the third week of MWM, Joan stated that her right thumb was much improved. She did not have pain when playing Mah-Jong, nor with any other previously painful activities such as lifting her shopping bag or using a knife when cooking. Instead, she would feel 'tired' in her thumb after activities. The ROM of her right thumb MPJ and the grip strength of her right hand were now as good as that for her left hand.

The flexion ranges of the MPJ and IPJ were 55° and 56° in the right thumb and 55° and 77° in the left, respectively. The mean grip strength across three trials was 18.6 kg (SD 0.5) in the right hand and 17.4 kg (SD 0.9) in the left. There was no pain with gripping. Passive motion testing of the right MPJ was also painless, including distraction, supination, pronation, abduction and adduction. There was occasional joint crepitus (not 'clicking') evident in the right thumb (3 times out of 10 trials of flexion with overpressure). The patient was instructed to discontinue the home exercises and then was re-evaluated by MRI 1 week later.

MRI scans after treatment

Using the same procedures as above (for the pre-treatment MRI scans), it was observed that the right proximal phalanx was found to be 9° relatively pronated to the right first metacarpal. Similarly, the left proximal phalanx was 5° relatively pronated to its neighbour.[1] Therefore, the proximal phalanx of the right thumb had the same amount of 'positional fault' as pre-treatment (i.e. 4° in pronation as compared to the left thumb). No reduction of the initial positional fault was found even though the patient now had no pain when flexing her right thumb and her grip strength had been restored.

AUTHORS' MULLIGAN CONCEPT COMMENTARY

The MWM provided an effective form of physical therapy for treating this patient with chronic pain and dysfunction of the thumb following trauma. The patient showed an immediate decrease of pain on active movement with MWM, a finding that has been demonstrated with other MWM techniques.[5–10] The success of MWM relies greatly on the selection of the direction for the sustained corrective glide (or other accessory movement). Mulligan states that the direction of correction is usually perpendicular to the plane of motion.[11] However, in practice, the process of determining the direction for the glide may be more of an iterative one in which a series of different directions of accessory movement are tested before settling on the most effective (Chapter 2).

In this case report, the authors employed MRI scans to study the positions of the phalanx and metacarpal bones and the effects of MWM on these bony positions. A small pronation positional fault was found in the axial plane of the MPJ of the right thumb, which appeared consistent with the mode of injury described by the patient. Interestingly, the supination MWM, which was chosen purely on a clinical reasoning basis (i.e. pain alleviation and improved ROM), addressed this positional fault during its application. It was not possible to establish if the immediate reduction of the patient's pain following application of the MWM was the direct result of correction of the positional fault. However, the finding that the direction of the effective MWM accessory movement (i.e. MPJ supination) was opposite to the MRI determined positional fault (i.e. MPJ pronation) and that the positional fault appeared consistent with the mechanism of injury, tends to suggest that selection of the direction of the glide in the MWM should also consider the mechanism of injury. That is, consideration should be given to the glide being in a direction opposite to that induced by the mechanism of injury.

The follow-up MRI scans taken after the completion of the treatment program showed no change from the positional fault seen on the pre-treatment MRI scans, even though there was an amelioration of pain and improvement in function. This finding indicates that 3 weeks of self-MWM may have produced its clinical effects through mechanisms other than a long-term correction of the positional fault. Interestingly, there was an immediate change in bony position during application of the MWM, as seen on repeat MRI scans. This initial effect may therefore be sufficient to stimulate longer-term changes in nociceptive and motor system (dys)function that are reflected in pain relief and improved function, possibly through a more complex mechanism(s) than implied by a simple and long lasting correction of bony alignment. Hypothetical and proposed mechanisms and effects are outlined in Chapters 4–7 and require further investigation.

References

1 Hsieh CY, Vicenzino B, Yang CH, et al. Mulligan's mobilization with movement for the thumb: a single case report using magnetic resonance imaging to evaluate the positional fault hypothesis. Manual Therapy. 2002;7(1):44–9.

2 Lucas G. Examination of the Hand. Springfield: Charles C. Thomas 1972.

3 Brukner P, Khan K. Clinical Sports Medicine (3rd edn). Sydney: McGraw-Hill Book Company 2007.

4 Gunther C, Burger A, Rickert M, et al. Grip strength in healthy Caucasian adults: reference values. Journal Hand Surgery (Am). 2008;33(4):558–65.

5 Abbott JH, Patla CE, Jensen RH. The initial effects of an elbow mobilization with movement technique on grip strength in subjects with lateral epicondylalgia. Manual Therapy. 2001;6(3):163–9.

6 Folk B. Traumatic thumb injury management using mobilization with movement. Manual Therapy. 2001;6(3):178–82.

7 O'Brien T, Vicenzino B. A study of the effects of Mulligan's mobilization with movement treatment of lateral ankle pain using a case study design. Manual Therapy. 1998;3(2):78–84.

8 Vicenzino B, Paungmali A, Buratowski S, et al. Specific manipulative therapy treatment for chronic lateral epicondylalgia produces uniquely characteristic hypoalgesia. Manual Therapy. 2001;6(4):205–12.

9 Vicenzino B, Wright A. Effects of a novel manipulative physiotherapy technique on tennis elbow: a single case study. Manual Therapy. 1995 Nov;1(1):30–5.

10 Vicenzino B, Paungmali A, Teys P. Mulligan's mobilization with movement, positional faults and pain relief: Current concepts from a critical review of literature. Manual Therapy. 2007;12(2):98–108.

11 Mulligan B. Manual Therapy — 'NAGS', 'SNAGS', 'MWMs' etc (6th edn). Wellington: Plane View Services 2010.

Chapter 15
A chronic case of fear avoidant low back pain

Toby Hall and Kika Konstantinou

HISTORY

At the time of assessment, Peter was 38 years old and married with two children, working as a draughtsman in an architect's office. He was able to work normally, but with low back pain (LBP), throughout the current episode. Prior to his present problem (9 months ago) he enjoyed cycling three times per week for up to 80 km but had been unable to do so since he hurt his back.

When asked what he thought the main problem was he replied that he had 'prolapsed a disc' in his back and this was preventing recovery. When asked what he thought therapy could do for him, he replied perhaps it could give him 'exercise to help the disc recover'. His stated goals were to be able to cycle regularly and return to home renovation.

Current history

Peter presented with a 9-month history of LBP as depicted on the body chart (Figure 15.1). The pain was described as an intermittent ache, localised to his lower lumbar spine and without any side dominance. There was no complaint of pain or other symptoms radiating to his legs. At its worst the pain could reach 7/10 on a numerical rating scale (NRS).

The problem had developed gradually over a number of weeks with no particular incident of onset. However, Peter had noticed the pain was related to sustained flexion loading activities, and was eased by activity involving extension. He associated the onset of his LBP with unaccustomed and heavy repetitive activity of home improvements on his recently acquired house. Notably he had started to renovate a few weeks prior to the onset of his back pain. He had been scraping up glued down floor coverings, shortly followed by de-nailing and laying wooden floorboards. This process took a number of days and involved either sustained end-range trunk flexion or repeated trunk flexion.

Following the onset of the problem he sought advice from his general practitioner who referred him to a physiotherapist. The physiotherapist had diagnosed a disc problem, possibly a prolapse, caused by a combination of the unaccustomed flexion activity, sustained flexion posture when cycling and poor office ergonomics. He was prescribed specific muscle retraining for multifidus and transversus abdominis to improve spinal stabilisation, as well as repeated extension exercise to help the disc. The therapist had also told him to maintain a neutral lumbar lordosis, particularly when performing trunk flexion activity. Peter's workstation had also been assessed and corrected to enable him to hold an upright lordotic posture at all times.

Peter had performed the exercises diligently for the first 2 months and continued to avoid flexion as much as possible. However, there had been little improvement in his symptoms and the only additional advice his general practitioner had given him was to remain active, take up walking rather than cycling and to learn to live with it. Having experienced such a poor response from mainstream medical treatment he sought relief from a chiropractor, acupuncturist and massage therapist. All had been unable to help him, although he reported short-term relief from the chiropractic manipulation, but after 10 treatment sessions he gave up.

Peter tried to return to cycling and to renovating his house but found that these activities exacerbated his back pain. Since then he had avoided all trunk flexion and had only been able to undertake home renovation that did not require repeated or sustained trunk flexion. This was of ongoing concern and prompted him to continue to seek treatment to find a solution to his problem.

Past history

Peter had experienced two previous episodes of LBP, 2 and 3 years earlier. Both episodes were less severe than the current one with the pain only lasting for 2 weeks, and did not require any treatment. In both cases the pain had started with cycling and had simply gone away by stopping this exercise for 2 weeks.

24-hour symptom behaviour

Aggravating activities and postures included sitting (particularly sitting slumped) for more than half an hour, driving a car for more than 20 minutes, cycling for more than 20 minutes, and repeated or sustained flexion associated with his house renovations. The provoked

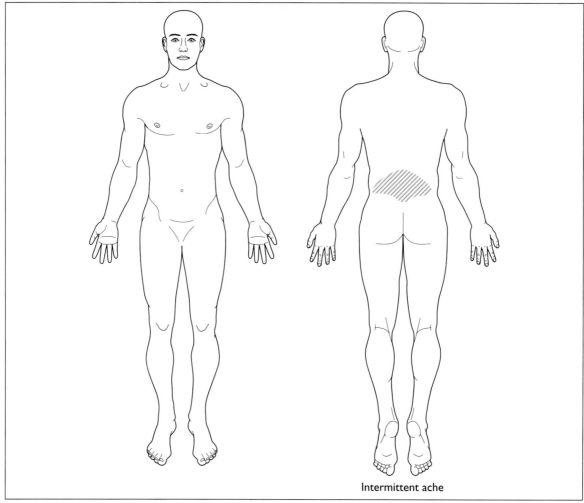

Intermittent ache

Figure 15.1 Body chart

pain usually quickly subsided once he stopped the aggravating activity.

The Patient Specific Functional Scale (PSFS) scores up to five activities that the patient is having difficulty performing. Each activity is rated from 0 to 10, with a score of 0/50 indicating maximum difficulty with activities while 50/50 indicates normal activity without any difficulty. The PSFS is a valid and reliable measure of disability and has been shown to be more sensitive to change following treatment than other measures of disability as well as pain and physical impairment.[1] Peter scored 20 out of a potential maximum of 40 for his four pain-provoking activities (5/10 each for sitting, cycling, home renovation and driving his car).

Avoiding sustained trunk flexion allowed the pain to subside. Peter had no difficulty sleeping and woke in the morning with no pain or back stiffness. Over a typical 24-hour period there appeared to be no pattern to his pain unless he undertook activities involving sustained flexion.

Medical history and investigations

Peter had a history of irritable bowel syndrome controlled by diet. In addition, he had complained of migraine headaches for most of his life, which he managed with anti-migraine medication at the onset of the symptoms. There was no evidence of other health issues and his general health was good. Prior X-ray films showed narrowing of the L5–S1 disc with no further abnormality detected.

EVIDENCE-INFORMED CLINICAL REASONING

1 What cues from the patient history may be of use in determining a prognostic hypothesis?

Clinician's response

On the positive side for Peter's prognosis, he was clearly an active participant in his rehabilitation. He maintained normal work activities, exercised and strictly followed medical advice. His stated goals seemed reasonable. In addition, there was no evidence of 'red flags' (e.g. no correlation with abdominal symptoms, no general malaise or weight loss) indicating serious spinal pathology. A further positive prognostic factor is that sustained flexion is a pain-provocative movement but the pain is quickly resolved when moving out of flexion. This would indicate a non-irritable disorder with a predictable pattern of pain provocation.

However, on the negative side, concern was raised by the initial physiotherapist's diagnosis of disc pathology and the explanation given to the patient. Misinterpretation of this diagnosis had caused some fear of flexion, to the point that Peter avoided flexion completely. Although no one prognostic factor has been shown to predict recovery from LBP,[2] fear avoidance was a potential contributing factor to the development of his chronic LBP[3] and to his poor response to treatment.[4] Great care needs to be taken in the way that a diagnosis is explained to the patient. Some patients become so focused on avoiding exacerbating their condition that they develop muscle guarding or bracing strategies with abnormal patterns of movement, which in itself can contribute to the development of chronic pain.[5, 6]

For this patient, flexion is the main pain-provocative movement and at first glance a symptomatic disc disorder appears a plausible explanation (on the basis of repeated or sustained flexion loading aggravating the pain, and avoidance of flexion helping manage the pain). However, the diagnosis given to the patient of disc pathology, together with the advice to limit all flexion activity, appears to have resulted in a patient fearful and avoidant of any flexion activities; behaviour consistent with a negative prognosis.

2 What patho-biological hypotheses were you considering at this stage and what case findings support these hypotheses?

Clinician's response

Based on the normal timeframe for tissue healing it is unlikely that any inflammatory changes associated with the tissue damage that occurred 9 months previously have not resolved,[7] particularly as the patient avoided the pain-provocative activities.[5] It is well known that commonly an episode of simple back pain will resolve but may recur. Chronic ongoing pain is more likely to be associated with some risk factors that are not yet clearly identified but may include fear avoidance.[2] In Peter's case at first glance it appears that following a traditional McKenzie treatment approach[8] of avoiding flexion, undertaking repeated extension exercises and maintaining a neutral lordosis had failed to improve his back pain, which is arguably inconsistent with a typical intervertebral disc derangement disorder.[9] However, it is more likely that the information

from the first physiotherapist and general practitioner was misinterpreted and has led to some fear and avoidance of flexion, possibly creating guarding behaviours with altered motor control and subsequent movement impairment.[5] In the authors' experience this is a common scenario that can be managed successfully with the Mulligan Concept. Acute back pain may lead to a lack of movement in a specific direction simply because of fear of aggravating the problem. This then feeds into and prolongs the disorder. If pain-free range of motion (ROM) is initially restored using the Mulligan approach this may be avoided.

PHYSICAL EXAMINATION

Posture and observation

On physical examination, Peter presented with an increase in the lower lumbar lordosis associated with an anterior pelvic tilt, both in standing and sitting. Observing the patient undress and remove his shoes revealed an unwillingness to flex his lumbar spine, he tended to move at his hips and knees maintaining his lower lumbar lordosis at all times. When asked why he did this he said that the previous physiotherapist had advised him to avoid flexing his back, as it would aggravate the disc problem.

Active movements

Active lumbar spine movements were full range and pain-free into extension and lateral flexion. However pain on lumbar flexion was rated at 7/10[10] and markedly restricted both in apparent segmental mobility (inability to reverse the lumbar lordosis in the lower lumbar spine) and overall ROM. The patient could only flex forward so that the fingertips were 32 cm from the floor. This technique has been shown to be a reliable method of measuring forward bending[11] although it does not only measure lumbar spine mobility.[12] Peter moved slowly and hesitantly into forward bending. Repeated movement into flexion revealed little change in ROM or pain. Repeated movement into extension did not change the flexion or extension ROM or pain. The combined movement of flexion/side flexion left was mildly more provocative than flexion/side flexion right. Rotation was not assessed due to the minimal amount of this movement in the lumbar spine.

Peter was subsequently asked to flex forward in standing with the addition of cervical spine flexion to assess the mechanosensitivity of the lumbosacral neural structures.[13] This movement was significantly more painful and restricted in range indicating some element of abnormal lumbar neural tissue mechanosensitivity. Lumbar spine flexion without cervical flexion, or with the knees slightly flexed, was greater in range and less painful.

Lumbar spine flexion and posterior pelvic tilt were assessed in sitting and provoked the usual back pain which was made worse when the patient had his cervical spine flexed. Posterior pelvic tilt and flexion in sitting were restricted in range, particularly in the lower lumbar spine where the patient was unable to reverse the normal lordosis. Moving from the resting position of anterior pelvic tilt to posterior tilt was difficult for the patient. The movement was jerky and poorly controlled, and he tended to substitute movement in the thoracic spine. Asking the patient simply to sit slumped demonstrated a limitation of lower lumbar flexion with an inability to 'let go' or relax the erector spinae muscles.

Neural tissue provocation tests and neurological function

Straight leg raise (SLR) was 75° on the right and 70° on the left. The addition of ankle dorsiflexion increased the back pain and reduced the SLR ROM slightly on both sides. The slump test was slightly more provocative but the movement was symmetrical between the two sides. Neurological function was not tested due to the localised nature of the pain without referral into the leg.

Passive segmental motion tests

Passive physiological intervertebral motion testing revealed limitation of flexion at L4–L5 and L5–S1 motion segments. Postero–anterior (PA) pressure applied centrally to the spinous process of L5, and to a lesser extent L4, provoked Peter's usual back pain. With the lumbar spine flexed as far as possible, with pillows placed under the abdomen, central PA pressure on L5 inclined cephalad provoked greater pain, whereas PA pressure on L4 in this position was unchanged. PA pressure applied unilaterally over the L5–S1 facet joints on the right and left was only mildly symptomatic, with no pain over the L4–L5 facet joints.

Muscle function

There was evidence of poor postural control in sitting and standing, together with an inability to attain a more neutral lumbar spine alignment. Furthermore, there was a notable increase in tone on palpation of the lower lumbar erector spinae muscles, particularly the multifidus palpated immediately adjacent to the lower lumbar spinous process. Peter had difficulty in relaxing these muscles. At this point of the examination, because of the significant joint hypomobility with direction specificity, further assessment of the local muscle system and motor control was not deemed necessary.

Response to Mobilisation with Movement

Given the apparent mechanical appearance of the patient's problem, as well as the non-irritable, localised, direction-specific nature, the condition appeared suited

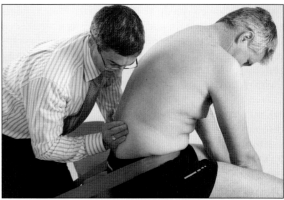

Figure 15.2 Lumbar flexion SNAG in sitting

to a lumbar spine sustained natural apophyseal glide (SNAG) technique.[14] A trial application of a lumbar SNAG was assessed in the sitting position. Sitting was chosen because of the reduced impact this would have over standing on the sensitised lumbosacral neuromeningeal structures. In addition, it is well known that there is increased load borne by the lumbar intervertebral discs in forward bending while standing in comparison to sitting.[15] A SNAG applied in sitting with contact on the L5 spinous process allowed the patient to flex without pain much further into range than he had been able to previously (Figure 15.2). Only moderate pressure was required on the spinous process to improve the movement.

EVIDENCE-INFORMED CLINICAL REASONING

1 How did the physical examination refine your diagnostic hypotheses?

Clinician's response

The direction specificity to the movement limitation and pain suggests an intervertebral disc disorder.[16] However, neither repeated flexion or extension increased or decreased the symptoms and probably points away from some ongoing inflammatory disorder or derangement of the intervertebral disc.[17, 18]

In addition to the apparent lower lumbar segmental hypomobility there was evidence of increased mechanosensitivity of lumbar neuromeningeal structures, probably the dura rather than a specific nerve root. This is based on the fact that there was only localised and central back pain, together with symmetry of pain provocation on SLR and increased pain with cervical flexion when sitting slumped.[17]

The overall interpretation of the information gained from the examination was that the patient's symptoms were consistent with a disorder of movement impairment[5] of the L4–L5 and L5–S1 functional spinal unit, associated with minor neuromeningeal mechano-sensitivity.

2 What were your thoughts for management, both with respect to any contributing factors maintaining the problem and the Mulligan Concept?

Clinician's response

It is apparent that Peter has a limitation of lumbar flexion in the symptomatic area. This restriction appears to be consistent whether the movement is performed in sitting or standing, from the top down or bottom up (posterior pelvic tilt in sitting or forward bending in standing). Peter avoids flexion because of both a fear of pain provocation and also a belief that this would harm his damaged intervertebral disc. He appeared to hold himself actively in extension and movements into flexion were poorly controlled. The disorder was chronic, static and not helped by Peter's fear of flexion secondary to some inappropriate advice from the initial physiotherapist. It would therefore be important to educate Peter about the anatomy and physiology of back pain and try to change his beliefs about his back problem, particularly with respect to his fears about his intervertebral disc[3] and flexion.

A lumbar SNAG technique is suggested to be most useful for patients with predominantly unisegmental, unidirectional loss of movement,[18] which is exactly the presentation in this case. This technique is a useful treatment approach as it can demonstrate to the patient that flexion can be pain-free and ROM quickly improved. The technique can also be progressively applied to gradually expose the patient to the painful movements of which they have become fearful. The aim of the SNAG with Peter was to encourage a gradually progressive resumption of normal activity, overcome fear avoidance and reduce anxiety.[3] When applying a lumbar SNAG it is important that the therapist quickly identifies the appropriate amount and direction of force required at the appropriate spinal level to gain the patient's confidence. Whilst a lumbar SNAG would appear ideally suited to manage the joint hypomobility problem, caution must be exercised in this case because of the evidence of lumbar neuromeningeal mechanosensitivity.

A recent study investigated the immediate effects of lumbar spine flexion SNAGs in a group of patients with LBP.[19] Patients responding best to this intervention (either pain reduction or increased ROM) presented with localised LBP, especially on flexion, with predominantly intermittent symptoms and restriction of flexion. The majority of positive responders reported flexion activities or postures as the main aggravating factors. The patients that did not seem to respond to the SNAGs had symptoms radiating to the leg and were reporting mostly a first-time LBP episode. All subjects had moderate functional restrictions as measured by the Roland-Morris Disability Questionnaire[20] but not high psychological distress as measured by the Distress and Risk Assessment Method Questionnaire.[21]

TREATMENT AND MANAGEMENT

Treatment 1

Due to the favourable response of the trial SNAG in sitting during the patient's assessment, this technique was chosen for the initial treatment. Table 15.1 details the lumbar SNAG technique. A number of features in both the patient history and physical examination suggested caution when applying this technique. Not least of which was the fact that Peter was afraid to flex. It was fortunate in this case that the symptomatic level was clearly indicated by the physical examination findings and that the disorder appeared to be localised to the L5–S1 segment. This enabled a very rapid change in the range of flexion, with an immediate reduction in pain. To err on the side of caution, only three sets of six repetitions of the SNAG technique were carried out in the first session and home exercises were not prescribed.

The immediate effect of the SNAG was to gain a pain-free range of flexion in sitting with some moderate improvement in the segmental mobility in the lower lumbar spine. In standing, the range of flexion improved by 5 cm after the Mobilisation with Movement (MWM). While changes in measures of physical impairment have been shown to be less responsive than pain and disability measures in the overall outcome of LBP,[1] intra-session changes in pain and ROM have been shown to predict a positive outcome to manual therapy.[23] So the immediate improvement in both pain and range of lumbar flexion boded well for recovery. Furthermore, survey research into the use and reported effects of lumbar SNAGs has shown that the most commonly reported changes are increased range and pain relief,[24] and this is consistent with the results observed after treating Peter.

Peter was instructed not to ride his bike or to do any home renovation until his next appointment. It was explained to him that this was a temporary measure and given time he should return to normal activity. Within the treatment session a considerable amount of time was also given to explaining to the patient about the physiology of back pain, healing of tissues, anatomy of the disc and fear avoidance behaviour. The aim was to reduce the patient's fear and anxiety regarding his back problem through education.

Treatment 2

The patient returned for reassessment and treatment 2 days later. He reported significant improvement in his confidence, less back pain and improved sitting tolerance. He now scored his sitting as 3/10 on the PSFS. Peter also noticed he could sit longer at work with less

Table 15.1	SNAG for lumbar spine flexion	
Indication	**Pain or loss of movement during lumbar spine flexion**	
Positioning	Patient	Patient sitting on the side of a treatment table.
	Treated body part	Lumbar spine in pain-free position.
	Therapist	Standing behind and slightly to the side of the patient with a manual therapy belt placed around the patient's pelvis and also around the back of the therapist's thighs. The therapist rests backwards on the belt to stabilise the patient on the treatment table.
	Therapist's hands	*Stabilising hand*: Anterior aspect of the patient's pelvis to provide counterforce for the gliding force. *Gliding hand*: The hypothenar eminence is placed on the inferior aspect of the spinous process of the superior vertebra.
Application guidelines	• Ensure that only sufficient force is used through the manual therapy belt to secure the patient on the treatment table. Excessive force can be very uncomfortable on the patient's abdomen. • The force generated through the gliding hand must be directed along the facet joint plane, which in the lumbar spine is generally orientated vertically.[22] • Hand contact tenderness can be minimised by the use of sponge rubber. • Ask the patient to flex forward and stop when they feel pain to avoid forcing a painful movement. • As a precaution apply gentle force initially, particularly if the disorder is acute. Stronger force is usually required when the lumbar movement is limited by stiffness. If the movement is moderately improved but still painful, stronger force can be employed. • Slightly alter the angle of force if pain-free flexion cannot be obtained. In some individuals variations in the anatomy of the facet joint may require an alteration in the direction of force to achieve pain-free movement. • Change the lumbar vertebral level at which the SNAG is applied if the movement is either unchanged or if it is made worse on the first application. • Attempt no more than four trials to obtain pain-free movement as failure to relieve pain over this number of trials will prove counterproductive. • Repeat the movement 6–10 times once pain-free movement is achieved. • Subsequent reassessment should reveal a significant improvement in pain-free ROM. • Three to five sets of further repetitions can be performed if improvement is evident on reassessment.	
Comments	• Maintain the glide force throughout the movement until the patient returns to the starting position. • It is important to encourage the patient to achieve the maximum end-range position.	
Variation	• SNAGs for lumbar flexion can be undertaken in a variety of different positions. When the patient gains full ROM in sitting (Figure 15.2) the technique can be progressed to standing (Figure 15.4). For the smaller therapist with a tall patient, SNAGs in standing or sitting may be difficult and the technique can be undertaken in 4-point kneeling with greater ease (Figure 15.5). • Self-treatment techniques are very important to reinforce the effectiveness of the SNAGs used in the clinic. A self-SNAG requires the use of a lumbar self-treatment strap or a cloth belt. The purpose of the strap is to replicate the force provided by the therapist's hand on the spinous process of the involved level. The patient pulls up on the strap in a vertical direction along the facet joint plane. The self-SNAG can be carried out in sitting (Figure 15.3) or standing. The exercise is usually repeated 10 times at least 3 times per day.	

discomfort and that the pain frequency over the previous two days had decreased.

On examination his flexion range was now 25 cm from the fingertips to the floor, with the same pain rated as 5/10. He moved more confidently into flexion and with less hesitation than on the previous occasion. Both lumbar flexion and posterior pelvic tilt in sitting were still more provocative with neck flexion than without it.

In view of the positive sustained response to the first treatment session the SNAG was repeated in sitting, but was progressed to five sets of 10 repetitions. The patient was also taught to perform a lumbar self-SNAG in sitting as a home exercise (Figure 15.3). Peter was shown how to place the lumbar self-SNAG strap on the

inferior aspect of the L5 spinous process. A small piece of sports tape was placed on the exact location so that he could easily find the correct placement each time. Peter was advised to alter the position of the strap in relation to the spine if he could not move into flexion without pain. He was advised to perform the exercise 10 times on five occasions during the day and that there should be no pain during the exercise.

At the end of the session lumbar flexion in standing had improved to 22 cm from the fingertips to the floor. In sitting, flexion was now pain-free, but the quality and range of the lower lumbar spine flexion, although improved, was still poor. Peter was asked to try a 20-minute cycling session, but told not to change his activities with respect to home renovation.

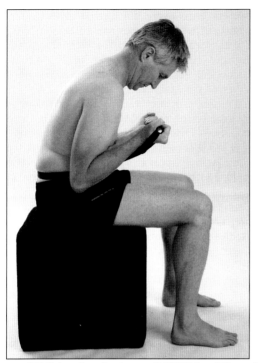

Figure 15.3 Lumbar flexion self-SNAG in sitting with a self-SNAG strap

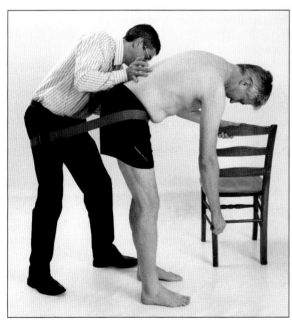

Figure 15.4 Lumbar flexion SNAG in standing

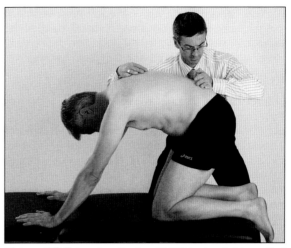

Figure 15.5 Lumbar flexion SNAG in 4-point kneeling

Treatment 3

Peter returned for reassessment and treatment 1 week later and reported further improvement as a result of the home exercise and the previous session's treatment. He was able to cycle for 20 minutes with only mild back pain, scored as 2/10 on the PSFS. Sitting was now down to 2/10 on this scale. Interestingly, although sitting was much improved Peter was still having difficulty driving for more than 20 minutes which was scored at the original 5/10 level.

Active lumbar flexion in standing was 22 cm from the fingertips to the floor with pain rated as 3/10. There were still significant signs of neuromeningeal mechanosensitivity as flexion in both standing and sitting was provoked by the addition of cervical spine flexion.

In light of the neuromeningeal mechanosensitivity the SNAG was progressed into a standing position for both the clinic treatment technique and home exercise, but with the knees flexed to 5°. Peter was instructed to continue with the self-SNAG exercise in sitting as well as the self-SNAG in standing with the knees flexed.

At the end of the third session lumbar flexion in standing had improved to 15 cm from the fingertips to the floor and was pain-free. The range of lower lumbar flexion was improving in both sitting and standing. Peter was asked to resume normal activity with respect to home renovation, but to do this gradually over weeks to allow his back muscle strength to increase with this activity.

Treatment 4

One week later Peter reported further improvement with all activities, with 8/40 scored on the PSFS. Driving appeared to be the most symptomatic activity, with pain after about 30 minutes forcing him to avoid further driving. Flexion in standing was pain-free but limited to 14 cm from the fingertips to the floor, and it was pain-free in sitting. Lumbar flexion in sitting was painful when the cervical spine was maximally flexed. The dominant feature now appeared to be neuromeningeal mechanosensitivity.[25, 26] Driving can be more provocative for neural structures than normal sitting because, when driving, the knees are more extended and the spine is generally more slumped. In addition, cervical flexion still elicited the back pain during flexion in sitting and standing, and the slump test was still positive for the back pain.

The lumbar SNAG technique in sitting was therefore progressed by pre-setting the cervical spine in flexion. Pain-free range was achieved by applying the SNAG at L5, during and after the application of the technique. The flexion range in standing improved to 10 cm from the fingertips to the floor. The home exercise was also modified accordingly.

Treatment 5

Two weeks later Peter reported almost no back pain with any activity, scoring 4/40 on the PSFS. This was only related to driving and renovating. He was still gradually building up his tolerance with these activities. Flexion in standing was 6 cm from the fingertips to the floor. The addition of cervical flexion did not provoke any symptoms but the slump test was still mildly provocative for the back pain, with movement of the left leg slightly more symptomatic.

The lumbar SNAG technique in sitting was progressed again by pre-setting the cervical spine in flexion and the left knee in 30° of flexion. Pain-free movement was achieved by applying the SNAG at L5. This SNAG was also given as a home exercise to replace all previous exercises. In light of the significant improvement the patient was discharged.

Final outcome

Peter was contacted by telephone 1 month later. He reported a return to all previous activities and no back pain.

AUTHORS' MWM COMMENTARY

A lumbar SNAG was successful in the management of this particular case. Pain, ROM and physical disability all improved as a direct result of the intervention. Peter had a clear history of localised chronic back pain. His disorder had been static for many months and improvement was highly unlikely to be due to natural resolution. It is, however, possible that improvement resulted because of a change in his understanding and beliefs regarding his back pain and improved self-efficacy.[27, 28] Empirical evidence indicates that exposure to fear stimuli and non-avoidance are crucial in fear reduction.[28] Furthermore, there is some evidence of a strong association between cognitive factors and the levels of pain and disability reported by patients with chronic LBP.[29] Exercise and mobilisation, together with patient education, that encourages resumption of normal activity, might help to break the fear avoidance/chronic pain cycle and should be incorporated in a modern treatment approach within the biopsychosocial model.[30]

A recent cross-over clinical trial investigating the immediate effects of lumbar spine flexion SNAGs in LBP patients concluded that the technique produced statistically significant increases in ROM but not pain reduction compared to a placebo intervention.[19] Analysis of the raw data indicates that 19 (73%) of the 26 patients demonstrated improvement in ROM or pain score with the SNAG treatment. On the other hand, only 9 (35%) of the 26 patients showed improvement in ROM or pain score with the placebo. Although this small study[19] provides preliminary support for the immediate effects of lumbar flexion SNAGs on ROM, the clinical significance remains to be determined.

It is not known which if any of the proposed effects are the mechanism of action for lumbar SNAGs as no studies have yet investigated this specifically (see Chapters 4–7). However, considering lumbar SNAGs specifically, there are some similarities between a PA pressure undertaken in prone lying and a SNAG applied through the spinous process. Lee and Evans[31] report that a PA pressure on the L5 spinous process induces anterior translation of the L5 vertebra and flexion at the L5–S1 segment. This is the same motion segment and limited direction of movement demonstrated in this case. The biomechanical effect of the SNAG may be enhanced by the cephalad direction of the glide along the facet joint plane, together with the active movement. Arguably this would facilitate gliding at the facet joint and reduce the articular surface compressive force. Interestingly, PA pressure inclined cephalad has been shown to be less stiff.[32]

Another possible explanation for the mechanism of action in this case may be through correction of a positional fault at the L5–S1 segment (see Chapter 4). In addition Mulligan hypothesised that lack of normal facet gliding in flexion may distort the disc[14] and provoke pain. An extended spine and lack of facet gliding may result from increased lumbar extensor muscle activity.[33] Lumbar flexion SNAGs may mobilise the stiff facet joints, which may have the effect of inhibiting extensor muscle and so relieving the provocative stress on the injured disc.

Zusman[34] has described a new rationale based on the theory of extinction and habituation for the pain relief provided by manual therapy. Pain is a form of aversive memory that once formed is recalled with increasing ease. Zusman (p 42)[34] states that:

> it is becoming increasing clear that many of the mechanisms known to be responsible for activity-dependent sensitisation of dorsal horn pain pathway neurones closely resemble those associated with supraspinal memory encoding long-term potentiation.

In simple terms, long-term potentiation occurs following a barrage of input from the periphery causing long-term changes of the postsynaptic neurone, a process known as central sensitisation.[35] Noxious stimuli from damaged tissues produces learning type changes or plasticity of the nervous system. The nervous system therefore 'learns' to respond to increasingly less powerful stimuli, a process similar to Pavlovian conditioning.[36]

Behaviourally, a conditioned fear response may be reduced in intensity through extinction; a form of learning characterised by a decrease in a conditioned response when the conditioned stimulus that elicits it is repeatedly non-reinforced.[36] In other words, we can extinguish the fear and memory of pain by overlaying a new memory through repeating the previously painful activity in a way that does not provoke pain. In terms of pain extinction, the aim is to encourage normal activity in a progressive, functional and pain-free manner.[34] In this case, flexion was the painful, fear avoidant activity/movement. The SNAG provided exposure to the feared movement in the absence of any overt danger, which is fundamental to interventions used in the extinction of aversive memories.[35, 36] Progressive mobilisation may also desensitise the nervous system through habituation. The mechanism involves a progressive decline in the ability of the presynaptic nerve terminal to transmit impulses. In Peter's case, nonnoxious sensory input from the repeated lumbar SNAG may have competed with and replaced pain sensitisation, returning the nervous system to a normal state.[34]

References

1 Pengel LH, Refshauge KM, Maher CG. Responsiveness of pain, disability, and physical impairment outcomes in patients with low back pain. Spine. 2004;29(8): 879–83.

2 Kent PM, Keating JL. Can we predict poor recovery from recent-onset non-specific low back pain? A systematic review. Manual Therapy. 2008;13(1): 12–28.

3 Vlaeyen JW, Linton SJ. Fear-avoidance and its consequences in chronic musculoskeletal pain: a state of the art. Pain. 2000;85(3):317–32.

4 Leeuw M, Goossens ME, Linton SJ, et al. The fear-avoidance model of musculoskeletal pain: current state of scientific evidence. Journal of Behavioural Medicine. 2007;30(1):77–94.

5 O'Sullivan P. Diagnosis and classification of chronic low back pain disorders: maladaptive movement and motor control impairments as underlying mechanism. Manual Therapy. 2005;10(4):242–55.

6 O'Sullivan PB, Beales DJ. Diagnosis and classification of pelvic girdle pain disorders — Part 1: a mechanism based approach within a biopsychosocial framework. Manual Therapy. 2007;12(2):86–97.

7 Waddell G. The physical basis of back pain. In Waddell (ed.) The Back Pain Revolution. Edinburgh: Churchill Livingstone 1998:135–54.

8 McKenzie R. The Lumbar Spine: Mechanical Diagnosis and Therapy. Waikanae: Spinal Publications, 1981.

9 McKenzie R, May S. The Lumbar Spine: Mechanical Diagnosis and Therapy (2nd edn). Waikanae: Spinal Publications 2003.

10 Breivik EK, Bjornsson GA, Skovlund E. A comparison of pain rating scales by sampling from clinical trial data. Clinical Journal of Pain. 2000;16(1):22–8.

11 Kippers V, Parker AW. Toe-touch test. A measure of its validity. Physical Therapy. 1987;67(11):1680–4.

12 Corben T, Lewis JS, Petty NJ. Contribution of lumbar spine and hip movement during the palms to floor test in individuals with diagnosed hypermobility syndrome. Physiotherapy Theory Practice. 2008;24(1):1–12.

13 Hall TM, Elvey RL. Management of mechanosensitivity of the nervous system in spinal pain syndromes. In: Boyling G, Jull G (eds) Grieves' Modern Manual Therapy (3rd edn). Edinburgh: Churchill Livingstone 2004:413–31.

14 Mulligan BR. Manual Therapy: 'NAGs', 'SNAGs', 'MWMs' etc (5th edn). Wellington: Plane View Services 2004.

15 Adams MA, Bogduk N, Burton K, et al. The Biomechanics of Back Pain. Edinburgh: Churchill Livingstone 2002.

16 Young S, April C, Laslett M. Correlation of clinical examination characteristics with three sources of chronic low back pain. Spine Journal. 2003;3(6):460–5.

17 Summers B, Malhan K, Cassar-Pullicino V. Low back pain on passive straight leg raising: the anterior theca as a source of pain. Spine. 2005;30(3):342–5.

18 Mulligan B. SNAGS: mobilisations of the spine with active movement. In: Boyling J, Palastanga N (eds) Grieves' Modern Manual Therapy: The Vertebral Column (2nd edn). Edinburgh: Churchill Livingstone 1994:733–43.

19 Konstantinou K, Foster N, Rushton A, et al. Flexion mobilizations with movement techniques: the immediate effects on range of movement and pain in subjects with low back pain. Journal of Manipulative and Physiological Therapeutics. 2007;30(3):178–85.

20 Stratford PW, Binkley J, Solomon P, et al. Defining the minimum level of detectable change for the Roland-Morris questionnaire. Physical Therapy. 1996;76(4):359–65; discussion 66–8.

21 Main CJ, Wood PL, Hollis S, et al. The distress and risk assessment method. A simple patient classification to identify distress and evaluate the risk of poor outcome. Spine. 1992;17(1):42–52.

22 Bogduk N. Clinical Anatomy of the Lumbar Spine (4th edn). Edinburgh: Churchill Livingstone 2004.

23 Tuttle N. Do changes within a manual therapy treatment session predict between-session changes for patients with cervical spine pain? Australian Journal of Physiotherapy. 2005;51(1):43–8.

24 Konstantinou K, Foster N, Rushton A, et al. The use and reported effects of mobilization with movement techniques in low back pain management; a cross-sectional descriptive survey of physiotherapists in Britain. Manual Therapy. 2002;7(4):206–14.

25 Hall T, Elvey RL. Evaluation and treatment of neural tissue pain disorders. In: Donatelli R, Wooden M (eds) Orthopaedic Physical Therapy (4th edn). New York: Churchill Livingstone 2009.

26 Schäfer A, Hall TM, Briffa K. Classification of low back related leg pain — a proposed pathomechanisms based approach. Manual Therapy. 2009;14(2): 222–30.

27 Moseley GL. Evidence for a direct relationship between cognitive and physical change during an education intervention in people with chronic low back pain. European Journal of Pain. 2004;8(1):39–45.

28 Tryon WW. Possible mechanisms for why desensitization and exposure therapy work. Clinical Psychology Review. 2005;25(1):67–95.

29 Woby S, Roach N, Urmston M, et al. The relation between cognitive factors and levels of pain and disability in chronic low back pain patients presenting for physiotherapy. European Journal of Pain. 2007;11(8):869–77.

30 Moseley L. Combined physiotherapy and education is efficacious for chronic low back pain. Australian Journal of Physiotherapy. 2002;48(4):297–302.

31 Lee R, Evans J. An in vivo study of the intervertebral movements induced by posteroanterior mobilisation. Clinical Biomechanics. 1997;12(6):400–8.

32 Allison GT, Edmondston SJ, Roe CP, et al. Influence of load orientation on the posteroanterior stiffness of the lumbar spine. Journal of Manipulative and Physiological Therapeutics. 1998;21(8): 534–8.

33 MacDonald DA, Moseley GL, Hodges PW. The lumbar multifidus: does the evidence support clinical beliefs? Manual Therapy. 2006;11(4):254–63.

34 Zusman M. Mechanisms of musculoskeletal physiotherapy. Physical Therapy Reviews. 2004;9(1):39–49.

35 Zusman M. Forebrain-mediated sensitization of central pain pathways: 'non-specific' pain and a new image for MT. Manual Therapy. 2002;7(2):80–8.

36 Myers KM, Davis M. Behavioral and neural analysis of extinction. Neuron. 2002;36(4):567–84.

Chapter 16
Restoration of trunk extension 23 years after iatrogenic injury

Mark Oliver

HISTORY

At the time of the intervention, John was a 48-year-old customs officer having previously served as a soldier. He presented with a 23-year history of symptoms as shown on the body chart (Figure 16.1). John experienced constant but variable pain in the right lumbosacral and sacroiliac region, slight pain in the right groin, marked limitation of trunk extension and an intermittent 'catching pain' in the right lumbosacral area. He also experienced episodic severe lumbosacral pain radiating into the right buttock and posterior thigh as far as the knee.

Past and present history

When he was 25 years of age, John sustained a severe fracture of the radius and the subsequent orthopaedic surgical procedure required bone graft material to be taken from the right anterosuperior pelvic brim. When John awoke after the procedure he experienced severe pain in the right lumbosacral and sacroiliac joint (SIJ) region. In addition, the right leg 'felt longer' and he had severe limitation of trunk extension. With multiple chiropractic interventions the lumbosacral and SIJ pain had somewhat lessened, but the perception of altered leg length and the limitation of trunk extension had remained unchanged since the procedure. John used a 1 cm heel raise in the left shoe as recommended by his chiropractor for the perceived leg length difference.

In recent years John had been given low back and trunk strengthening exercises by a fitness instructor as part of an exercise-based rehabilitation program, but had been unable to achieve any significant improvement in spinal function, trunk mobility or pain. He was very motivated and undertook weight training and cardiovascular exercise within the limits of his problem, but was frustrated by his inability to effectively strengthen muscles around the low back and pelvis.

Acute exacerbations most often occurred after weight training, vigorous exercise or heavy lifting. When pain was acute spinal flexion became severely limited, the lumbosacral catching pain became significantly worse and the pain would radiate into the right buttock and posterior thigh as far as the knee. The acute episodes occurred at least once every 2–3 months, always related to activity, and eased over 3–4 days after chiropractic manipulation of the low back. Acute symptoms were not present on the day of examination.

Symptom behaviour

The right SIJ and lumbosacral pain was aggravated by moderate–heavy weight training and exercise, so John was forced to keep weights reasonably light and avoid some exercises completely. Jarring activities such as running on hard surfaces or jumping also aggravated symptoms, so he confined running to grassed surfaces and used an orbital trainer.

Pain was increased significantly by lying supine on a hard surface for more than 30 minutes or sleeping supine on a firm bed. When moving out of the supine lying position, John experienced significant right SIJ and lumbosacral pain that eased to a constant low level ache over 30–60 minutes. The lumbosacral and SIJ pain was aggravated by sustained standing, even for relatively short periods, and John preferred to position himself in step-standing to minimise symptoms. As part of his duties as a customs officer, John was at times required to wear heavy body armour that caused a marked increase in pain around the right SIJ region.

Sustained sitting was not a problem, but if symptoms were acute John had difficulty straightening from the flexed position after sitting for more than 30 minutes or so. Half bent positions such as leaning over a basin to clean his teeth would often result in the catching pain in the right lumbosacral region when straightening up.

If the pain was felt to radiate into the buttock, John could obtain some relief by rolling a tennis ball deep into the painful region. Coughing and sneezing produced some 'tenderness' in the right low back region if lumbar symptoms were acute.

Radiological investigations

Plain radiographs had been taken by a chiropractor many years ago, but were not available for review. John's understanding was that the chiropractor felt that they showed a leg length difference (right leg longer than left). No further investigations had been undertaken.

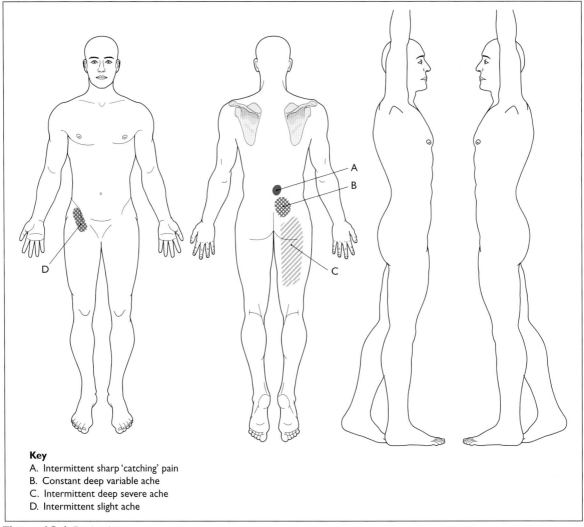

Figure 16.1 Body chart

EVIDENCE-INFORMED CLINICAL REASONING

1 What factors did you hypothesise contributed to the onset of the pain 23 years ago?

Clinician's response

Harvesting donor bone from the iliac crest for a bone graft involves hammering a hollow punch into the innominate bone to extract bone marrow. The patient is anaesthetised and the amount of force involved in hammering and extracting is significant. Complication rates are much greater at the donor site than at the operative site,[1] and have been extensively reported.[2–9] Most attention is paid to the immediate post-operative pain at the donor site but little mention is made of the likelihood of long-term morbidity.[10] Coventry and Tapper[11] described six patients in whom 'SIJ instability'

developed many years after bone graft harvesting from the posterior iliac crest. They postulated that the posterior sacroiliac ligaments must have been transected during the harvest, but this has not been confirmed by investigative studies.

In John's case, the bone graft procedure was very clearly the reason for the onset of the lumbosacral and SIJ pain, but as the bone material was taken from the anterosuperior iliac crest the integrity of the SIJ ligaments was not affected directly by the extraction. With the patient anaesthetised the forces involved in extraction of bone graft material may have been strong enough to derange the SIJ. Of particular interest was that the pain was accompanied by an immediate marked loss of trunk extension that had persisted unchanged for more than 20 years. On questioning, John clearly differentiated the episodic acute lumbosacral symptoms from the chronic pain in the SIJ region and long-standing trunk extension limitation. Chiropractic intervention had assisted in relieving the acute lumbosacral symptoms, but except for immediately after the injury, manipulation had not altered the SIJ pain or the trunk extension loss at all. This suggested the possibility that two closely related problems were present, but that only one had been influenced by the treatment.

2 Did you have any thoughts as to why the problem had not resolved over this long period?

Clinician's response

John was a highly motivated, intelligent individual who exercised regularly and appropriately. However, despite strengthening and other exercise rehabilitation he had been unable to overcome the trunk movement limitation and pain, nor strengthen key muscles in the lumbosacral and pelvic regions. The limitation of trunk extension and alteration in muscle function was present immediately after the bone graft procedure. Possible causative mechanisms considered at this stage included altered relative flexibility[12] between the hips, pelvis and lumbar spine and altered nociceptive and mechanoreceptor neural afferent activity from lumbospinal structures[13–16] or SIJ structures[17–20] changing muscle recruitment and movement patterns.

PHYSICAL EXAMINATION

Posture and observation

In standing, John had a 'flat back' posture[21] with the pelvis in a neutral position in the sagittal plane. Weight-bearing through the legs appeared fairly symmetrical, but the right leg was externally rotated and the right knee slightly more flexed than the left. There was a concavity in the right posterolateral buttock and slightly less muscle bulk in the right medial thigh, right buttock and right low lumbar spine compared to the left. Otherwise, general muscle definition and tone appeared to be very good.

When walking, there was a slight positive Trendelenburg sign with displacement of the trunk to the right when weight-bearing through the right leg. The external rotation of the right femur observed in standing was also present when walking, and when asked to walk with the right leg in the same amount of rotation as the left the Trendelenburg sign increased and John found it necessary to decrease his stride length.

On observation and palpation in standing and in supine lying, the right anterior superior iliac spine (ASIS) was slightly higher and more laterally positioned than the left. John had previously observed and felt this asymmetry and was of the opinion that it had been present since the bone graft procedure. In relaxed standing the right greater trochanter was palpably more posteriorly located than the left, consistent with external rotation of the femur. With active assisted repositioning of both femurs so that the greater trochanters were in the most lateral position (i.e. neutral hip rotation about the longitudinal axis of the femur), there was significantly more tissue resistance to repositioning the right compared to the left.

Trunk active movements

For consistency, the terminology proposed by Lee[22] is used to describe the various components of spinal, pelvic and hip motion. When both innominates and the sacrum rotate as a unit (pelvic girdle) about a coronal axis through the hip joint, this is termed anterior or posterior pelvic tilt. It is important to be aware when movement of the entire pelvic girdle is being described, as opposed to specific movement between one innominate and the sacrum.

On forward bending, as the pelvis tilted forwards, there was significant posterior displacement of the pelvis with contributions to movement from the hips and the lumbar spine relatively proportional. John could easily touch his toes using this movement strategy. Forward bending appeared to be slightly limited at the lower lumbar levels, while there was slight hyperflexion from the mid-lumbar to the mid-thoracic spine. A small arc of pain was experienced over the right lumbosacral region on return to the upright position. There was no observable or palpable difference between left and right posterior superior iliac spine (PSIS) movement and no asymmetry of movement in the lower lumbar levels. The painful arc that occurred on the first movement was not evident on repeated movements.

Backward bending was severely limited with marked restriction of lower lumbar extension and posterior pelvic tilt. A marked increase in the right SIJ pain and bilateral 'stiffness' in the lumbar spine was reported. Normal movement was evident above the lower two lumbar levels. There was a significant knee flexion component to the movement. End of range (EOR) overpressure increased right SIJ and lumbosacral symptoms.

Trunk right lateral bending appeared to be slightly restricted at the right lower lumbar spine and pelvis, with significant pain reported in the lumbosacral region with EOR overpressure. Left lateral bending was slightly limited with tightness reported in the right lower lumbar spine. Lumbar left and right lateral gliding was not restricted, but EOR overpressure on right lateral gliding produced low grade right lumbar pain. Standing trunk axial rotation was slightly stiff in both directions but did not alter lumbosacral or SIJ symptoms.

Combining trunk backward bending with right lateral bending markedly increased right lower lumbar and SIJ pain, while the addition of trunk left lateral bending to backward bending did not significantly alter symptoms.

Hip physiological movements

On full squat, there was a sensation of tightness in the right anterior hip region and the right lower limb was forced to externally rotate to allow EOR movement to occur. On active hip and knee flexion in standing, application of EOR overpressure (achieved by pulling the flexed knee to the chest) was full range and pain-free on the left, while on the right there was slight restriction of hip movement with external rotation of the thigh, and tightness experienced in the right groin. When John was asked to maintain neutral hip rotation and repeat the movement, the range of hip flexion became slightly more limited, with mild discomfort experienced in the groin. Standing hip extension was restricted on the right compared to the left with some obvious compensatory external rotation of the lumbar spine, pelvis and hip.

In relaxed supine lying, the right leg was externally rotated from the hip compared to the left. When hip rotation was tested passively, the right hip demonstrated significantly greater range of external rotation than the left. Right hip internal rotation in supine lying was restricted compared to the left and exhibited significant passive resistance from the neutral hip position onwards. No pain was experienced on these movements. Hip adduction was reasonably equal in range, but greater tension was noted in the right tensor fascia latae. Right hip flexion/adduction produced moderate anterior hip pain and was slightly restricted compared to the left. The range of hip abduction was slightly greater on the right than the left, both with the knee extended and flexed. Left hip flexion/abduction/external rotation (FABER) was normal range, while right hip FABER was approximately 20% more flexible than the left, both being symptom-free.

Combined left hip and pelvic flexion in supine lying was to 120°, whereas right hip and pelvic flexion began to feel restricted at just over 90° and produced slight groin pain and a feeling of stiffness in the hip. If the right hip was allowed to externally rotate then 110° was possible before there was significant resistance to movement and similar EOR groin pain was produced.

SIJ mobility tests

Relative movement between the innominate and the sacrum was palpated and observed during the 'Stork test' (also known as the Gillet test). Hungerford et al[23] demonstrated that physical therapists were able to reliably palpate and distinguish between anterior rotation and no movement of the innominate in relation to the sacrum on the supporting leg side during the Stork test. In John's case, when standing on the left foot and flexing the right hip to 90°, the right innominate and the left innominate visibly and palpably rotated posteriorly in relation to the sacrum. When standing on the right foot and flexing the left hip to 90°, the left innominate rotated posteriorly in relation to the sacrum, but the right innominate visibly and palpably rotated anteriorly in relation to the sacrum.

In unsupported sitting, John habitually sat with the lumbar spine in a flexed position. He found it difficult to move into a neutral spine position and was near EOR of lower lumbar extension when trying to do so. In sitting, he had poor voluntary recruitment of the transversus abdominis and right low lumbar multifidus muscles. The sitting forward flexion test demonstrated symmetrical PSIS movement.

Muscle function

While standing on both feet, dropping the right side of the pelvis into lateral pelvic tilt was relatively normal and symptom-free. Dropping the left side of the pelvis into lateral pelvic tilt while standing on both feet demonstrated a slightly greater range of pelvic drop, as well as somewhat greater lateral displacement and anterior rotation of the pelvis compared to the opposite side.

Single leg stance (modified Trendelenburg test[24]) on the left leg was relatively normal, but when weight-bearing on the right leg there was significantly greater lateral sway of the pelvis with poor stability and control of lower limb rotation. The pelvis remained relatively horizontal when standing on either leg. Sitting hip hitch was difficult on the right. Functional hamstring length and thoraco-dorsal fascia length tests described by Lee[22] were normal.

In supine lying, voluntary activation of transversus abdominis, although performed correctly according to the criteria of Richardson et al[25] was difficult, weak and harder to perform on the right than the left. When both femurs were positioned in neutral hip rotation (with the greater trochanter in the most lateral position) active recruitment of transversus abdominis was significantly easier bilaterally, but still weaker on the right. Whilst actively maintaining the right femur in neutral rotation an automatic contraction of transversus abdominis occurred, but still not as strong as that on the left.

On active straight leg raise (ASLR) in supine lying,[26, 27] the right leg felt 'heavier' and required a little more effort to lift than the left, with slight right rotation of the pelvis relative to the lumbar spine. The leg felt a little easier to lift if medially directed pressure was applied to each ASIS, but if forces were applied to the pelvis in other locations and directions the ASLR response did not change. Addition of resisted isometric trunk flexion/right rotation did not alter the ASLR response. Resisted isometric left and right hip flexion in neutral rotation at 90° flexion tested with normal strength. Right adductor muscle strength (tested with the hip in neutral rotation in 45° hip flexion) was slightly weaker on the right than the left. Active hip hitching and lengthening on the right was significantly more difficult than on the left and the movements on the right were observed to be more restricted.

Compared to the left, right ASLR performed in prone lying was slightly restricted with what appeared to be compensatory movement, in the middle and upper lumbar spine and of external rotation at the hip. John commented that the right leg felt 'heavier' than the left. Medially directed pressure applied to the pelvis at the ASIS, between the greater trochanter and the iliac crest above and over the posterior iliac crest did not change the ASLR response. Recruitment of latissimus dorsi[22] did not change the ASLR response. When the femur was placed in neutral rotation and held there by the examiner, it was much more difficult for the patient to lift the right leg.

Functional hip abduction tests confirmed weakness of the right hip abductors and John had difficulty holding the right leg against gravity in side lying with the hip and spine in neutral. If resistance to abduction was applied, John recruited the trunk right side flexors and hitched the pelvis laterally. He was able to produce more right hip abduction force if the hip was permitted to externally rotate.

Palpation

Palpation of the posterolateral buttock concavity behind the greater trochanter extending to the sacrum elicited significantly more local tenderness on right than the left. The anterior hip joint at the level of the inguinal ligament was tight and tender to palpation, but the left was not. There was also some tenderness to palpation in the region of the right interosseous ligament at the PSIS and at the long dorsal sacroiliac ligament, with greater tenderness elicited at the sacrotuberous ligament. There was local tenderness to palpation over the right L5–S1 zygapophyseal joint which was greater if palpation was performed with the spine in prone lying passive extension.

The right piriformis, obturator internus/gemelli, (posterior) gluteus medius and (medial) gluteus maximus muscles were all tender to palpation. There was also tenderness on palpation of the gluteus minimus, tensor fascia latae and the fascia of the lateral hip and lateral thigh, as well as the right hip adductors, notably adductor longus.

Passive movement tests

Testing of SIJ passive accessory movement was performed using the techniques described by Lee.[22] Ultrasound imaging shows that the stiffness value of the SIJ can vary according to muscle activity.[28, 29] Hold-relax techniques were used to relax the hip external rotators and abductors, but there was no noticeable difference in the results of the passive accessory tests after the hold–relax procedures compared to before.

Passive accessory movements of the left SIJ were normal. Passive anteroposterior translation of the right innominate in relation to the sacrum (directed along the SIJ plane) was moderately limited compared to the left, but the movement did not elicit symptoms. Passive accessory posterior rotation of the right innominate on the sacrum was severely restricted and elicited a slight increase in the right SIJ pain. Passive anterior rotation of the right innominate was slightly limited compared to the left but did not alter the symptoms. Inferior translation provoked pain in the right SIJ and lumbosacral regions, and felt mildly restricted compared to the left. Superior translation also felt slightly restricted compared to the left side.

In prone lying, postero–anterior (PA) pressure applied to the right side of the sacrum in line with the SIJ plane to test right SIJ PA translation showed moderate restriction compared to the left, and elicited low grade discomfort in the right SIJ region. Although there are normally differences in the amount of SIJ motion between the dominant and non-dominant sides of asymptomatic individuals,[30] the difference in this case was considered very significant.

Hip joint accessory movements were normal, and in the lumbar spine there was no indication of significant restriction on either passive accessory or passive physiological movements.

Passive 'leg pull' on the right produced pain in the right SIJ region and felt restricted compared to the left (to the clinician and the patient). No abnormality was detected on pubic symphysis movement testing, but the anterior surface of the right pubic bone adjacent to the symphysis was slightly tender on palpation. Transverse anterior distraction and posterior distraction SIJ pain provocation tests were negative.

Other tests

The slump test and passive straight leg raise neural provocation tests did not elicit significant symptoms.

Leg length was measured from the tip of the lateral malleolus to the greater trochanter and also to the ASIS. With the femur aligned so that the greater trochanter was in the most lateral position, leg length was not significantly different, despite the previously noted asymmetrical positions of the left and right ASIS.

EVIDENCE-INFORMED CLINICAL REASONING

1 What did you consider were the key findings from the physical examination and how did they promote your understanding of the case?

Clinician's response

Hungerford et al[31] compared relative movement of the innominate and sacrum when performing the Stork test between subjects experiencing SIJ pain and matched controls with no pain. They found that on the side of hip flexion the innominate rotated posteriorly in relation to the sacrum both in the pain group and the control group. However, on the supporting leg side the control group demonstrated posterior rotation of the innominate in relation to the sacrum, while the pain subjects were found to demonstrate anterior rotation of the innominate in relation to the sacrum. When standing on the right leg, John also demonstrated anterior rotation of the right innominate in relation to the sacrum.

An electromyography (EMG) study of the same patient population demonstrated evidence of altered lumbopelvic muscle recruitment in the presence of SIJ pain.[17, 18] In the control subjects, activation of the internal oblique and multifidus muscles occurred prior to initiation of weight transfer to the supporting limb. In pain subjects, activation of internal oblique, multifidus and gluteus maximus was delayed on the symptomatic side, whereas for biceps femoris it was earlier. The researchers concluded that this alteration in the strategy for lumbopelvic stabilisation could disrupt load transference through the pelvis. John's presentation was consistent with the study findings in that he had consistently experienced difficulty recruiting deep abdominal muscles, right low lumbar multifidus and gluteus maximus when exercising.

John's SIJ dysfunction presented as limited joint motion, but whether presenting as excessive joint motion or limited joint motion, involvement of the SIJ can affect muscle activity by altering neural afferent activity, particularly proprioceptive and nociceptive information from the SIJ ligaments and joint capsule. Stimulation of nerves and mechanoreceptors in the SIJ and joint capsule of pigs substantially alters muscle function of multifidus, gluteus maximus and quadratus lumborum.[14, 19, 20] This may have been one of the mechanisms limiting John's ability to restore appropriate muscle function.

2 Were there any cues in the physical examination as to the application of Mobilisation with Movement (MWM) in this case?

Clinician's response

The SIJ was considered to be the major problem in the alteration of both relative flexibility and muscle function. It was hypothesised that an appropriate MWM of the SIJ would not only restore trunk extension and lessen associated pain, but would also remove the SIJ as a cause of abnormal muscle function.

In John's case, the most symptomatic and limited physiological movements were lumbar extension and posterior pelvic tilt, so these were chosen together as the initial movement direction for the MWM. The Stork test demonstrated that when weight-bearing on the right leg, the right innominate was not rotating posteriorly in relation to the sacrum and on accessory movement testing posterior rotation and posterior translation of the right innominate in relation to the sacrum were the most restricted movements, so these were selected as initial directions for the mobilisation component of the MWM.

On the ASLR medially directed pressure on the ASIS significantly improved the ASLR and on muscle function testing rotation of the right femur to a neutral rotation position facilitated transversus abdominis function. Consequently, these were also considered to be useful components of an effective MWM technique. It is interesting to note that hip flexion movements are less restricted and less painful in lateral rotation compared to neutral but a neutral femoral rotation posture facilitates transversus abdominis activity. This could be considered paradoxical; that is, correction of hip rotation during flexion produces pain in this patient, but generally pain tends to have an inhibitory effect on 'core' muscles. It is possible that there are two different issues being addressed by the MWM. Firstly, the limitation of posterior rotation of the innominate subsequently compromises the hip joint during flexion, forcing the femur to externally rotate. Secondly, normalisation of the position and movement of the innominate allows a neutral femoral rotation posture facilitating an appropriate motor pattern.

The SIJ plane is variable between individuals, between sides and in the transverse and coronal planes.[32] As established previously (Chapter 2) the direction of the MWM glide appears critical in optimising the outcome, so therefore, it is vital to establish the angle of the SIJ plane relative to the sagittal plane when considering SIJ MWM (Figure 16.2).[33] The joint plane is parallel to the applied line of anteroposterior force where the greatest amount of movement with the least amount of resistance is elicited (e.g. Figure 2.6).

TREATMENT AND MANAGEMENT

Treatment 1

No physical treatment was performed after the examination. The patient was given advice regarding modification of sleeping position as he was sleeping in three-quarter prone lying, usually on the left side with

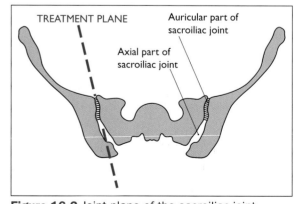

Figure 16.2 Joint plane of the sacroiliac joint

the right hip in a FABER position or in supine lying with the right hip in a FABER position. Sustained EOR loading in these positions may result in significant abnormal stress of the hip joint and SIJ.

Treatment 2 (1 week later)

Modification of the sleeping position had not altered symptoms, and the physical presentation was unchanged since the day of the initial examination.

A SIJ MWM for painful limitation of trunk extension (Table 16.1 and Figure 16.3) was applied as a trial treatment. With the patient standing, a passive anterior rotation force was applied to the sacrum using the

heel of the right hand just medial to the right SIJ and a counter-rotating posterior rotation force was applied to the innominate using the left hand over the right ASIS. The forces were applied parallel to the SIJ plane and sustained as the patient extended the lumbar spine and posteriorly tilted the pelvis. The technique was not successful and the patient reported that the movement felt blocked.

A combination of anterior rotation and anterior translation was then applied to the right side of the sacrum, with posterior rotation again applied to the innominate. There was some improvement in the range of extension and less pain was experienced, but the movement

Table 16.1	Sacroiliac joint MWM for trunk extension (Figure 16.3)	
Indication	**Pain or loss of movement on trunk extension**	
Positioning	Patient	Standing.
	Treated body part	Pelvis in relaxed upright position.
	Therapist	Standing to the side of the patient, opposite the side to be treated.
	Therapist's hands	If applying the technique to the right SIJ the left hand is placed over the anterior aspect of the right ASIS, with the thenar and hypothenar eminences of the right hand over the sacrum as close as possible to the right SIJ.
Application guidelines	• The clinician applies posterior rotation, medial rotation (around a vertical axis) and posterior translation forces to the right innominate with the hand over the ASIS, and anterior rotation/inferior translation/anterior translation forces to the sacrum through the thenar and hypothenar eminences over the sacrum. • The forces are applied parallel to the SIJ treatment plane. • If the joint plane is found to be orientated slightly oblique to the sagittal plane, the hand over the sacrum will direct force anterolaterally and the hand over the ASIS will direct force posteromedially, parallel to each other and to the plane of the SIJ. • To apply the posterior translation component to the ASIS, the clinician must elevate the elbow of the left arm, directing the pressure along the line of the forearm towards the SIJ. • The patient is instructed to hold the clinician's left forearm for support and then to extend the spine actively with the knees slightly flexed. • The left lateral aspect of the clinician's head, neck and upper shoulder should provide light support for the patient as the spine is extended. • The patient is instructed to avoid cervical extension during the manoeuvre. • To avoid stress on the clinician and to ensure effectiveness of the technique, it is important that the patient posteriorly tilts the pelvis while extending the spine and does not just lean backwards. The therapist's hands can help guide the pelvis into posterior pelvic tilting. Sometimes asking them to 'drop the tail-bone then extend' helps. • Full range and pain-free lumbar extension should be possible. • As a trial treatment, two sets of three movements are initially performed and trunk extension retested. • If the initial treatment is successful, 2–3 sets of 6–8 movements are performed.	
Comments	• The weight and leverage of the trunk is sufficient to apply end of range overpressure. • The patient can assist by applying the medial rotation component of the mobilisation. The patient places one hand over each ASIS and 'squeezes' the ASIS towards each other. The clinician then places one hand over the patient's hand on the side to be treated and applies the remaining mobilisation components.	
Variation	• The SIJ MWM can be performed for painful limitation of trunk movement in any direction. • The point of application of force to the sacrum can be varied according to response. • The MWM can be performed in four-point kneeling, sitting or in supine/prone lying. • If necessary, the innominate can be taped into posterior or anterior rotation, medial or lateral rotation. • The MWM can be performed as a self-treatment. • The MWM can be performed as the patient performs an exercise and may improve muscle function. • Often maintaining the hip neutral rotation position during the MWM facilitates appropriate muscle function, particularly transversus abdominis activity. • If there is a restriction of trunk flexion as well as extension, it is likely that the same combination of mobilisation forces will improve movement in both directions. • If it is difficult to improve trunk extension, a SIJ MWM into trunk flexion may assist restoration of extension, even if flexion was not restricted.	

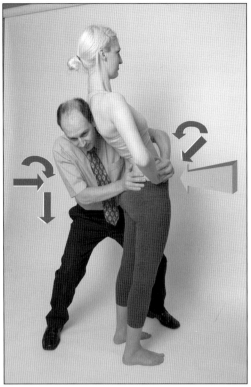

Figure 16.3 SIJ MWM for painful limitation of trunk extension with force direction vectors and movements

was still significantly restricted. Different directions of force were tested until it was found that a combination of anterior rotation/anterior translation/inferior translation applied to the sacrum and posterior rotation/posterior translation applied to the innominate produced a marked improvement in the range of trunk extension and eliminated pain during the movement. While the hands on the sacrum and innominate were applying the accessory movements, both hands were together encouraging posterior tilting of the pelvis. The MWM was repeated six times.

On retesting, there was a significant improvement in the range of extension and John reported that he could 'feel the spine bending'. There was still a feeling of stiffness in the lumbar spine, but less pain was experienced in the right SIJ and lumbosacral region.

A medially directed force applied to the ASIS was then added to the existing mobilisation combination, resulting in further improvement in the extension range. The technique was then repeated eight times, extension retested and another set of eight MWMs was performed. As no pain was experienced, the patient was asked to move further into range and then experienced only a stretching sensation in the upper right thigh at EOR.

On retesting there was a significant increase in the range of trunk extension with much improved quality of movement. The entire pelvis could be seen to tilt posteriorly and the lumbar spine extended much more freely than it had prior to the treatment intervention. Left and right lateral bending mobility was also improved, but some lower lumbar stiffness was still evident on right lateral bending with discomfort in the right lumbosacral region. On right side single leg standing, there was much less lateral sway and John felt more stable. On the Stork test the right innominate continued to rotate anteriorly in relation to the sacrum, but right ASLR was easier to perform.

Treatment 3 (16 days later)

John reported that his back and pelvis had been 'the best in years', but still felt 'a bit niggly around the area'. On prolonged supine lying John was still experiencing 'a little bit of pain', but there was 80–90% less discomfort on waking. He felt stronger and more stable when exercising, and had been able to increase his level of exercise without additional discomfort. John no longer experienced lumbosacral pain bending over a sink or bench, and when lifting at work did not feel the need to steady himself to bend. Subjectively, prior to the intervention John had experienced a painful arc on forward bending during some functional activities but now had no pain at all ('I can now bend over and the stomach seems to support it').

On examination, forward bending in standing was full range and pain-free while backward bending/posterior pelvic tilt was slightly limited. John reported 90% less pain on backward bending and reported it as mostly stiffness across the lumbar spine. Left lateral bending did not produce significant symptoms, while right lateral bending was still slightly limited and produced a low grade ache in the right lumbosacral and upper SIJ region. Right leg standing showed less pelvic lateral sway, but the right innominate was still rotating anteriorly in relation to the sacrum on the Stork test. ASLR was similar to when tested at the completion of the previous treatment session.

Passive accessory posterior rotation of the right innominate in relation to the sacrum was slightly–moderately restricted but did not elicit pain. Passive antero-posterior translation of the right innominate was also still slightly restricted compared to the left. Inferior translation was only minimally restricted compared to the left and did not produce symptoms. There was still slight limitation of hip flexion on the right and the hip was externally rotating, but less than before.

Because there had been a significant improvement in lumbar extension/posterior pelvic tilt and SIJ accessory joint movements, the SIJ MWM was repeated using the same combination of forces. Three sets of eight SIJ MWMs were performed, and on retesting lumbar extension/posterior pelvic tilt, the movement was easier to perform. For the last two sets, the patient was asked to rotate the right hip to the neutral rotation position. This was done because of the observation in the physical examination that this hip position facilitated an improved contraction of transversus abdominis compared to the externally rotated hip position. John did not feel the need to bend his knees and reported that he felt 'strong' during the movement. On retesting, lumbar extension/posterior pelvic tilt felt a little stiff, but when repeated was comfortable and pain-free. Right lateral bending produced a slight pain in the right lumbosacral region.

John was asked to perform 2–3 sets of six SIJ self-MWMs into lumbar extension/posterior pelvic tilt. Because the right SIJ was now moving well, the technique was applied centrally over the sacrum and directed at both joints. The clenched right fist was placed centrally over the sacrum and reinforced with the left hand. A gentle PA force with anterior rotation was applied as the patient performed lumbar extension/posterior pelvic tilt painlessly.

Although John had stopped attending a gymnasium because the heavy exercises aggravated his pain, he had been performing an exercise routine on a regular basis at home for many years, and continued to do this throughout the treatment period. It consisted of gym-ball work, free weights and specific exercises for abdominals, lumbar multifidus and gluteus maximus. Some modifications were made to this routine.

Treatment 4 (20 days later)
As long as John did not lie supine, lumbosacral stiffness and pain was no longer present on waking and John could bend forwards immediately without any catching. He was able to stand for a significantly longer period without discomfort, although after several hours there was 'still a little niggle' in the right lumbosacral region and he needed to place one foot on a low step to ease the symptoms. Interestingly, John commented that before treatment started he felt that his 'hips were out of line'. If he observed himself in a mirror using the waist of his underpants as a reference he had needed to lift the left side of the pelvis to be level, but now he was level without correction. Observation and palpation confirmed both ASIS were more symmetrical than when first examined.

Spinal and pelvic movements were full range and symptom-free, except for a feeling of tightness and minimal pain in the right lumbosacral region at EOR extension and right side bending. This pain was marginally increased on combined extension/right side bending. On right leg standing, balance was significantly improved but the right limb was still slightly externally rotated. The range of trunk extension was no longer reduced by repositioning the hip to neutral rotation, but active hip and knee flexion in standing with EOR overpressure remained slightly restricted with an external rotation component and discomfort experienced in the right groin. When John was asked to maintain neutral hip rotation the range of hip flexion became more limited with increased groin discomfort. These results were reproduced on passive pelvic and hip flexion in supine lying. On the Stork test with left hip flexion standing on the right foot, the right innominate was now rotating posteriorly in relation to the sacrum. Right SIJ accessory movements were comparable to the left, except for minimal restriction of posterior rotation and posterior translation of the innominate.

A trial SIJ MWM combining hip flexion with SIJ posterior rotation was performed in step standing (Table 16.2 and Figure 16.4). Using this technique it was possible to reach EOR hip and pelvic flexion (in neutral hip rotation) without pain. The MWM was repeated six times, following which hip flexion in standing and in supine lying were both significantly better with only slight limitation remaining. A further two sets of eight MWMs were performed and on retesting full range pain-free flexion in standing and hip/pelvis flexion in lying were possible without external rotation of the hip. The patient was given a SIJ self-MWM for hip flexion in step standing to ensure that the range of motion (ROM) was maintained (Figure 16.5).

Treatment 5 (3 weeks later)
Symptoms were minimal and John felt that he was moving much better with almost no pain. The ache and stiffness were now occurring in the morning only if he had slept in supine lying, and this was significantly less than before. Prolonged standing, even wearing body armour was much less of a problem. General and specific exercises were much easier.

Spinal and hip movements were normal except for slight lumbosacral pain at EOR trunk backward bending combined with right lateral bending. Passive accessory movements of the SIJ, hip joint and lumbar spine and ASLR tests were all normal. On retesting muscle function, the ability to specifically recruit transversus abdominis, lumbar multifidus, gluteus maximus and the hip abductors was significantly better, as was John's ability to adopt and maintain a neutral spine position in sitting. Palpation revealed slight tenderness at the right L5–S1 zygapophyseal joint, but joint movement was normal. There was much less tenderness of the deep hip external rotators, the anterior hip joint and the SIJ ligaments.

Treatment consisted of modification and progression of specific functional exercises and integration of the hip neutral rotation position into a strength and conditioning program. No manual therapy was required.

Table 16.2 Sacroiliac joint MWM for hip and pelvic flexion (Figure 16.4)		
Indication	**Pain and limitation of hip and pelvic flexion due to restriction of SIJ movement**	
Positioning	Patient	Step standing with one foot on chair or lowered plinth.
	Treated body part	Pelvis in relaxed upright position.
	Therapist	Standing to the side of the patient, opposite the side to be treated.
	Therapist's hands	If applying the MWM to the right SIJ, the left arm passes across the patient's abdomen so that the hand is on the left ASIS. The thenar eminence of the right hand is placed over the upper right quadrant of the sacrum as close as possible to the right SIJ.
Application guidelines	• Anterior rotation/anterior translation forces are applied to the sacrum through the right hand and a posterior rotation force is applied to the innominate through the left. • The forces are applied parallel to the treatment plane of the SIJ. • Ensure that the hip joint is in neutral hip rotation. • As the clinician maintains the forces, the patient is asked to flex at the hip and knee. • EOR is held for 1–2 seconds, and the patient then returns to the starting position. • The clinician can guide the patient's pelvis with their hands. • The patient can rest one hand on the flexed thigh and a flexed elbow on the therapist's shoulder for support. • Initially, two sets of three movements are performed and hip flexion is retested. • If the initial treatment is successful, 2–3 sets of 6–8 movements are performed.	
Comment	• The clinician's hand on the ASIS is used to prevent the hip joint from reaching EOR flexion. This helps protect the joint and assists localisation of movement to the SIJ.	
Variation	• If the pelvis is wide or the therapist finds that applying forces to the opposite SIJ is difficult, the clinician can stand on the same side as the SIJ to be treated. • If focussing on hip and SIJ movement, the patient maintains a neutral spine position. • If inclusion of spinal flexion is indicated, the patient can be encouraged to flex the spine while flexing the hip. • The MWM can be performed as a self-treatment procedure (Figure 16.5). The left arm passes medial to the left inner thigh so that the left hand is wrapped inferiorly and posteriorly around the right ischial tuberosity. The first web space of the right hand is spread over the right ASIS. The patient then pulls the right ischial tuberosity forwards and pushes the right ASIS backwards to produce posterior rotation of the right innominate. As the position is held, the patient then flexes the right hip by leaning forwards with additional EOR overpressure applied by flexing the trunk.	

Final outcome

A 6-month review was conducted and John reported that he had experienced no significant symptoms and was able to run on the pavement without pain. He was not concerned with the remaining issues which were slight right lumbosacral pain with prolonged standing, and slight stiffness in the same area on waking if he had slept in supine lying. There had been no acute episodes despite increased exercise and activity.

John demonstrated full range pain-free movement in the lumbar spine, pelvis and hip.

There was marked improvement in muscle tone in the right low lumbar multifidus and gluteus maximus, as well as the right hip adductors and abductors. Tenderness over L5-S1 was very difficult to elicit.

John had resumed supervised gymnasium based exercise and it was deemed no further treatment was necessary. On follow-up phone calls at 12 and 24 months no significant problems were reported.

AUTHOR'S MWM COMMENTARY

The sudden loss of SIJ mobility over 20 years ago appeared to have placed abnormal stress on the adjacent lumbar spine segment and hip joint to the point that they became symptomatic. Innervated structures of the SIJ and pelvis also appeared to be pain generators. Limitation of SIJ movement may also have disturbed lumbosacral joint function by altering tension on the iliolumbar ligaments. Cutting the anterior band of the iliolumbar ligament (bilaterally) in cadavers significantly increases SIJ rotation in the sagittal plane,[34] suggesting a relationship between iliolumbar ligament tension and SIJ movement.

A study of lumbar spine extension creep using fresh cadaveric material indicated that passive EOR loading for just 20 minutes was sufficient to cause significant soft tissue deformation.[35] This may explain why John experienced pain in prolonged standing and supine lying, with the SIJ MWM restoring sufficient range in the lumbar spine and pelvis to allow him to avoid EOR loading in these positions. He was then also able to maintain a comfortable neutral spine position in sitting.

When pain-free SIJ movement was restored, specific exercise that prior to the MWM had been ineffective, was now useful in restoration of muscle function, particularly of transversus abdominis, lumbar multifidus, gluteus maximus and the hip abductors. Recent studies[14,19,20] demonstrate relationships between SIJ loading, stimulation of SIJ

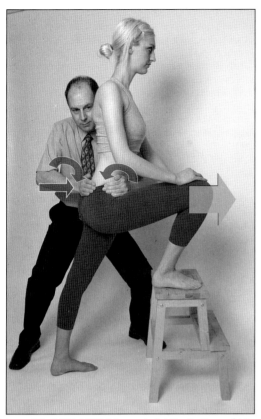

Figure 16.4 SIJ MWM for painful limitation of hip and pelvic flexion

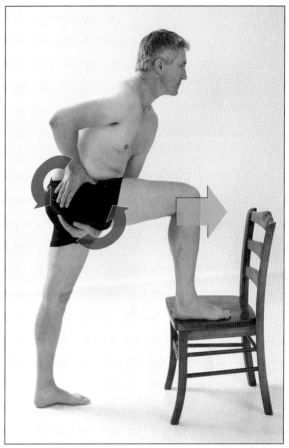

Figure 16.5 Self-MWM for posterior rotation of the innominate for painful limitation of hip and pelvic flexion in step standing

mechanoreceptors and nociceptors, and muscle activity in the pelvis, hip and spine. Hungerford et al[18] demonstrated altered muscle timing and recruitment in the presence of SIJ pain.

Hungerford et al[31] found that during the Stork test with subjects who were not experiencing SIJ pain the supporting leg demonstrated innominate posterior rotation and posterior, medial and superior translation relative to the sacrum. In this case study, the successful SIJ MWM comprised this combination of rotation and translation components. Relative superior translation of the innominate in relation to the sacrum was achieved by gliding the sacrum inferior relative to the innominate, and although postero–inferior translation was applied to the innominate, anterior translation was simultaneously applied to the sacrum. In subjects with SIJ pain, the innominate rotated *anteriorly* and translated posteriorly, medially and *inferiorly* relative to the sacrum in single leg standing on the supporting leg.[31] This case highlights the relatively subtle adjustment in the direction of the glide component of a MWM sometimes required to optimise improvement in the CSIM (see Chapter 2). A process colloquially referred to as 'fiddling' by Brian Mulligan.

In this case where the SIJ was hypomobile, it appears that as well as reducing pain on movement the MWM restored restricted movement between the innominate and the sacrum. However, if the SIJ was hypermobile or unstable, in addition to gently and painlessly freeing a 'locked joint', the SIJ MWM may hypothetically encourage normal movement and control abnormal movements, thereby facilitating normal sensory afferent information and avoiding painful stimuli that may trigger protective neuromuscular responses. The MWM in this case would need to be used in combination with strategies to stabilise the SIJ, including passive supports[22, 36, 37] and appropriate stabilising exercises.[12, 22, 25, 38]

Although trunk extension had been painfully restricted for over 20 years, simple but specific SIJ MWM resulted in rapid resolution of lumbar spine, pelvis and hip symptoms. This case study highlights that failure to recognise and effectively treat a significant mechanical SIJ disorder may render exercise completely ineffective.

References

1 Whitecloud TS. Complications of anterior cervical fusion. Instructional Course Lectures. 1978;27: 223–7.

2 Arrington ED, Smith WJ, Chambers HG, et al. Complications of iliac crest bone graft harvesting. Clinical Orthopaedics and Related Research. 1996;(329):300–9.

3 Banwart JC, Asher MA, Hassanein RS. Iliac crest bone graft harvest donor site morbidity: a statistical evaluation. Spine. 1995;20(9):1055–60.

4 Chan K, Resnick D, Pathria M, et al. Pelvic instability after bone graft harvesting from posterior iliac crest: Report of nine patients. Skeletal Radiology. 2001;30(5):278–81.

5 Fernando TL, Kim SS, Mohler DG. Complete pelvic ring failure after posterior iliac bone graft harvesting. Spine. 1999;24(20):2101–4.

6 Kurz LT, Garfin SR, Booth RE, Jr. Harvesting autogenous iliac bone grafts: a review of complications and techniques. Spine. 1989;14(12):1324–31.

7 Russell JL, Block JE. Surgical harvesting of bone graft from the ilium: point of view. Medical Hypotheses. 2000;55(6):474–9.

8 Seiler JG, III, Johnson J. Iliac crest autogenous bone grafting: donor site complications. Journal of the Southern Orthopaedic Association. 2000;9(2):91–7.

9 Younger EM, Chapman MW. Morbidity at bone graft donor sites. Journal of Orthopaedic Trauma. 1989;3(3):192–5.

10 Robertson PA, Sherwood MJ. The morbidity of autogenous bone graft donation. In: Lewandrowski K-U, Wise DL, Trantolo DJ, Yaszemski MJ, White III AA (eds) Advances in Spinal Fusion: Molecular Science, Biomechanics, and Clinical Management. New York: Marcel Dekker; 2004:683–97.

11 Coventry MB, Tapper EM. Pelvic instability: a consequence of removing iliac bone for grafting. The Journal of Bone and Joint Surgery. 1972;54(1):83–101.

12 Sahrmann SA. Diagnosis and Treatment of Movement Impairment Syndromes. Sydney: Elsevier 2001.

13 Holm S, Indahl A, Solomonow M. Sensorimotor control of the spine. Journal of Electromyography and Kinesiology. 2002;12(3):219–34.

14 Indahl A, Holm S. The sacroiliac joint: Sensory-motor control and pain. In: Vleeming A, Mooney V, Stoekart R (eds) Movement Stability and Lumbopelvic Pain: Integration of Research and Therapy. Edinburgh: Churchill Livingstone 2007:101–11.

15 Indahl A, Kaigle AM, Reikeras O, et al. Interaction between the porcine lumbar intervertebral disc, zygapophyseal joints, and paraspinal muscles. Spine. 1997;22(24):2834–40.

16 van Dieen JH, Selen LP, Cholewicki J. Trunk muscle activation in low-back pain patients: an analysis of the literature. Journal of Electromyography and Kinesiology. 2003;13(4):333–51.

17 Hungerford B, Gilleard W. The pattern of intrapelvic motion and lumbopelvic muscle recruitment alters in the presence of pelvic girdle pain. In: Vleeming A, Mooney V, Stoekart R (eds) Movement Stability and Lumbopelvic Pain: Integration of Research and Therapy. Edinburgh: Churchill Livingstone 2007:361–76.

18 Hungerford B, Gilleard W, Hodges P. Evidence of altered lumbopelvic muscle recruitment in the presence of sacroiliac joint pain. Spine. 2003;28(14):1593–600.

19 Indahl A, Kaigle A, Reikeras O, et al. Sacroiliac joint involvement in activation of the porcine spinal and gluteal musculature. Journal of Spinal Disorders and Techniques. 1999;12(4):325–30.

20 Indahl A, Kaigle A, Reikeras O, et al. Pain and muscle responses of the sacroiliac joint. Fourth Interdisciplinary World Congress on Low Back and Pelvic Pain. Montreal 2001.

21 Kendall FP, McCreary EK, Provance PG, et al. Muscles: Testing and Function with Posture and Pain. Philadelphia: Lippincott Williams & Wilkins 2005.

22 Lee DG. The Pelvic Girdle: An Approach to the Examination and Treatment of the Lumbopelvic-hip Region (3rd edn). Edinburgh: Churchill Livingstone 2004.

23 Hungerford BA, Gilleard W, Moran M, Emmerson C. Evaluation of the ability of physical therapists to palpate intrapelvic motion with the Stork test on the support side. Physical Therapy. 2007;87(7):879–87.

24 Albert H, Godskesen M, Westergaard J. Evaluation of clinical tests used in classification procedures in pregnancy-related pelvic joint pain. European Spine Journal. 2000;9(2):161–6.

25 Richardson C, Jull G, Hodges P, et al. Therapeutic Exercise for Spinal Segmental Stabilization in Low Back Pain: Scientific Basis and Clinical Approach. Edinburgh: Churchill Livingstone 1999.

26 Mens JM, Vleeming A, Snijders CJ, et al. Validity of the active straight leg raise test for measuring disease severity in patients with posterior pelvic pain after pregnancy. Spine. 2002;27(2):196–200.

27 Mens JM, Vleeming A, Snijders CJ, et al. The active straight leg raising test and mobility of the pelvic joints. European Spine Journal. 1999;8(6):468–73.

28 Richardson CA, Snijders CJ, Hides JA, et al. The relation between the transversus abdominis muscles, sacroiliac joint mechanics, and low back pain. Spine. 2002;27(4):399–405.

29 van Wingerden JP, Vleeming A, Buyruk HM, et al. Stabilization of the sacroiliac joint in vivo: Verification of muscular contribution to force closure of the pelvis. European Spine Journal. 2004;13(3): 199–205.

30 Bussey MD, Milosavljevic S, Bell ML. Sex differences in the pattern of innominate motion during passive hip abduction and external rotation. Manual Therapy. 2009;14(5):514–9.

31 Hungerford B, Gilleard W, Lee D. Altered patterns of pelvic bone motion determined in subjects with posterior pelvic pain using skin markers. Clinical Biomechanics. 2004;19(5):456–64.

32 Solonen KA. The sacroiliac joint in the light of anatomical, roentgenological and clinical studies. Acta Orthopaedica Scandinavica, Supplementum. 1957;27:1–127.

33 Mulligan BR. Manual therapy 'NAGS', SNAGS', 'MWMs' etc (5th edn). Wellington: Plane View Services 2004.

34 Pool-Goudzwaard A, Van Dijke G, Mulder P, et al. The iliolumbar ligament: Its influence on stability of the sacroiliac joint. Clinical Biomechanics. 2003;18(2):99–105.

35 Oliver MJ, Twomey LT. Extension creep in the lumbar spine. Clinical Biomechanics. 1995;10(7):363–8.

36 Damen L, Spoor CW, Snijders CJ, et al. Does a pelvic belt influence sacroiliac joint laxity? Clinical Biomechanics. 2002;17(7):495–8.

37 Mens JM, Damen L, Snijders CJ, et al. The mechanical effect of a pelvic belt in patients with pregnancy-related pelvic pain. Clinical Biomechanics. 2006;21(2):122–7.

38 Mosely GL. Motor control in chronic pain: new ideas for effective intervention. In: Vleeming A, Mooney V, Stoekart R (eds). Movement Stability and Lumbopelvic Pain: Integration of Research and Therapy. Edinburgh: Churchill Livingstone 2007:513–25.

Chapter 17
Hockey hip, a case of chronic dysfunction

Wayne Hing and Brian Mulligan

HISTORY

Bree is a 27-year-old single female working in a law firm presenting with anterior left hip (groin) pain. She has a very busy lifestyle outside work, mainly occupied with training for and playing her primary sport of field hockey. She currently plays as a goalie in club, national and international field hockey which involves up to six training sessions per week, along with playing games and attending gym training sessions.

Bree's main symptom was localised left anterior hip pain which did not extend further afield. She described this pain (pain A) as sharp and which, on a numerical rating scale, reached 7/10 at its worst. She also reported a second pain (pain B) which was a residual dull ache associated with a 'weak' feeling that lingered after undertaking aggravating activities. The symptoms are outlined on the body chart (Figure 17.1). Pain A was aggravated by general use of the hip and leg, including activities such as running and stair climbing, but also by end-range hip movements, such as squatting and lunging. Pain B was aggravated by prolonged sitting. Bree commented that she felt better in the mornings and did not complain of any symptoms of pins and needles, clicking or catching in the hip. There were no issues with her hip related to her work.

Current history

The anterior hip pain initially started 8 months previously when Bree felt a progressive 'tightness' over the front of her hip during one of her hockey games. After that game, Bree was able to continue training and playing hockey, however, she noticed a gradual increase in intensity and severity of symptoms with time. She also noted that the tightness in her left hip area, which would normally disappear or diminish once she had warmed up, was now starting to remain and worsen with time. Bree particularly felt her symptoms during kicking and lunging movements. She had been assessed by the local regional team physiotherapist and diagnosed with a strained left hip flexor muscle. The initial management provided by the team physiotherapist consisted of local soft tissue treatment, exercise and stretching, specifically for a muscle problem.

Bree sought treatment on game days and weekends, however the effects were not long lasting, leading to a point where she felt she had to reduce the amount of hockey she was playing. Treatment continued over the next 4–6 months, which resulted in a reduction of symptoms with Bree able to run small distances and commence some gym-based exercise, however, she was unable to resume training and playing hockey. Local anaesthetic injections administered by the team's sports physician to the hip flexor muscle trigger points were used as a diagnostic test to investigate her symptoms of pain during exercise. The injections did not give her complete resolution of symptoms, which was interpreted as an indication that this was not the only cause of her pain. A provisional diagnosis of hip flexor tendinosis was given at this stage.

Treatment was progressed to include eccentric loading of the hip flexors, acupuncture and deep soft tissue massage to the associated flexor muscle region and tensor fasciae latae. As well as the aforementioned soft tissue management, hip joint mobilisations consisting of longitudinal traction[1] were performed by the treating physiotherapist. At this stage Bree felt that she had made some improvement, however, once she returned to training and playing she still needed to take 75 mg Diclofenac medication once a day and felt minimal relief, with pain A (7/10) and pain B (3/10) still very evident.

At this stage, 9 months on from the original onset of injury, Bree was still unable to play or train fully and in particular was complaining of being unable to perform full deep lunges or squat, and was unable to kick a hockey ball without considerable pain. Prior to this current episode of hip pain, Bree had no other relevant conditions or complaints relating to her left hip or pelvic regions.

Symptom behaviour

Aggravating activities included any training involving the hip and leg. This related to gym-based exercise, running and hockey training, especially activities involving hip flexion such as lunging, squatting, sprinting, and running up or down steps or a steep hill. Of particular concern to Bree were the specific actions

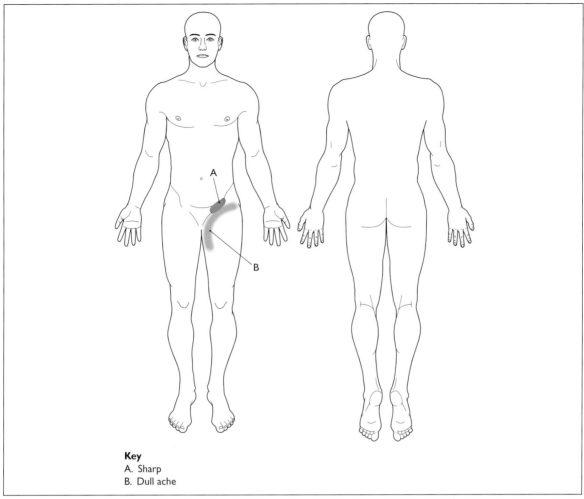

Key
A. Sharp
B. Dull ache

Figure 17.1 Body chart

related to her hockey goalkeeping role which involved a considerable amount of kicking, lunging and pivoting on either leg while wearing significant padding for protection, and which added weight and contributed to the movement patterns associated with goalkeeping. She reported that once pain A (7/10) was aggravated it resolved immediately once the aggravating activities ceased, however the residual ache (pain B) would take up to 4–6 hours to ease. Bree felt now that pain B was taking longer to resolve and was getting worse. She was now finding that sitting for extended periods of time (for example, long-haul plane flights) brought on pain B.

Bree did not experience morning stiffness upon waking, however, she occasionally experienced pain at night and associated this with lying in one position for too long and twisting awkwardly while turning in bed. Over a typical 24-hour period there appeared to be no pattern to her pain unless she undertook the activities that aggravated her symptoms.

Medical history and investigations

There was no history of medical or other conditions that would impact on Bree's condition, nor influence management. Bree had taken Diclofenac in the earlier stages of her history to control pain, however, had taken no other prescribed medications for this or any other condition. An earlier X-ray was normal and no other investigations had been performed to date.

EVIDENCE-INFORMED CLINICAL REASONING

1 At the end of the history, what were your thoughts or hypotheses regarding the source of Bree's hip pain?

Clinician's response

The information from the history suggests that Bree may have suffered a strain of her left hip flexor muscle(s). A number of reported signs and symptoms were consistent with having a soft tissue strain, including the sharp localised pain without referral. Muscle strain is by far the most common muscle injury suffered in sport, and frequently involves muscles which cross two joints and act mainly in an eccentric fashion, such as the hip flexors.[2] Hip flexor strain can occur from overuse of the muscles that help you flex your hip or perform high kicks.[3] This type of strain may result from an explosive hip flexion manoeuvre, such as sprinting or kicking, or from eccentric overload as the hip is extended.[4] It is a condition that commonly occurs in athletes who undertake forceful kicking activities.[3] These factors are very much consistent with Bree's history and symptoms.

However, a number of features in the history are not consistent with this injury. Against the muscle strain hypothesis is the fact that Bree had not responded to conservative management for this type of injury, as well as failing to fully respond to the local anaesthetic injections. In general, the timeframe for healing of a muscle strain injury is directly related to the severity of injury. Minor muscle strain injuries may be healed in 1 week, whereas severe injuries may require 4–8 weeks.[2] Bree's symptoms have well exceeded this timeframe strongly suggesting that there is another cause. Although the outcome of a muscle strain is generally good it also depends on the severity of the injury. A full return to activity with no residual disability is usually possible after healing of a minor injury. However, a major injury can result in limited range of motion (ROM) and weakness.[2]

With the above in mind, consideration of other structures as a source of symptoms is warranted. Anterior hip pain can indicate pathology of the hip joint (e.g. degenerative arthritis) or sacroiliac joint, as well as iliopsoas bursitis.[5] The history suggests a loading component to Bree's symptoms, and along with the fact that sustained positions, such as sitting at work, going to the movies and driving the car, aggravated her pain, this supports a hip joint hypothesis. Sacroiliac joint dysfunction also refers pain to the groin in 14% of patients.[6] Sacroiliac joint dysfunction can also produce pelvic instability and predispose other pelvic and hip structures to injury through functional overload.[7] Although iliopsoas bursitis typically presents with anterior hip pain aggravated by activity, it is usually associated with a painful snapping sensation[8] which was absent in this case.

Femoroacetabular impingement can also cause hip pain and is most commonly seen in active young adults. The exacerbating activities often include stair climbing, athletic events and prolonged sitting, all consistent with this case. Physical examination and radiologic studies are needed to rule out the diagnosis of femoroacetabular impingement. The impingement test, which consists of passive hip flexion, adduction and internal rotation, should reproduce the patient's pain with this condition.[9]

In summary, multiple tissue involvement is likely in Bree's case with consideration of the chronic nature and lack of resolution of pain with treatment of the soft tissues, and the poor response to medication.

2 Did you have any treatment hypotheses under consideration at this early stage? If so, what factors in the patient's history, based on your experience and the scientific evidence, support your treatment hypothesis?

Clinician's response

Treatment hypotheses consisted of further treatment to the soft tissues but also extending treatment to the underlying hip joint. It is recognised that anterior hip pain may arise from several possible causes.[5] Whether the dysfunction be intra-articular (e.g. labral tear or femoroacetabular impingement) or extra-articular in origin to the hip joint (e.g. hip flexor muscle strain or tendinosis, or iliopsoas bursitis), a thorough physical examination is first needed to confirm the diagnosis.

Bree described specific movements and activities that provoked her symptoms, with the intermittent sharp hip pain provoked by dynamic loading and stressing of the anterior joint structures. This apparent mechanical nature to the symptoms appears favourable for a trial of manual therapy intervention. In addition, the poor response to treatment thus far indicates a need to reconsider treatment options. Over the 9-month period Bree did not respond well to conservative management for the hip flexors and standard traction of the hip joint, with only short-term relief and symptoms returning soon after returning to activity and training.

The manual therapy management to date, consisting of traditional longitudinal hip traction in the resting position of slight flexion and abduction,[1] appears limited and it can be hypothesised that progressive manual therapy intervention is warranted.

PHYSICAL EXAMINATION

Posture

On observation in standing, Bree had a slightly reduced lumbar lordosis and an appearance of an anteriorly displaced pelvis relative to her upper trunk. Functionally, Bree tended to bend more at the hips and appeared to initiate movement less from the lumbar spine. There was no marked observable abnormality during walking.

Active and functional movement tests

Lumbar spine flexion, extension and lateral flexion all displayed normal range and rhythm with no symptoms provoked.

Specific to her left hip, active flexion (100°) and both external (40°) and internal (25°) rotation were reduced due to resistance and pain with overpressure. Combined movement of flexion, abduction and external rotation

(FABER test) was limited to approximately 40% of normal range. The active movement of adduction was also limited at the very end of range although this was associated with a feeling of resistance rather than pain. The left anterior hip pain (pain A) was reproduced with active squatting and lunging with the left leg forward. When lunging with the right leg forward, Bree described a 'tightness' in the anterior left hip region rather than pain.

Passive movement tests

Passive physiological movement testing of Bree's left hip revealed end-range restriction and discomfort into flexion (105°), and external (40°) and internal (30°) rotation. All other movements were normal in range. Additionally, the left hip quadrant was limited to 100–105° flexion and was painful (5-6/10), whilst her right hip ROM tested normal in all directions.

Assessment of the sacroiliac joint was performed using pain provocation tests[10] and these were negative. Passive accessory glides applied to the lumbar spine were also unremarkable and did not reproduce any of her symptoms.

Muscle assessment

General length testing was normal for the left and right gastrocnemius, soleus, quadriceps, hamstring and right hip flexor muscles. The left hip flexors were found to be reduced in length by at least 20°, with reproduction of Bree's anterior left hip 'tightness' on end-range passive overpressure. This sensation was also reproduced on resisted hip flexion, whilst resisted abduction was normal, with the patient in the Thomas test position.[11] On palpation, the rectus femoris, sartorius and anterior tensor fasciae latae muscle insertions, near the anterior superior iliac spine were all uncomfortable.

EVIDENCE-INFORMED CLINICAL REASONING

1 At the end of the physical examination, what were your hypotheses for Bree's symptoms and what findings supported these?

Clinician's response

At the end of the physical examination, the primary hypothesis of an anterior hip flexor muscle complex injury associated with hip joint involvement appeared to be the most likely.

There was a lack of evidence for pathology of the lumbar spine or sacroiliac joint with all testing of these structures negative.

There was evidence that supported an articular contribution to Bree's symptoms, with marked restriction in passive ROM of all movements of the hip. Cyriax[12] states that testing of the inert structures (i.e. joint capsules and ligaments) requires a passive stretch of the joint tested. The decreased ROM, the pattern

of movement loss and the end-feel of the joint range found in Bree's assessment may be suggestive of an articular dysfunction.[9, 12, 13] The articular signs and symptoms potentially signal the presence of osteoarthrosis particularly considering their relationship with the loss of ROM.[14]

The possibility of a labral pathology could also be an option with its diagnosis in athletes becoming more common as technology to identify such lesions becomes more advanced. A past history of vague, recurrent groin or thigh symptoms should alert the clinician to the possibility of a labral lesion.[15] There is also evidence of tendinopathy of the associated hip musculature which is supported by the chronic nature of Bree's recovery.[16]

2 Was Mobilisation with Movement (MWM) indicated for treatment? If not, were there alternative Mulligan Concept treatment hypotheses you were considering?

Clinician's response

From the history presented above it is apparent that MWM has not been trialled as a joint mobilisation technique for Bree. Although lacking for the hip joint, there is strong evidence in the literature of the success of MWM as a joint mobilisation treatment for other joints.[17–19] Additionally, the limited and short-term response that Bree illustrated, in response to the previously described management, supported the need to progress the mobilisation component in its range and function (i.e. weight-bearing).

TREATMENT AND MANAGEMENT

Treatment 1

Table 17.1 details the hip MWM techniques that were performed within this case. These included the lateral glide of the hip MWM for improving hip flexion (Figure 17.2a and b). It was decided at this stage to treat Bree's flexion restriction before addressing the other movement limitations that were established in her assessment. The rationale for this was because Bree's main complaint was the lunge and squat limitation.

The immediate effect of the lateral glide hip MWM during application was an increase in the range of passive hip flexion to full range (–120°) with no pain on passive overpressure performed by Bree, pulling her knee to her chest. Two sets of 10 repetitions were applied. Flexion remained full range and pain-free after the application of this MWM dose. Testing of the functional tests of squat and lunge showed improvement with an increase in range, however there was still some restriction and end-range pain in these weight-bearing positions. Bree tolerated the hip MWM with no report of any side-effects.

Additional treatment was delivered within this session consisting of stretches to the hip flexor muscle

Table 17.1	Lateral glide MWM during hip flexion	
Indication	**Groin and/or anterior hip pain and/or loss of movement during hip flexion or associated movements**	
Positioning	Patient	Supine lying near side of treatment table.
	Treated body part	Hip on symptomatic side flexed to 90° (or less if pain is provoked).
	Mobilisation belt	Belt placed around the therapist's waist and also around the patient's femur and positioned as close to the groin as comfortable.
	Therapist	Standing beside the patient's symptomatic leg next to the patient's flexed knee. A lateral distraction force is applied perpendicular to the femur by the therapist by moving their pelvis away from the bed and the patient's leg.
	Therapist's hands	One hand is placed inside the mobilisation belt on the patient's iliac crest near the anterior superior iliac spine to help stabilise the pelvis. The therapist's other hand and arm is used to support and guide the patient's femur to provide stability and maintain control of the thigh position as the MWM is performed.
Application guidelines	• The hip joint MWM can be performed for the physiological movements of hip flexion, internal rotation, external rotation and extension only. • The lateral distraction glide is sustained for the duration that the physiological movement is carried out. • While the glide is maintained the hip is moved further into the desired physiological ROM (Figure 17.2a and b). • This process is repeated approximately 6–10 times with any required 'fine-tuning' to gain maximal range undertaken by subtly changing parameters (e.g. glide direction or force). • If hip pain is not eliminated or is made worse the glide parameters should be modified or another glide trialled. • Subsequent reassessment of passive physiological or active hip movement should reveal a significant improvement in pain-free ROM. • The MWM technique can be progressed in subsequent treatment sessions by applying the technique in weight-bearing with a gradually increasing ROM as the condition allows.	
Comments	• The glide is achieved initially as a pure lateral glide, however modification and 'tweaking' of the glide may be required to obtain a pain-free glide and an improvement in the physiological joint ROM. This can be achieved by altering parameters such as the angle and force of the glide. • Maintain the glide throughout the procedure, until the patient returns to the starting position. • Overpressure must be applied at the end of the available range and sustained for a few seconds. • The aim is to achieve maximal, pain-free hip movement.	

group and soft tissue massage to the rectus femoris and psoas muscles. This resulted in a more comfortable and maintained gain in her initial increased ROM and muscle length. Bree was also instructed to cease taking her non-steroidal a anti-inflammatory medication at this stage of her management. This was because such medication is associated with a risk of adverse gastrointestinal and other effects [20, 21] and also because of the need to monitor the response to management without masking of pain by the medication.[22]

Bree was asked to limit her hockey training to every 3 days rather than daily until the following treatment session to facilitate reassessment of her progress and symptom response. This reduction in training was also intended to limit the degree of loading of the hip joint and associated structures.

Treatment 2

Bree was reassessed 4 days later. She reported significant improvement in both the level of discomfort and pain and her level of function. The sharper anterior hip pain A was reduced (4/10) and less frequently felt, whilst pain B was not occurring. Bree was now able to squat lower before pain and lunging was much improved with end-range discomfort of a lesser intensity. On physical reassessment, her left hip passive flexion range of movement had maintained most of the initial improvement (115°) but was still limited at the end of range. Despite this improvement in flexion, the movements of passive internal (30°) and external (40°) rotation were still limited and painful on passive overpressure.

In view of the positive and sustained response to the first treatment session, lateral glide hip MWM for flexion was repeated using the same dosage. In addition, two sets of 10 repetitions of lateral glide MWM were performed for hip internal rotation and also for FABER movement. These resulted in improvements in available pain-free range for these movements. Further progression of the lateral glide MWM into flexion in a weight-bearing position in four-point kneeling and then in a lunge position were carried out. At the end of the second treatment session Bree had gained full range of hip flexion (120°) and was pain-free to overpressure. She was able to fully lunge without pain and both internal and external rotation had markedly improved to be nearly full range (40°). Furthermore, Bree was able to achieve a full squat with only end-range 'tightness'.

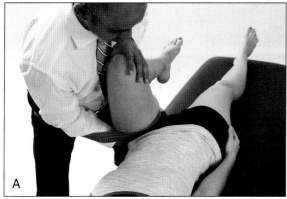

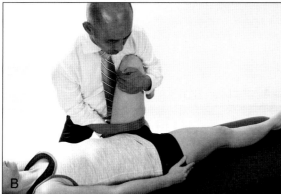

Figure 17.2 Lateral glide MWM of the hip in (a) flexion and (b) internal rotation of the hip

Bree's home exercise program was continued with stretches for her hip joint and associated musculature to maintain her newly available ROM.

Treatment 3

A week later Bree returned for treatment and reported sustained improvement since the last treatment. She was now able to run comfortably and noticed no pain with her general gym sessions. During her hockey training (including general warm up, running and hockey-specific activities such as kicking and lunging during her goal-keeping drills) she was nearly pain-free (pain A 2/10) and experienced little residual ache (pain B 1/10) after training.

On examination, Bree had maintained the hip ROM gained last session with end-range flexion (120°) and external rotation (45°) full in range and with no end-range overpressure discomfort. However, internal rotation (40°) was still limited with discomfort experienced on overpressure. Isometric contraction of the hip flexor muscles was not painful, nor was eccentric contraction.

In view of the continued improvement from the previous session the hip MWMs were repeated for flexion, both internal and external rotation, extension and FABERS to ensure full range and normal joint end-feel were achieved.

At the end of the third treatment session all active hip movements were full range (including internal rotation) and pain-free with overpressure. Now that pain-free, full hip ROM had been restored it was possible to manually test Bree's hip flexor strength. A small decrease in strength was present with a more noticeable tendency to fatigue with repeated testing present. Bree was thus advised to perform specific hip flexor strengthening exercises along with general flexibility exercises. Bree was also advised to progressively increase her training load and hockey-specific goal-keeping drills and return to playing hockey.

Treatment 4

Two weeks later Bree reported further improvement with all activities. She was able to run for up to 5 km without hip discomfort, train in the gym with her squats and lunge weight training exercises painless and full in range, and also train for hockey fully. On physical examination, Bree's hip ROM for flexion, internal and external rotation, and the FABER test were full and pain-free. Tested in the Thomas position, there was no pain or restriction on assessment of the hip flexor and iliotibial band muscle length, nor with eccentric contraction. Bree was given advice regarding progression of her training tolerance. She was also advised to maintain key recovery components after her running and training program with icing, flexibility exercises and warming down strategies. No further treatment sessions were planned.

Outcome of intervention

Bree was followed up 2 weeks and a further 1 month after the final treatment session. She had made steady progress with her training and playing and was able to run comfortably and without any problem.

Bree was followed up for the last time 3 months after the final treatment session. Her left hip symptoms were now completely resolved and she was back playing hockey and training fully.

AUTHORS' MWM COMMENTARY

This chapter presents a case history of an elite athlete with a prolonged history of left anterior hip pain initially diagnosed as a hip flexor muscle strain. It illustrates a complex pathology which has elements of muscle dysfunction with both strength and flexibility components, associated with an underlying joint dysfunction. The response to treatment and ongoing nature of the symptoms appears to have not improved until the joint dysfunction was addressed with appropriate joint management using a MWM.

Bree's case illustrates how the Mulligan Concept techniques of hip MWM can facilitate the rapid resolution of chronic, complex groin and thigh pain involving local myofascial injury with associated joint dysfunction. It is possible that the muscle pathology and inhibition could have been intimately related to the involvement of the associated hip joint with its movement restriction and pain.[13, 23, 24] The manual traction techniques initially applied in this case may not have been successful due to the sustained static nature of the stretch whereby limited joint movement occurred. That is, any gains in muscle relaxation or pain inhibition could have been immediately lost as soon as the traction was ceased.

In general, manual therapy assessment, where possible, should be directed towards formulating a specific diagnosis. However, in some cases this may be difficult as multiple pathologies affecting a number of different structures are present. For instance, hip pain and restriction may be the result of a number of disorders, such as hip flexor muscle pathology[25] and underlying joint degeneration,[26–28] a similar situation to the present case. The pain-free nature of MWM allows for the application of manual therapy despite the need to consider several pathologies and the irritability and severity of the accompanying pain. In Bree's case, MWM achieved full hip ROM and ultimately pain-free hip joint and overlying muscle function.

References

1 Kaltenborn F. Mobilisation of the Extremity Joints (3rd edn). Oslo: Olaf Norlis Bokhandel 1980.

2 Noonan T, Garrett W, Jr. Muscle strain injury: diagnosis and treatment. Journal of the American Academy of Orthopaedic Surgeons. 1999;7(4):262–9.

3 Rouzier P. Hip flexor strain. Sports medicine advisor 2009. Online. Available from: http://www.med.umich.edu/1libr/sma/sma_iliopsoa_sma.htm (cited May 2010).

4 Anderson KM, Strickland SM, Warren R. Hip and groin injuries in athletes. The American Journal of Sports Medicine. 29(4):521–33.

5 Margo K, Drezner J, Motzkin D. Evaluation and management of hip pain: an algorithmic approach. Journal of Family Practice. 2003;52(8):607–17.

6 Slipman CW, Jackson HB, Lipetz JS, et al. Sacroiliac joint pain referral zones. Archives of Physical Medicine and Rehabilitation. 2000;81(3):334–8.

7 Macintyre J, Johnson C, Schroeder EL. Groin pain in athletes. Current Sports Medicine Reports. 2006;5(6):293–9.

8 Webner D, Drezner JA. Lesser Trochanteric Bursitis: a rare cause of anterior hip pain. Clinical Journal of Sport Medicine. 2004;14(4):242–4.

9 Wisniewski SJ, Grogg B. Femoroacetabular Impingement: An overlooked cause of hip pain. American Journal of Physical Medicine & Rehabilitation. 2006;85(6):546–9.

10 Laslett M, Young SB, Aprill CN, et al. Diagnosing painful sacroiliac joints: a validity study of a McKenzie evaluation and sacroiliac provocation tests. Australian Journal of Physiotherapy. 2003;49(2):89–97.

11 Peeler J, Anderson JE. Reliability of the Thomas test for assessing range of motion about the hip. Physical Therapy in Sport. 2007;8(1):14–21.

12 Cyriax H, Cyriax PJ. Illustrated Manual of Orthopedic Medicine (2nd edn). Edinburgh: Butterworth Heinemann 1993.

13 Pua YH, Wrigley TV, Cowan SM, et al. Hip flexion range of motion and physical function in hip osteoarthritis: mediating effects of hip extensor strength and pain. Arthritis & Rheumatism. 2009;61(5):633–40.

14 Cibulka MT, White DM, Woehrle J, et al. Hip pain and mobility deficits—hip osteoarthritis: clinical pratice guidelines linked to the international classification of functioning, disability, and health from the orthopaedic section of the American Physical Therapy Association. Journal Orthopedic and Sports Physical Therapy. 2009;39(4):A1–A25.

15 Binningsley D. Tear of the acetabular labrum in an elite athlete. British Journal of Sports Medicine. 2003;37(1):84–8.

16 Manning M, Barron D, Lewis T, et al. Soft tissue injuries: hip and thigh. Emergency Medicine Journal. 2008;25(10):679–85.

17 Mulligan B. Mobilisations with movement (MWMs) for the hip joint to restore internal rotation and flexion. Journal of Manual and Manipulative Therapy. 1996;4(1):35–6.

18 Bisset L, Beller E, Jull G, et al. Mobilisation with movement and exercise, corticosteroid injection, or wait and see for tennis elbow: randomised trial. British Medical Journal. 2006;333(7575):939–44.

19 Abbot JH. Mobilization with movement applied to the elbow affects shoulder range of movement in subjects with lateral epicondylalgia. Manual Therapy. 2001;6(3):170–7.

20 Graumlich JF. Preventing gastrointestinal complications of NSAIDs. Risk factors, recent advances, and latest strategies. Postgraduate Medicine. 2001;109(5):117–20.

21 Biederman RE. Pharmacology in rehabilitation: nonsteroidal anti-inflammatory agents. Journal of Orthopaedic and Sports Physical Therapy. 2005;35(6):356–67.

22 MEDSAFE. Information for Health Professionals: Non-selective NSAIDS — Cardiovascular, skin, and gastrointestinal risks. Online. Available: http://www.medsafe.govt.nz/profs/PUArticles/NSAIDSRisks.htm (cited May 2010).

23 Hopkins JT, Ingersoll CD. Arthrogenic muscle inhibition: a limiting factor in joint rehabilitation. Journal of Sports Rehabilitation. 2000;9(2):135–59.

24 Hurley MV. The effects of joint damage on muscle function, proprioception and rehabilitation. Manual Therapy. 1997;2(1):11–7.

25 Di Lorenzo L, Jennifer Y, Pappagallo M. Psoas impingement syndrome in hip osteoarthritis. Joint Bone Spine. 2009;76(1):98–100.

26 Klassbo M, Harms-Ringdahl K, Larsson G. Examination of passive ROM and capsular patterns in the hip. Physiotherapy Research International. 2003;8(1):1–12.

27 Sims K. Assessment and treatment of hip osteoarthritis. Manual Therapy. 1999;4(3):136–44.

28 Hoeksma HL, Dekker J, Ronday HK, et al. Manual therapy in osteoarthritis of the hip: outcome in subgroups of patients. Rheumatology. 2005:1–4.

Chapter 18
Thigh pain: a diagnostic dilemma

Toby Hall

HISTORY

Peter is a 46-year-old accountant who works in his own accountancy business and is married with four children. His work is sedentary and sometimes 'bothers' his back and causes thigh pain, although not sufficiently so to force him to take time off work. Peter has a very busy lifestyle, mainly occupied by transporting his children to various sporting activities after school. He is also the coach for his youngest son's athletics team, which involves two training sessions per week. No medical help had been sought for his condition and he self-referred for treatment. When asked what he thought was the problem, Peter stated 'chronic hamstring tightness'. When asked what he thought therapy could do to help, he suggested he needed 'exercise or stretching' for the specific muscle problem.

Current history

Peter's main complaint was a sharp pain felt in his posterior right thigh along with an intermittent, right-sided low back pain radiating into the posterior thigh as a mild dull ache (Figure 18.1). On a numerical rating scale (NRS), the thigh pain at its worst had an intensity of 5/10 and the low back pain 3/10. Peter denied any pain or other symptoms in the lower leg or foot, or on the opposite side. The sharp posterior thigh pain appeared to be completely independent of both the low back pain and the ache in the posterior thigh, with different activities causing each symptom.

The sharp posterior thigh pain started about 3 years previously when Peter tore his right hamstring muscle in the mid-belly while running. He attempted a 400 metre race, and was three-quarters of the way around the track when the hamstring tear occurred. The severity of the pain forced him to stop running. Over the next week there was significant bruising and swelling of the hamstring muscle and he was forced to limp, making walking very difficult. At that time Peter did not seek treatment and simply waited for the problem to recover. Although the bruising and swelling subsided, and the pain slowly reduced over the next 2 weeks, he continued thereafter to experience sharp pain in the posterior thigh. He tried sports massage therapy, which consisted of deep tissue massage to the posterior thigh, but this had not helped and he stopped after three sessions. One of the parents in his son's athletics team was a physiotherapist who recommended he try physiotherapy on this occasion. Peter's goal was to be able to run with the children in his son's athletics team without pain.

Previous history

Prior to this current episode of hamstring pain, Peter had experienced numerous episodes of hamstring tears as a teenager, all while playing Australian Rules football. In addition to the current symptoms of sharp posterior thigh pain, Peter also reported a 5-year history of right-sided low back pain radiating to the right posterior thigh. This again had been episodic in nature, which Peter assumed was related to his sedentary occupation. The frequency, but not the intensity of the back pain had increased in the last 3 years. His back pain tended to flare up for a few days when he sat for longer periods, such as when he was busy at work preparing reports. On average, this generally now occurred every month, but was only mild in nature and depended on the nature of his work. He had not sought any medical advice regarding his back problem, instead tending to wait for the pain to settle on its own accord.

Symptom behaviour

Aggravating activities and postures for the sharp thigh pain included walking briskly, jogging and sitting, particularly sitting in an erect position. Hamstring stretches provoked the pain immediately. Aggravating activities for the low back pain and dull thigh ache were sustained sitting for more than 2 hours (slumped sitting was particularly painful, as was driving a car for more than 30 minutes) and any task where he had to flex his lumbar spine in standing. The Patient Specific Functional Scale (PSFS) is a valid and reliable measure of disability and has been shown to be more sensitive to change following treatment than other measures of disability, pain and physical impairment.[1, 2] Peter recorded a combined score of 20/50 for sitting, driving, walking, running and forward flexion. A score of 50/50 would indicate ability to perform activity at the same level as before the onset of the problem. The lower the

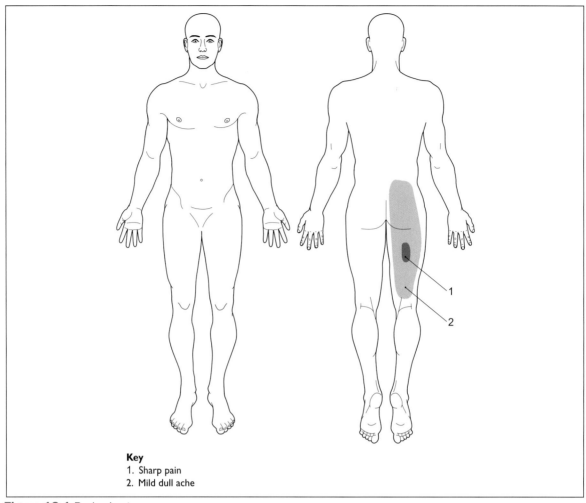

Key
1. Sharp pain
2. Mild dull ache

Figure 18.1 Body chart

score the greater the perceived interference caused by pain in those activities.

Peter reported that the back-related pain usually subsided quickly once he stopped the provocative action, indicating low irritability. A similar finding of low irritability was determined for the sharp thigh pain. Standing up and walking around reduced the back pain and thigh ache. He had no difficulty sleeping and woke in the morning with no pain or back stiffness. Over a typical 24-hour period there appeared to be no pattern to his pain other than the provocation of symptoms following the aforementioned activities.

Medical history and investigations
There was no history of medical or other conditions that might impact on Peter's clinical presentation or would influence management. He was not taking any medications for the presenting problem or any other condition.

EVIDENCE-INFORMED CLINICAL REASONING

1 From the history, the symptoms appear to be unrelated. Did you hypothesise that you would find two separate clinical problems on physical examination?

Clinician's response
Peter has presented with two areas of symptoms that at first glance appear completely unrelated. Both sets of symptoms are provoked and eased by different activities and come on at different times. In addition, the mechanism of injury and subsequent pain and thigh bruising associated to the latest injury points to a hamstring strain in the mid-belly, probably a grade 2 muscle tear based on the significant disability at the time.[3] As the low back pain was present prior to the hamstring injury, this logically indicates two separate tissue sources of pain.

It has been reported that injuries to the hamstring tendon or muscle-tendon junction are more severe and take longer to heal.[4] However, 3 years is well beyond the known biological healing time for muscle injuries, even those involving the muscle-tendon unit.[5] Ongoing pain might therefore suggest dysfunction of structures remote from the hamstring muscle including the lumbar spine, sacroiliac joint, lumbosacral neuromeningeal tissues and the posterior fascial system, anywhere from the cranium to the foot.[6] Dysfunction of all of these structures has been associated with recurrence and prolongation of hamstring problems.[7]

In Peter's case, two areas of interest for the physical examination are the lumbar spine and sacroiliac joint. Hamstring injuries and failure to recover may be due to poor functioning of the lumbar spine.[7] An association has been demonstrated in patients with low back pain of restricted range of lumbar spine and pelvic motion and decreased extensibility of the hamstring muscles.[8] Furthermore, a past history of low back injury has been correlated with an increased risk of referred pain and back-related hamstring injury.[9] Hence, physical examination of a number of possible contributing structures to Peter's hamstring pain is required.

2 Peter has experienced symptoms for several years. What did you consider was his prognosis at this point? What findings in his history were favourable and unfavourable for manual therapy in this regard?

Clinician's response

Peter describes very specific movements and activities that provoke his symptoms, with the sharp hamstring pain provoked by dynamic loading and the low back pain by sustained postures. This apparent mechanical nature to the symptoms is favourable for manual therapy intervention.

In terms of his account of his symptoms, and favourably for his prognosis, there appears to be no psychosocial issues or 'yellow flags', and no 'red flags' indicating serious spinal or other pathology. Peter's stated goals seem reasonable, but the long-term nature of the problem may warrant caution in terms of prognosis.

PHYSICAL EXAMINATION

Postural observations

On physical examination in standing Peter exhibited a normal lumbar lordosis but significant 'sway back' posture, with the pelvis anteriorly displaced relative to the upper trunk. Walking revealed no markedly observable abnormal motions. He tended to sit with a posterior pelvic tilt and was very close to the end-range of lumbar flexion. When asked to actively correct his posture in sitting he tended to initiate movement in the upper lumbar spine, remaining in a posterior pelvic tilted position and lower lumbar flexion. Passive correction

of neutral pelvis position could be achieved. Peter's pelvis further tilted posteriorly when he attempted single hip flexion in sitting and when he performed knee extension on the right more so than the left side, which Peter could not consciously prevent. These features have been associated with back pain.[10–12]

Active and combined movement tests

In standing, Peter's lumbar spine flexion was painful and reduced segmental mobility was observed throughout the lumbar spine. Range was limited to fingertips 20 cm above the floor and the limiting factor appeared to be stiffness, with mild back pain (3/10 on the NRS) and a pulling sensation in the posterior right thigh. Extension was of normal range and asymptomatic. Lateral flexion was mildly restricted towards the left side but was asymptomatic. Lateral flexion to the right was normal in range and asymptomatic. Lower quarter screening tests for increased peripheral nerve sensitisation were positive. Lumbar flexion was more restricted and provoked more pain in the back and posterior right thigh with the addition of right ankle dorsiflexion together with cervical spine flexion. This was not the case with left ankle dorsiflexion.

Combined movement testing was most provocative with the combination of lumbar spine flexion and left side flexion, which increased the back pain and provoked mild posterior thigh pain. No active or combined lumbar spine movements provoked the sharp hamstring pain.

The Stork test revealed a normal pattern of control with posterior rotation of the innominate relative to the sacrum on the weight-bearing side for both sides of the pelvis.[13]

Neural tissue provocation tests and neurological function

Straight leg raise (SLR) was 45° on the right, provoking a feeling of pain and tightness in the posterior thigh, and 65° on the left with only stretching pain provoked. The addition of ankle dorsiflexion on the right increased the posterior thigh pain and reduced the range of motion (ROM) significantly, which was not the case on the left. The slump test was provocative for the back and thigh pain and with the spine fully flexed there was a reduction of 20° knee extension on the right compared to the left leg. Furthermore, knee extension was also restricted and painful on the right side when the pelvis was positioned in end-range of anterior tilting. This movement provoked a mild version of the sharp hamstring pain. The sciatic and tibial nerves on the right side, in contrast to the left, were markedly tender to gentle direct manual pressure. Neurological examination was unremarkable with no signs of loss of axonal conduction.

Sacroiliac joint pain provocation and other tests

'Compression' and 'distraction' testing (applied via the anterior superior iliac spines) and the thigh thrust test were not pain provocative. No further testing was undertaken for the sacroiliac joints.[14] Hip flexion mobility was bilaterally normal and asymptomatic.

Passive segmental mobility tests

With the lumbar spine in a combined position of flexion and left side flexion, postero–anterior (PA) pressure applied unilaterally over the right L5–S1 and to a lesser extent L4–L5 facet joints provoked Peter's usual back pain. Passive physiological intervertebral motion testing revealed no limitation of flexion at either the L4–L5 or L5–S1 motion segments.

Hamstring muscle tests

Hamstring muscle length testing in supine lying (90/90 test[15]) provoked the posterior thigh pain and was reduced by 25° on the right compared to the left side. Hamstring muscle contraction in a lengthened position also provoked the posterior thigh pain. Similarly, palpation of the right medial hamstrings in the mid-belly provoked pain in the posterior thigh. In a supine position, pain provocation on palpation was increased during hamstring eccentric contraction.

EVIDENCE-INFORMED CLINICAL REASONING

1 After the physical examination, what were your hypotheses for the two pains and what findings supported this?

Clinician's response

Peter's lumbar spine disorder appears to be consistent with some aspects of a flexion pattern of motor control dysfunction.[16] Lumbar flexion activities and postures provoke his pain, he sits at end-range of lumbar flexion/posterior pelvic tilting, and he has difficulty correcting his seated posture to a neutral lordosis. A number of studies have shown similar patterns of control impairment in low back pain populations.[10, 11] For example, industrial workers with low back pain related to flexion activities choose to sit with less hip flexion and with their spines significantly closer to end of range of lumbar flexion in 'usual' sitting than do healthy controls.[11] A flexion control impairment may explain the back and posterior thigh ache, but not the sharp posterior thigh pain as this was provoked by isolated stretching of the hamstring muscle during anterior pelvic tilting.

Although lumbar spine movement appeared to be full range in sitting, in standing there was significant limitation of forward bending, which might indicate an inability of the lumbar articular structures to bear load, consistent with a control impairment. Negating the loading hypothesis are the strong signs of peripheral nerve sensitisation involving the sciatic nerve and lumbosacral plexus,[17] as well as hamstring muscle tightness.

Involvement of the right sacroiliac joint as a possible pain source is unlikely as a normal pattern of movement was found on the stork test. Patients with posterior pelvic pain arising from the sacroiliac joint typically demonstrate an altered pattern of movement of the weight bearing innominate relative to the sacrum when standing on the symptomatic side.[13] This test has recently been shown to be reliable[18] and aids in the early identification of sacroiliac joint dysfunction. The findings of the pain provocation tests also do not support a sacroiliac joint (nor hip joint) problem. Laslett et al[14] reports that if the thigh thrust test and anterior superior iliac spine 'distraction' and 'compression' tests are all negative then this indicates the sacroiliac joint is unlikely to be the source of pain.

There is evidence of strong fascial connections between biceps femoris and peroneus longus at the fibula.[19] Hence it has been postulated that SLR with dorsiflexion may stress the myofascial structures of the posterior leg.[4] However, it is unlikely in this case that the symptoms arise from dysfunction of the fascia in the leg as there were no other findings implicating the fascia, but there was consistent evidence of peripheral nerve sensitisation on a range of tests.

Although a specific diagnosis of the tissue of pain origin is not always achievable, identification of the responsible segment should be made where possible.[20] In Peter's case, the pain source for the low back pain and dull posterior thigh pain appears to be the L4–L5 and L5–S1 segments, based on the reproduction of his pain on applying PA pressure at these motion segments. The assessment findings are consistent with a maladaptive flexion pattern of control impairment.[16] In simple terms this classification is based on three key points. Firstly, symptom reproduction is consistently associated with lumbar spine flexion movements or postures. Secondly, the lumbar spine is held in a flexed position, constantly provoking pain. Finally, although there is normal segmental mobility at the symptomatic level, the patient finds it difficult to 'lordose' the spine to reduce the provocative stress on the sensitised segments. This pattern of poor posture and altered motor control sets in process a closed loop whereby end-range lumbar flexion stresses the sensitised structures, which then contributes to the maintenance of the sensitised pain state.[11] This closed loop may explain the ongoing chronic pain, which is peripherally driven through ongoing sensitisation of nociceptors in the stressed motion segments (see Chapter 6).

Central sensitisation is an inevitable consequence of tissue injury.[21] In this case, however, there was no strong evidence that the pain was centrally mediated given the pain was intermittent in nature, within distinct anatomical locations, and relieved by specific activities that unload the symptomatic structures.[22] Moreover, there were no features in the examination that suggested psychosocial factors were enhancing the chronic pain state.[23]

In contrast to the low back related thigh pain, the sharp posterior thigh pain appears localised to the hamstring muscle as there is pain on both isolated hamstring stretching and isometric contraction. In addition, there is also evidence of a localised area of abnormal sensitivity to palpation of the hamstring, and pain provocation is further increased during hamstring lengthening and eccentric contraction.[24] There are no known biological mechanisms (other than changes in central sensitivity and pain processing) pertaining to ongoing hamstring pathology that can explain these signs. Muscle trauma usually heals within a well defined period.[25] However, muscle injuries heal with scar tissue rather than by regeneration. Since the initial hamstring trauma was moderately severe (haematoma with leg bruising), it is inevitable that scar tissue and probably adhesions were formed.[4] If the scar tissue was not sufficiently stressed during the stages of recovery it may have become 'functionally disabling'.[25] This may potentially explain the recurring pain in the region of the previous hamstring tear.

In some ways the hamstring muscle problem exacerbates the lumbar flexion pattern and vice versa. Limited extensibility of the right hamstring promotes increased posterior pelvic tilt and lumbar flexion, thereby increasing the stress on the L4–L5 and L5–S1 segments. In reverse, attempting to adopt an upright posture with a more neutral lumbar and pelvic position potentially increases the stress on the shortened, sensitised hamstring muscle. Hence, it was decided to address the hamstring problem, which would also address aspects of the low back control problem. Attempting to hit two birds with one stone.

2 Was Mobilisation with Movement (MWM) indicated for treatment? If not, were there alternative Mulligan Concept treatment hypotheses you were considering?

Clinician's response

Mulligan[26] recommends a trial application of each of four techniques for patients with low back related leg pain referred to the posterior thigh. These include the gate technique, the bent leg raise (BLR) technique, the traction SLR technique (TSLR) and the compression SLR technique. These techniques fulfil the criteria of MWM and can be very effective mobilisation techniques in certain clinical situations. To date there have been no studies examining the relative efficacy of these procedures. Both the BLR and TSLR have been investigated and have been shown to have immediate

effects to improve hamstring muscle length and range of SLR,[27–29] but no studies have investigated the long-term efficacy. It is the clinical experience of the author that patients with significant peripheral nerve sensitisation respond most favourably to the BLR technique, and this may also address the hamstring extensibility problem. The BLR technique can be likened to a nerve 'slider'[30, 31] where the mechanosensitised nerve is gently mobilised along its length without tensioning the nerve. Rozmaryn et al[32] showed the benefits of adding nerve-gliding exercises to the standard conservative management of carpal tunnel syndrome. Furthermore, there is some evidence that incorporating nerve-sliding manoeuvres can be effective in reducing pain and improving function in patients with low back related leg pain.[33] In contrast the TSLR will effectively tension the sciatic nerve, and may potentially exacerbate pain in the presence of sensitisation of the lumbosacral or sciatic neural tissues. Hence the BLR technique was the first technique chosen to help manage this case.

TREATMENT AND MANAGEMENT

Treatment 1

Table 18.1 details the BLR technique (Figure 18.2) used in the first treatment session. Due to the low irritability and chronic nature of both the back pain and hamstring problem the technique was carried out to the maximum range of hip flexion, but the knee was positioned so as to maintain the comfort of the patient. In addition, the resistance to the isometric contraction was applied gently to avoid pain from contracting the hamstring muscle. Peter tolerated the technique with no report of either back or thigh pain. Three repetitions of the technique were carried out.

The immediate effect of the BLR technique was an increase in forward bending in standing of 5 cm. Moreover, right SLR increased by 15° to 60° and was only mildly painful. The 90/90 hamstring extensibility test was no longer painful but the range was still reduced when compared to the left side.

Peter was taught a home exercise designed to mimic the BLR technique (Table 18.1 and Figure 18.2). He was asked to do 10 repetitions of the exercise three times per day.

In addition to the BLR technique, some time was spent on retraining proprioceptive awareness of the neutral pelvic position. As Peter found this difficult in sitting with the hips in 90° flexion, the chair height was raised to reduce the hip flexion. After some practise Peter was able to achieve a neutral pelvic position. He was asked to carry out five repetitions of this exercise on a high stool at least five times per day, holding the position for 5 seconds each time.

Peter was advised to maintain his current physical activity levels and not to jog or attempt hamstring stretches.

Table 18.1	Bent leg raise MWM to improve straight leg raise	
Indication	**Low back/posterior thigh pain and/or loss of movement during straight leg raise (SLR); limitation of hamstring extensibility**	
Positioning	Patient	Supine lying near side of treatment table.
	Treated body part	Hip on symptomatic side flexed to 90° (or less if pain is provoked). Ipsilateral knee flexed to 90° (or more if pain is provoked).
	Therapist	Standing beside the patient's symptomatic leg with the patient's flexed knee resting on the therapist's shoulder. Traction force is applied along the line of the femur by the therapist extending their trunk, lifting the leg resting over their shoulder, while pushing down through the support arm.
	Therapist's hands	One hand rests on the treatment table to provide stability, the other grasps the patient's femur to control the thigh position.
Application guidelines	• An isometric contraction of the hamstring muscles is sought by asking the patient to simultaneously flex the knee and extend the hip against the therapist's body. The contraction is sustained for 5 seconds. While the traction force is maintained the hip is moved further into the range of flexion, where the isometric hamstring contraction is performed again (Figure 18.2). This process is repeated approximately five times at arbitrary points in the hip flexion range, until the maximum range of hip flexion is achieved. • If leg or back pain is provoked the knee should be further flexed or the hip abducted. • Repeat the entire procedure three times. • Subsequent reassessment of SLR or forward bending in standing should reveal a significant improvement in pain-free range of movement. • The BLR technique can be progressed in subsequent treatment sessions by applying the technique with a gradually increasing range of knee extension as the condition allows. • Self-treatment techniques (Figure 18.3) are very important to maximise the effectiveness of the BLR. One exercise is for the patient to stand with the foot on the affected side resting on a chair or stool. The patient slides both hands down the medial side of the leg until the flexed knee reaches their shoulder. If symptoms are provoked the patient is instructed to stop short of pain and perform an isometric contraction of the hamstring muscles (by extending the hip and flexing the knee against the resistance of the chair) for 5 seconds and then try to move further. This process can be repeated a number of times. Alternatively, the therapist may choose to apply sustained natural apophyseal glides (SNAGs) to the lumbar spine to try to relieve symptoms on forward bending. The exercise is usually repeated 10 times on at least three occasions during the day.	
Comments	• Be careful not to compress the hip joint and provoke groin pain. • Traction is applied along the line of the femur, which should cause the pelvis to posteriorly rotate, thus reducing stress on the hip joint. • Maintain the traction throughout the procedure, until the patient returns to the starting position. • Aim to achieve maximum, pain-free hip flexion.	

Treatment 2

Peter returned for re-evaluation and treatment 3 days later. He reported significant improvement in both the back and thigh symptoms. The sharp posterior thigh pain was no longer present during brisk walking and the back pain had not been as noticeable.

On reassessment, his forward bending range in standing was now 15 cm from fingertips to the floor. Right SLR was 55° and the hamstring 90/90 test was unchanged from the end of the previous treatment. Seated lumbopelvic posture was improved in both a normal chair, and in a high sitting position.

In view of the positive and sustained response to the first treatment session the BLR technique was repeated and progressed to five repetitions. In addition, there was some refinement of the anterior pelvic tilt dynamic control exercise in high sitting.

At the end of the second treatment session forward bending in standing had improved to 10 cm from fingertips to the floor. Right SLR was now 65° and the hamstring 90/90 test was only 10° less in range than

the left side. Furthermore, Peter was able to achieve a neutral pelvic position in a normal chair. His home exercise program was accordingly progressed (Figure 18.3). He was also asked to sit with a neutral pelvic tilt while gently extending his right knee from 90° to 70° knee flexion and back. On initial assessment it was apparent that knee extension in sitting invoked posterior pelvic tilt due to the relative hamstring tightness.

Treatment 3

Peter reported further improvement as a result of treatment 2. He was able to sit more comfortably at work and had noticed little in the way of back or either posterior thigh pain.

Forward bending in standing was now 10 cm from fingertips to the floor. Right SLR was 65° and there was a side to side difference of only 5° on the hamstring 90/90 test. Peter's posture in sitting was much improved. He was able to move independently in and out of a neutral lordotic and neutral pelvic tilt position in sitting. He was also able to control knee extension

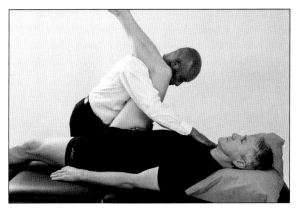

Figure 18.2 Bent leg raise technique

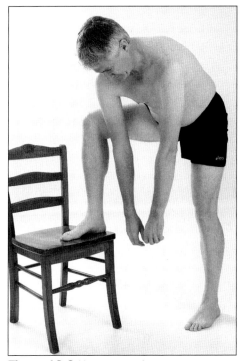

Figure 18.3 Home exercise

from 90° to 70° knee flexion without losing control of his pelvis. Palpation of the lumbar spine at L4–L5 and L5–S1, as well as the right hamstring revealed less tenderness than at the initial session. Isometric contraction of the hamstring muscle was not painful, nor was eccentric contraction.

In view of the continued improvement from the previous session the BLR technique was repeated and was progressed with the knee now in 70° knee flexion. In addition, there was some further refinement of the anterior pelvic tilt dynamic control exercise in high sitting.

At the end of the third treatment session forward bending in standing had improved to 5 cm from fingertips to floor and remained pain-free. The hamstring

90/90 test was symmetrical in range between both sides. Peter was advised to start a gentle walking/jogging program, gradually progressing to full but gentle jogging. Re-education of hamstring extensibility continued by gradually progressing the range of knee extension as the condition allowed, while ensuring pelvic tilt and lumbar lordosis were maintained in a neutral position during the stretch.

Treatment 4

Three weeks later Peter reported further improvement with all activities. He was able to jog for approximately 1 km without hamstring discomfort, sit with minimal discomfort (2/10) during the day at work and drive for at least 1 hour before the onset of back discomfort (2/10). Disability was rated as 40/50 on the PSFS.

Forward bending in standing was 5 cm from fingertips to floor and pain-free. Right SLR was 70° on the left and the right. The hamstring 90/90 test was symmetrical. There was no pain on palpation of the hamstring muscle, even on eccentric contraction. Peter's posture in sitting and his ability to control the neutral pelvic position while gradually extending the knee was excellent.

Peter was given advice about gradually progressing his jogging exercise tolerance. He was also advised to start hamstring flexibility exercises (while ensuring a neutral lordosis was maintained) as part of a daily routine of flexibility. No further treatment sessions were planned.

Peter was contacted by telephone 3 months after the final treatment session. He had made gradual progress with his jogging and stretching program and was able to run comfortably for 5 km without any problem. His low back symptoms were completely managed by careful attention to his sitting posture.

AUTHOR'S MULLIGAN CONCEPT COMMENTARY

Peter's case illustrates how a Mulligan Concept technique can facilitate the rapid resolution of chronic, complex back and thigh pain arising from multiple structures and involving issues of motor control, peripheral nerve sensitisation and myofascial dysfunction.

The Mulligan Concept has been criticised for failing to be specific.[34] However, many disorders are complex, involving multiple structures. For instance, posterior thigh pain following a football injury may involve hamstring muscle pathology and sciatic nerve sensitisation,[35] a situation similar to this case. A single Mulligan Concept technique has been shown to improve SLR range where limitation is due to either a low back articular disorder or to peripheral nerve sensitisation.[29] This duality of technique application is arguably a strength of the Mulligan Concept rather than a weakness.

The intention of the BLR technique is to restore normal mobility as well as reduce pain and other physical impairments. Dixon and Keating[36] contend that an improvement in the range of SLR must be greater than 6° in order to state that a real change has occurred. In Peter's case, after four treatment sessions there was a 25° change in the range of SLR, meeting this criterion. The range improved concurrently with symptoms and disability as measured by the PSFS.

To date only one study has investigated the effect of the BLR technique on low back related pain and impairment.[27] This small, double-blind, randomised, placebo controlled trial evaluated the immediate effects of the BLR technique. The adjusted mean difference in range of SLR between the two groups, 24 hours after intervention, was 7° and pain scores were significantly reduced in the intervention group on a NRS.

In this case, symptoms changed from 5/10 to 2/10 on the NRS after four treatment sessions, exceeding the bounds of measurement error for clinically meaningful change.[37] One mechanism underlying this change may be through mobilisation of the sensitised nerve tissues, similar to a 'slider' technique,[38, 39] which has been shown to be beneficial in a nerve sensitisation disorder.[40] In Peter's case, there were significant signs of peripheral nerve sensitisation probably contributing to the low back and thigh pain. However, it is unlikely that this is the only treatment effect of the BLR technique (see Chapters 5–7).

Another mechanism underlying the beneficial effects of the BLR technique might be a change in stretch tolerance of the hamstring muscle. It seems reasonable to hypothesise that increased hamstring extensibility is closely connected to central neurophysiological processing (see Chapters 5–7) and that the BLR technique triggers neurophysiological responses influencing muscle stretch tolerance. An increase in hamstring extensibility might reduce stress on painful lumbar tissues, in this case because of an increase in anterior pelvic rotation resulting in less stress on the sensitised lower lumbar motion segments.

Other mechanisms of pain relief may include habituation and extinction, described by Zusman.[41] Stimulation from damaged tissues produces learning type changes or plasticity of the nervous system. The nervous system therefore 'learns' to respond to increasingly less powerful stimuli, a process similar to Pavlovian conditioning.[42] In terms of pain extinction, the aim is to encourage normal activity in a progressive, functional and pain-free manner.[41] In Peter's case, forward bending and hamstring contraction were both painful. The BLR technique may have provided exposure to the previously painful movement in the absence of any overt danger, which is fundamental to interventions used in the extinction of aversive memories.[42]

Progressive mobilisation may also desensitise the nervous system through habituation. This mechanism involves a progressive decline in the ability of the pre-synaptic nerve terminal to transmit impulses. In this case study, non-noxious sensory input from the repeated BLR technique may have competed with and replaced pain sensitisation, returning the nervous system to a more normal state.[41]

References

1 Donnelly C, Carswell A. Individualized outcome measures: a review of the literature. Canadian Journal of Occupational Therapy. 2002;69(2):84–94.

2 Pengel LH, Refshauge KM, Maher CG. Responsiveness of pain, disability, and physical impairment outcomes in patients with low back pain. Spine. 2004;29(8):879–83.

3 Ekstrand J, Gillquist J. Soccer injuries and their mechanisms: a prospective study. Medicine and Science in Sports and Exercise. 1983;15(3):267–70.

4 Hoskins W, Pollard H. The management of hamstring injury — part 1: issues in diagnosis. Manual Therapy. 2005;10(2):96–107.

5 Jarvinen TA, Jarvinen TL, Kaariainen M, et al. Muscle injuries: optimising recovery. Best Practice and Research in Clinical Rheumatology. 2007;21(2):317–31.

6 Hoskins W, Pollard H. Hamstring injury management — part 2: treatment. Manual Therapy. 2005;10(3):180–90.

7 Hoskins WT, Pollard HP. Successful management of hamstring injuries in Australian Rules footballers: two case reports. Chiropractic and Osteopathy. 2005;13(4).

8 Halbertsma JP, Goeken LN, Hof AL, et al. Extensibility and stiffness of the hamstrings in patients with non-specific low back pain. Archives of Physical Medicine and Rehabilitation. 2001;82(2):232–8.

9 Verrall GM, Slavotinek JP, Barnes PG, et al. Clinical risk factors for hamstring muscle strain injury: a prospective study with correlation of injury by magnetic resonance imaging. British Journal of Sports Medicine. 2001;35(6):435–9; discussion 40.

10 Burnett AF, Cornelius MW, Dankaerts W, et al. Spinal kinematics and trunk muscle activity in cyclists: a comparison between healthy controls and non-specific chronic low back pain subjects — a pilot investigation. Manual Therapy. 2004;9(4):211–9.

11 O'Sullivan PB, Mitchell T, Bulich P, et al. The relationship beween posture and back muscle endurance in industrial workers with flexion-related low back pain. Manual Therapy. 2006;11(4):264–71.

12 Smith A, O'Sullivan P, Straker L. Classification of sagittal thoraco-lumbo-pelvic alignment of the adolescent spine in standing and its relationship to low back pain. Spine. 2008;33(19):2101–7.

13 Hungerford B, Gilleard W, Hodges P. Evidence of altered lumbopelvic muscle recruitment in the presence of sacroiliac joint pain. Spine. 2003;28(14):1593–600.

14 Laslett M, Aprill CN, McDonald B, et al. Diagnosis of sacroiliac joint pain: validity of individual provocation tests and composites of tests. Manual Therapy. 2005;10(3):207–18.

15 Hartig DE, Henderson JM. Increasing hamstring flexibility decreases lower extremity overuse injuries in military basic trainees. American Journal of Sports Medicine. 1999;27(2):173–6.

16 O'Sullivan P. Diagnosis and classification of chronic low back pain disorders: maladaptive movement and motor control impairments as underlying mechanism. Manual Therapy. 2005;10(4):242–55.

17 Hall TM, Elvey RL. Management of mechanosensitivity of the nervous system in spinal pain syndromes. In: Boyling G, Jull G (eds) Grieves Modern Manual Therapy (3rd edn). Edinburgh: Elsevier Churchill Livingstone 2005:413–31.

18 Hungerford BA, Gilleard W, Moran M, et al. Evaluation of the ability of physical therapists to palpate intrapelvic motion with the Stork test on the support side. Physical Therapy. 2007;87(7):879–87.

19 Weinert CR, Jr., McMaster JH, Ferguson RJ. Dynamic function of the human fibula. American Journal of Anatomy. 1973;138(2):145–9.

20 Phillips DR, Twomey LT. A comparison of manual diagnosis with a diagnosis established by a uni-level lumbar spinal block procedure. Manual Therapy. 1996;1(2):82–7.

21 Zusman M. Forebrain-mediated sensitization of central pain pathways: 'non-specific' pain and a new image for MT. Manual Therapy. 2002;7(2):80–8.

22 O'Sullivan PB, Beales DJ. Diagnosis and classification of pelvic girdle pain disorders — Part 1: a mechanism based approach within a biopsychosocial framework. Manual Therapy. 2007;12(2):86–97.

23 Waddell G. The Physical Basis of Back Pain. The Back Pain Revolution. Edinburgh: Churchill Livingstone 1998:135–54.

24 Hopper D, Deacon S, Das S, et al. Dynamic soft tissue mobilisation increases hamstring flexibility in healthy male subjects. British Journal of Sports Medicine. 2005;39(9):594–8; discussion 8.

25 Jarvinen TA, Jarvinen TL, Kaariainen M, et al. Muscle injuries: biology and treatment. American Journal of Sports Medicine. 2005;33(5):745–64.

26 Mulligan BR. Manual therapy, Nags, Snags, MWMS etc (5th edn). Wellington: Plane View Services 2004.

27 Hall T, Hardt S, Schafer A, et al. Mulligan bent leg raise technique — a preliminary randomized trial of immediate effects after a single intervention. Manual Therapy. 2006;11(2):130–5.

28 Hall TM, Cacho A, McNee C, et al. Effects of the Mulligan traction straight leg raise technique on range of movement. Journal of Manual & Manipulative Therapy. 2001;9(3):128–33.

29 Hall TM, Beyerlein C, Hansson U, et al. Mulligan traction straight leg raise: A pilot study to investigate effects on range of motion in patients with low back pain. Journal of Manual & Manipulative Therapy. 2006;14(2):95–100.

30 Butler D. The sensitive nervous system. Adelaide: NOI Group Publications 2000.

31 Shacklock M. Clinical Neurodynamics. Edinburgh: Elsevier 2005.

32 Rozmaryn LM, Dovelle S, Rothman ER, et al. Nerve and tendon gliding exercises and the conservative management of carpal tunnel syndrome. Journal of Hand Therapy. 1998;11(3):171–9.

33 Schafer A, Hall TM, Briffa K, Ludtke K, Mallwitz J. Outcomes differ between subgroups of patients with low back and leg pain following neural manual therapy — a prospective cohort study (submitted for publication).

34 Cornwall J. Commentary. New Zealand Journal of Physiotherapy. 2005;13(3):113–4.

35 Kornberg C, Lew P. The effect of stretching neural structures on grade one hamstring injuries. Journal of Orthopaedic and Sports Physical Therapy 1989;10(12):481–7.

36 Dixon JK, Keating JL. Variability in straight leg raise measurements: Review. Physiotherapy. 2000;86(7):361–70.

37 Childs J, Piva S, Fritz JM. Responsiveness of the Numeric Pain Rating Scale in patients with low back pain. Spine. 2005;30(11):1331–4.

38 Coppieters MW, Alshami AM. Longitudinal excursion and strain in the median nerve during novel nerve gliding exercises for carpal tunnel syndrome. Journal of Orthopaedic Research. 2007;25(7):972–80.

39 Coppieters MW, Butler DS. Do 'sliders' slide and 'tensioners' tension? An analysis of neurodynamic techniques and considerations regarding their application. Manual Therapy. 2008;13(3):213–21.

40 Coppieters MW, Bartholomeeusen KE, Stappaerts KH. Incorporating nerve-gliding techniques in the conservative treatment of cubital tunnel syndrome. Journal of Manipulative Physiological Therapy. 2004;27(9):560–8.

41 Zusman M. Mechanisms of musculoskeletal physiotherapy. Physical Therapy Reviews. 2004;9:39–49.

42 Myers KM, Davis M. Behavioral and neural analysis of extinction. Neuron. 2002;36(4):567–84.

Chapter 19
Two single case studies of lateral ankle sprain in young athletes

Bill Vicenzino, Toby Hall and Tracey O'Brien

Note: This study is revised and adapted from O'Brien and Vicenzino[1]

PREAMBLE

Previous chapters report patient cases that were managed with Mobilisation with Movement (MWM) and dealt in depth with the clinical thinking and reasoning that the practitioners underwent. This chapter consists of a previously published paper[1] and takes a different approach to the foregoing case report chapters. It is different in that it presents two cases in the framework of a case study design, but with some additional clinical reasoning commentary included. The single case study design is the next level of evidence up from case reports (as presented in the previous chapters) and provided that the patient is willing it is a feasible and practical design that can be used by practitioners to report the outcomes of their treatments in specific patients. One or more case studies may then be combined to provide guidance to practitioners in managing patients or they can be used in the development of other experiments, grant applications and randomised clinical trials, all of which lead to the development of the evidence base. For example, the lateral glide MWM for tennis elbow was first described in Mulligan's textbook and several case reports, then in a single case study[2] and a series of clinical and laboratory experiments,[3–10] before being used as the basis for a National Health and Medical Research Council project grant application (#252710) that funded a full randomised clinical trial (n = 198), which has been recently published in several high standing medical and evidenced-based health care journals.[11–15]

In order to provide readers with an example of a case study design within this book, two male patients, Rohan and Cameron, who each had sustained a recent plantarflexion and inversion ankle injury and had no previous history of ankle sprains, are presented as single case studies. After a brief description of their presentation and description of the MWM being studied, this chapter then outlines the key elements of the single case study design methods that were applied. In detailing the elements of the study, we first describe the treatment and management that was adopted and then the outcome measures of pain, impairment and function used, before outlining the specific case design features and the outcomes of management for Rohan and Cameron. We also include clinical reasoning comments so as to maintain a linkage with clinical translation and the theme of the other case reports in this book.

HISTORY

Rohan was a 17-year-old basketball player who presented with pain about the lateral malleolus (Figure 19.1a) 3 days post-injury to his right ankle. He presented non-weight-bearing (NWB) on crutches, with pain on all ankle movements and marked swelling around the lateral malleolus and mid-foot. No fracture was evident on X-ray.

Cameron was an 18-year-old football player who presented two days post-injury to his left ankle. His main signs and symptoms were difficulty walking up stairs, reduced ankle movement, pain about his lateral malleolus and marked swelling of the ankle (Figure 19.1b). He was full weight-bearing but with reduced dorsiflexion and time in the stance phase of gait.

CONSIDERATIONS FOR EVIDENCE-INFORMED CLINICAL REASONING

1 What are the hypothesised patho-mechanical causes of lateral ankle pain at this early stage in these two similar cases?

Clinician's response

Forced plantarflexion/inversion is the most common mechanism of injury at the ankle. It frequently results in damage to the anterior talofibular ligament (ATFL), although other structures may be involved.[3] The anterior inferior tibiofibular ligament sprain or 'high' ankle sprain is reported as being relatively unusual[4] and only occurring in more severe ankle sprains.[3] Nevertheless, there is anecdotal clinical evidence to the contrary, that these injuries are more common than previously thought.[4] Other reported causes of lateral ankle pain and dysfunction include: fractures around the ankle joint; osteochondral fractures of the talar dome; dislocation of the peroneal tendons; chronic synovitis; anterior, posterior

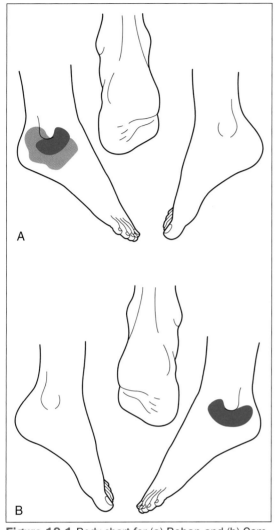

Figure 19.1 Body chart for (a) Rohan and (b) Cameron
Both had swelling about the ankle and into the foot

or anterolateral impingement; reflex sympathetic dystrophy;[3] subtalar joint instability;[5] degenerative arthritis; osteophytic impingement; loose bodies and subtalar joint impingement.[6] The presence of any of these conditions can complicate the management of ankle pain and may lead to chronic ankle pain and dysfunction.

2 What is the underlying premise regarding the pathophysiology of lateral ankle sprain according to the Mulligan Concept? What evidence is there to support such a proposal?

Clinician's response
Mulligan[7] claims that when a person rolls their ankle, as in an inversion sprain, that instead of the ATFL tearing, the force is transmitted via this ligament to the lateral malleolus and causes the distal fibula to sublux anteriorly and inferiorly. There is evidence, which on balance indicates, that there may be an anteriorly positioned fibula in sub-acute and chronic ankle instability in some patients. However, measuring such a subluxation is not currently possible in the clinical setting. See Chapter 4 for further information in this regard.

3 Does the Mulligan Concept have a role to play in managing lateral ankle sprain?

Clinician's response
Lateral ankle sprains are common and are frequently treated by health care practitioners. The conventional treatment approach includes electrotherapy, manual therapy and mobilisation, as well as strengthening, proprioceptive and sports specific exercises.[3] MWM is a relatively recent clinical development and is not yet employed as a standard manual therapy treatment for acute ankle pain. As a result it has not been thoroughly investigated.

TREATMENT AND MANAGEMENT
The treatment technique under investigation in the two single case studies was a MWM for the lateral malleolus. The technique involves the manual application of a sustained postero-lateral and superior glide of the distal end of the fibula, while the subject actively inverts the ankle to the end of pain-free range (Table 19.1). If full pain-free range is achieved then the therapist applies passive overpressure (Figure 19.2). In both cases, the MWM was repeated four times during treatment and followed up by the application of a simple taping technique that sought to replicate the glide, and so optimise the effect of the MWM (Figure 19.3).

CONSIDERATIONS IN EVIDENCE-INFORMED CLINICAL REASONING

1 What is the evidence underpinning the clinical efficacy of the MWM? Why would you consider applying a technique without empirical evidence?

Clinician's response
We could not find any investigation or clinical trial that studied the clinical efficacy of this MWM applied manually, hence the aim of this single case study report; that is, to describe the clinical effects of MWM where there is an absence of high level clinical trial evidence. Whilst there is no study on the manually applied MWM, there is a study that evaluated the preventative capacity of the MWM taping technique to prevent ankle sprains. Moiler et al[8] studied 125 basketball players who underwent 433 exposures (Control 209, Taped 224) and sustained 11 ankle sprains. Only two sprains occurred in the taped group, which was statistically significant in favour of fibular taping (odds ratio

Table 19.1	Instructions for the application of the distal fibula repositioning MWM	
Indication	**Pain and limitation primarily of ankle inversion after plantarflexion/inversion sprain. Secondary limitation includes ankle plantarflexion and dorsiflexion**	
Positioning	Patient	Patient lays supine.
	Treated body part	The leg is raised slightly off the treatment table and supported by the therapist's hands to allow free movement of the foot and ankle into plantarflexion and inversion.
	Therapist	The therapist stands at the foot of the table facing the patient.
	Therapist's hands	The therapist stabilises the tibia with their medial most hand. The fingers of this hand are placed on the posterior aspect of the tibia to allow free movement of the fibula. The therapist's mobilising hand is placed with the thenar eminence in contact with the anterior/inferior aspect of the distal fibula. The fingers of this hand wrap around the posterior aspect of the lower leg to rest posterior to the fingers of the other hand stabilising the tibia. A lumbrical action of the mobilising hand on the fibula (metacarpophalangeal joint flexion of the 2nd–5th fingers together with flexion at the carpometacarpal joint of the thumb) is directed at the fibula in an effort to glide the fibula in a posterior, superior and lateral direction. If the correct glide is applied the patient will be able to actively invert through a larger range without pain.
Application guidelines	• The force applied to the fibula is directed in a posterior, superior and lateral direction. • With correct application of the fibula glide, the foot will be seen to move towards slight eversion. • While the fibula glide is maintained the patient is instructed to actively move the foot into inversion. • If the technique is indicated, the patient will be able to achieve considerably greater range inversion without pain. • If pain persists, even after modifications are tried, the technique should not be used. • Repeat the movement several times before reassessing the active movement independent of the glide. Reassessment should reveal a significant improvement in pain-free range of movement. • If full range and pain-free active inversion can be achieved with the fibula glide, the therapist then applies gentle, passive, inversion overpressure for 1–2 seconds. It is important that this movement is also pain-free.	
Comments	• Ensure that gentle and not excessive force is applied to the fibula. Excessive force may cause discomfort or pain preventing application of the technique. This is particularly true for an acute ankle sprain where there may be significant local tenderness and swelling. It is advisable to use a thick piece of sponge rubber to soften the contact on the fibula in all cases. • The patient must experience no pain or other symptoms at any stage of the mobilisation or active movement. Should pain occur the technique should be modified by subtly altering the direction of the mobilisation force on the fibula or the amount of force applied.	
Variation	• Taping of the lateral malleolus in order to simulate this MWM is frequently beneficial (Figure 19.3). • Once inversion range is fully restored and pain-free it is possible to progress the technique by combining plantarflexion and inversion. • In some cases dorsiflexion may also be limited and painful post ankle inversion sprain. Following treatment for plantarflexion and inversion, dorsiflexion may also be restored using the same mobilisation procedure. Dorsiflexion may be further progressed by repeating the procedure in a weight-bearing position.	

[OR] 0.2; 95% confidence interval [CI]: 0.04 to 0.93; number needed to treat [NNT] 22; 95% CI: 12–312).

2 What is the underlying rationale regarding this MWM?

Clinician's response

The rationale underlying the manually applied MWM treatment technique for lateral ankle sprain is based on a patho-anatomical mechanism (Chapter 4) of anteroinferior subluxation of the distal fibula.[9, 10] It has been hypothesised that the MWM treatment technique (and the accompanying taping technique) achieves its effects by repositioning the subluxed fibula. There have been no direct investigations of this repositioning hypothesis, yet it seems conceivable that applying a force in the opposite direction to the subluxation would seem appropriate.

While there has been little mechanism-based research for the manually applied MWM, East et al[11] recently studied possible mechanisms of the fibular repositioning tape in landing from a jump (n = 30, 10 with fibular repositioning tape, 10 with placebo tape and 10 controls). They reported that the fibular tape limited plantarflexion at ground contact and reduced tibialis anterior EMG activity prior to contact, suggesting the ankle was in a more stable position when, in respect to ankle inversion sprains, it was at the most vulnerable phase of landing. The relationship between a subluxing stress (force) on the distal fibula and these kinematic effects of the tape are uncertain at this stage, but provide a platform for further work.

Further study is required to investigate the mechanisms of action of MWM, either manually applied or through taping, with respect to the anteriorly subluxed fibula.

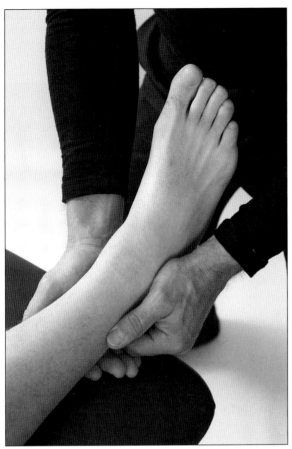

Figure 19.2 Distal fibula repositioning MWM (see Table 19.1 for instructions)

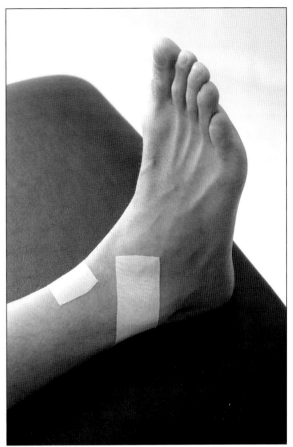

Figure 19.3 Taping of the ankle to mimic the glide component of the MWM

3 So if there is little in the way of evidence underpinning the clinical efficacy of MWM in the management of ankle sprains or showing that it reduces anteroinferiorly displaced distal fibulae, what reasoning did you employ in selecting it as a treatment technique?

Clinician's response

MWM techniques are implicitly assessment techniques in that if a patient with ankle sprain presents to the clinic, following the interview and in conjunction with physical examination findings consistent with the diagnosis, the practitioner may apply a trial MWM as per Chapter 2. If the patient's specific impairment measure improved substantially during the MWM application then this would serve as patient-specific evidence on which to proceed with MWM in the management of the ankle injury. Likewise if a trial of MWM did not change substantially the patient's main problem or client specific impairment measure then other management approaches should be considered. Within this consideration would be the possibility of more serious pathology

(e.g. fractures, impingement syndrome, loose bodies, peroneal tendon subluxation) that will not respond to physical treatments and thus require referral to other health care practitioners.

OUTCOME MEASURES

Pain and function visual analogue scales

The level of current pain perception was measured using a visual analogue scale (VAS). The pain VAS consisted of a 10 cm horizontal line anchored at one end by the words 'no pain' and at the other end by the words 'worst pain imaginable'. The function VAS was used to measure the patient's perceived function level over the previous 24-hour period.[12] A 10 cm horizontal line was anchored at one end by the words 'no function (could not walk)' and at the other end by 'full function (could return to sport)'. At the time of completing the pain and function VASs, both the patient and the therapist were blind to the scores made on previous occasions. The clinical utility and reliability of these scales has been previously demonstrated.[12, 13]

Inversion range of motion

Inversion was measured using a modified pedal goniometer (Figure 19.4), which has demonstrated intra-tester reliability.[14] The patient sat on a bed in a long sitting position and the leg and foot were secured to the pedal goniometer using velcro straps. The pedal goniometer's foot-plate was maintained in 42° plantarflexion, so as to closely approximate the axis of the goniometry to that of inversion of the rear foot axis.[15]

Dorsiflexion range of motion

Dorsiflexion was measured in weight-bearing with the patient facing a wall. The distance between the great toe and the wall, while the knee was in contact with the wall, was used as an index of dorsiflexion. A tape measure was used to measure this distance. Heel contact with the floor was maintained throughout the test. This method of measuring weight-bearing dorsiflexion has been shown to be reliable.[16]

Ankle performance test scale

The test described by Kaikkonen et al[17] for ankle performance was used with a minor modification because it was appropriate for the clinical situation

and it provided a valid and reliable index of ankle function (Table 19.2). Therapist input was standardised between both patients and measurement times.

Table 19.2	The Kaikkonen et al[17] scale, comprising the criteria and associated numerical rating scale	
Question		**Score**
1 Do you have any of the following symptoms during activity? Pain, swelling, stiffness, tenderness, or giving way?		
	No symptoms of any kind	15
	Mild symptoms (only one of these symptoms is present)	10
	Moderate symptoms (two or three of these symptoms are present)	5
	Severe symptoms (four or more of these symptoms are present)	0
2 Can you walk normally?		
	Yes	15
	No	0
3 Can you run normally?		
	Yes	15
	No	0
4 Walking down the stairs.		
	Under 13.5 seconds	10
	13.5–15 seconds	5
	Over 15 seconds	0
5 Rising on heels with the injured leg.		
	Over 40 times	10
	30–39 times	5
	Under 30 times	0
6 Rising on toes with the injured leg.		
	Over 40 times	10
	30–39 times	5
	Under 30 times	0
7 Single-limbed stance with the injured leg.		
	Over 55 seconds	10
	50–55 seconds	5
	Under 50 seconds	0
8 Laxity of the ankle joint (clinical anterior drawer sign [ADS]).		
	Stable (< or = 5 mm)	10
	Moderate instability (6-10 mm)	5
	Severe instability (10 mm)	0

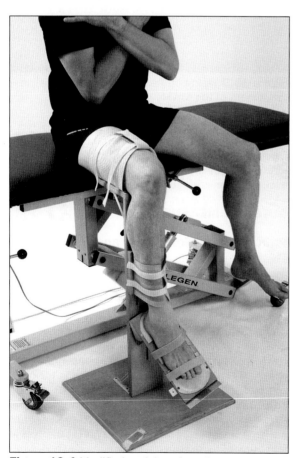

Figure 19.4 Modified pedal goniometer

(Continued)

Table 19.2 The Kaikkonen[17] scale, comprising the criteria and associated numerical rating scale—cont'd

Question	Score
9 Dorsiflexion range of motion (non-weight-bearing with a goniometer).	
> or = 10 degrees	10
5-9 degrees	5
<5 degrees	0

Explanatory notes
(a) An overall score is calculated by adding the scores obtained for each individual criterion. Kaikkonen et al[17] determined that for their population the ankle rated as excellent if the score was over 85, the ankle rated as good between 70 and 80, the ankle rated as fair between 55 and 65, and the ankle rated poorly if scored lower than 50.
(b) Kaikkonen et al[17] suggested that a staircase of 44 steps should be walked down and the performance timed by a stopwatch and recorded. Each step in the study by Kaikkonen et al[17] was 18 cm in height and 22 cm in depth. Walking down the stairs was performed one step at a time with the sole of the foot having full contact with the stair. Kaikkonen et al[17] found that the patient with an ankle that was functioning well could walk the stairs in less than 18 seconds; the ankle that demonstrated average function performed this activity in 18–20 seconds; and the patient with a poorly functioning ankle took more than 20 seconds to complete the stair-walking exercise. Due to the environs of the practice at which the present study was performed, a staircase with 33 steps, each of 17 cm height and 28 cm depth, was used. Hence the rating scale times were proportionally modified to less than 13.5 for the well functioning ankle, 13.5–15 for the average ankle, and over 15 seconds for the poor ankle.
(c) Rising on the heel and then the toes of the injured leg was performed at a rate of 60 times per minute using a metronome. A minimum of 1 cm of free movement was required to be measured as a rise.
(d) The single-limb stance with the injured leg is a balance test, which is performed on a square beam in one-legged stance, weight on the forefoot with the knee of the opposite side flexed and the hands behind the back.

CASE STUDY DESIGN PROCEDURE

The case study design for each of the two individual cases differed. Conventionally, the single case study design includes a number of different phases, all of which are represented by a letter. For example, A is usually a baseline or no-treatment phase, B is usually an intervention phase in which the subject of interest is tested, and C is usually a post-intervention no-treatment phase. The two single case study designs used herein were ABAC and BABC.

Rohan was assigned the BABC protocol and Cameron the ABAC protocol. The first treatment phase B for Rohan and the only treatment phase for Cameron involved six treatment sessions over a 2 week period. Rohan received two B phases; the second involved three sessions over 1 week. The no-treatment phase A for Rohan involved three measurement sessions over

1 week, whereas the initial no-treatment phase A for Cameron included five measurement sessions over 1 week. This 1-week observation period was used as an indication of the natural progression of the injury without treatment for Cameron, whereas for Rohan, it reflected the history following several sessions of treatment. Ideally, a 2-week no-treatment observation period for Cameron would possibly have provided a better comparison with the first treatment phase for Rohan. This was difficult to justify because he was attending the clinic for treatment. The post-treatment evaluation C phase involved three measurement sessions over 1 week. The study took place over a 5-week period.

Each session commenced with the administration of the ankle performance test,[17] pain and function VASs, and measurements of range of inversion and dorsiflexion. In the B phases, the MWM was performed after the battery of tests. A measurement of inversion range was taken pre-, during and post-MWM and a pain VAS measurement was taken pre- and post-application of MWM during inversion testing. A measurement of dorsiflexion range was taken pre- and post-MWM in weight-bearing. The patients did not receive feedback on any of the outcome measures during the study. Two strips of 35 mm rigid strapping tape (BDF Australia) were applied following treatment to mimic the MWM (Figure 19.3).

Outcome of treatment

Characteristic patterns of the treatment effect on the outcome measures during individual treatment sessions (pre-, during and post-application of treatment) and over the course of the study (phases A, B and C) are graphically presented in Figures 19.5 to 19.8.

Range of inversion and pain

The application of the MWM treatment technique improved inversion range of motion (ROM) (Figure 19.5a) while it was applied and to a lesser extent after it was applied. It also reduced pain immediately after its application (Figure 19.5b). This was the case for both Rohan and Cameron. The gain in inversion was between 2° and 6° (9% and 17%, respectively) and the magnitude of the pain reduction immediately following MWM was greatest in the first treatment session at 3 and 2.4 cm or 38% and 60% reduction in pain from pre-MWM, respectively.

Function

Perceived level of function increased at a greater rate over the treatment phase (B) for both patients when compared to phases A and C (Figure 19.6).

Range of dorsiflexion

Dorsiflexion improved following the application of the MWM treatment technique (Figure 19.7). The maximum increase in the dorsiflexion index with any one MWM treatment session was about 1 cm.

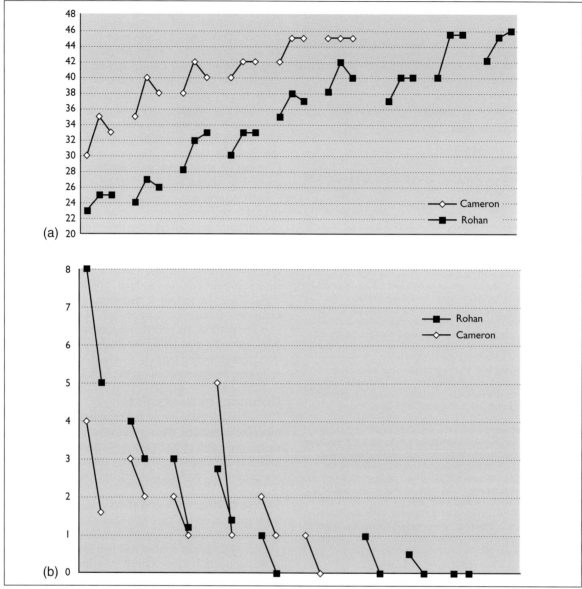

Figure 19.5 (a) Inversion range of motion data recorded before, during and after the application of the MWM treatment technique. Only data from the days on which treatment was administered are presented. Each group of three data points for each treatment represent pre-application, during and post-application data as consecutively linked by a line from left to right

(b) Pain VAS data recorded during inversion before and after the application of the MWM treatment technique on the days on which treatment was administered

Note that Cameron had only one treatment phase (B).

Ankle performance test

The test score in both patients' first treatment phase B showed an improvement over the six sessions (Figure 19.8). The slope of the line representing the first B phase for Rohan (BABC design) was 7.4 (P = 0.0006; R^2 = 0.95) and the slope of the B phase for Cameron (ABAC design) was 5.3 (P = 0.0003; R^2 = 0.97). The

natural rate of progression was 1.5 (P = 0.058) for phase A (pre-treatment phase) for Cameron.

Relationship between outcome measures

Strong correlations existed between the ankle performance test score and function (r = 0.92), ankle performance test score and pain (−0.90), ankle performance

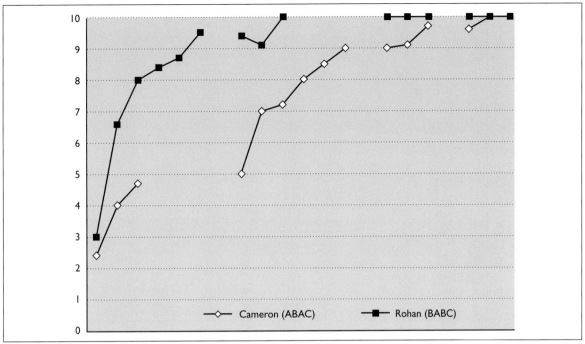

Figure 19.6 Perceived functional ability over the previous 24 hours for both patients during all phases of the study

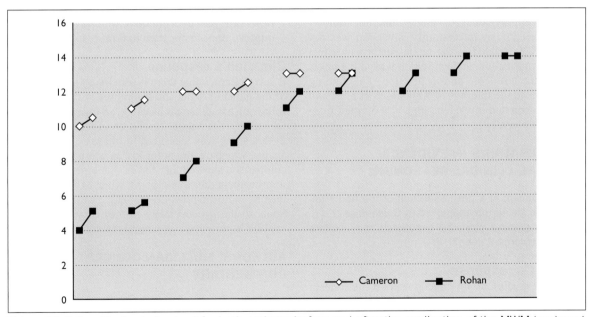

Figure 19.7 Dorsiflexion index (cm) for both patients before and after the application of the MWM treatment technique. Pre- to post-application data are paired and joined by a line.
Note that only the treatment phase is presented.

test score and dorsiflexion (0.87) and between dorsiflexion and function (0.80). Significant but weaker correlations were present between pain and function (−0.72), inversion and dorsiflexion (0.60), ankle performance test score and inversion (0.59), inversion and function (0.52), and between pain and inversion (−0.48). All correlations were significant at the 0.01 level.

All outcome measures were correlated with each other using the Pearson correlation coefficient, supporting that they are valid measures to make in

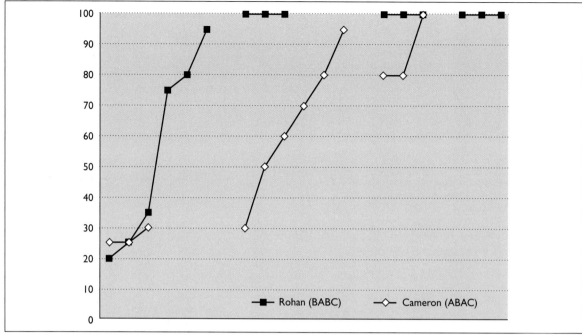

Figure 19.8 The results for both patients from the ankle performance test protocol
Note only measures from three alternate days of the five days of phase A for Cameron appear here.

assessing improvement of ankle function following an ankle injury. Interestingly, inversion was not as strongly correlated to the ankle performance test score and to function as dorsiflexion was to the ankle performance test score and to function. This finding was similar to the findings of Kaikkonen et al[17] and was the reason that inversion range was omitted from their test protocol.

CONSIDERATIONS IN EVIDENCE-INFORMED CLINICAL REASONING

1 Is the concept of a positional fault of the fibula following ankle sprain supported by these cases? What alternative plausible hypothesis may explain the improvement seen?

Clinician's response
These case studies do not directly support the concept of a positional fault of the fibula, for two reasons: (1) positional fault was not measured in these cases, and (2) it remains to be shown that positional faults can be measured in the acute stage of ankle injuries. Research to date showing positional faults has only investigated patients with sub-acute and chronic ankle injury, not acute. There are several other plausible explanations for the outcomes reported in these two cases, which are not readily discerned from this research methodology. Some of these other plausible explanations have been detailed in previous chapters (Chapters 4–7).

2 How can you be confident that MWM produced improvement faster than natural resolution?

Clinician's response
It is well known that there is usually a rapid resolution of the patient's signs and symptoms in the initial days following a traumatic injury (e.g. an inversion sprain of the ankle). The natural resolution of the ankle injuries in this study was measured in phase A for Cameron, against which treatment for Rohan was compared. This comparison showed that for all outcome measures the improvement rate was superior when MWM was used, thereby indicating that the technique's effects are additional to the improvements witnessed when no intervention is provided (i.e. natural resolution).

AUTHORS' MULLIGAN CONCEPT COMMENTARY

These two case studies have demonstrated the immediate effects of applying a Mulligan MWM treatment technique to acute lateral ankle sprains and substantiates Mulligan's claim of rapid and significant improvement.[10] There were observable rapid and clinically meaningful improvements in ROM of inversion and dorsiflexion, and immediate decreases in pain that translated into improvements in more global outcome measures such as the ankle performance test score of Kaikkonen et al[17] and function VAS. Most importantly, these two acute stage ankle injury cases demonstrate that in the first week after commencement of MWM the rate of improvement in measures of pain, function and impairments is far superior to that of natural resolution.

There are two characteristics of the effects of MWM techniques that were demonstrated in this study. They are the immediate and rapid improvement in pain and movement, and the progressively cumulative improvement over a number of days. These characteristics of the MWM technique have been discussed in Chapter 4.

References

1 O'Brien T, Vicenzino B. A study of the effects of Mulligan's mobilization with movement treatment of lateral ankle pain using a case study design. Manual Therapy. 1998;3(2):78–84.

2 Vicenzino B, Wright A. Effects of a novel manipulative physiotherapy technique on tennis elbow: a single case study. Manual Therapy. 1995;1(1):30–5.

3 Brukner P, Khan K. Clinical Sports Medicine (2nd edn). Sydney: McGraw-Hill 2001.

4 Briner W, Carr D, Lavery K. Anteroinferior tibiofibular ligament injury: not just another ankle sprain. Physician and Sports Medicine. 1989;17(11):63–9.

5 Martin DE, Kaplan PA, Kahler DM, et al. Retrospective evaluation of graded stress examination of the ankle. Clinical Orthopaedics and Related Research. 1996;(328):165–70.

6 Meislin R, Rose D, Parisien S, Springer S. Arthroscopic treatment of synovial impingement of the ankle. American Journal of Sports Medicine. 1983;21(2):186–9.

7 Mulligan BR. Manual Therapy: 'NAGS', 'SNAGS', 'MWMs' etc (5th edn). Wellington: Plane View Services 2004.

8 Moiler K, Hall T, Robinson K. The role of fibular tape in the prevention of ankle injury in basketball: A pilot study. Journal of Orthopaedic and Sports Physical Therapy. 2006;36(9):661–8.

9 Hetherington B. Lateral ligament strains of the ankle, do they exist? Manual Therapy. 1996;1(5):274–5.

10 Mulligan BR. Manual Therapy. 'NAGS', 'SNAGS', and 'MWMs' etc. Wellington: Plane View Services 1995.

11 East MN, Blackburn JT, DiStefano LJ, et al. Effects of fibular repositioning tape on ankle kinematics and muscle activity. Athletic Training & Sports Health Care. 2010;2(3):113–22.

12 Stratford P, Gill C, Westaway M, et al. Assessing disability and change on individual patients: a patient specific measure. Physiotherapy Canada. 1995;47:258–63.

13 Melzack R, Katz J. Pain measurement in persons in pain. In: Wall P, Melzack R (eds) Textbook of Pain. Edinburgh: Churchill Livingstone 1994:337–51.

14 Tweedy R, Carson T, Vicenzino B. Leuko and Nessa Ankle braces: effectiveness before and after exercise. Australian Journal of Science and Medicine in Sport. 1994;26(3–4):62–6.

15 Boyle J, Negus V. Joint position sense in the recurrently sprained ankle. Australian Journal of Physiotherapy. 1998;44(3):159–63.

16 Bennell KL, Talbot RC, Wajswelner H, et al. Intra-rater and inter-rater reliability of a weight-bearing lunge measure of ankle dorsiflexion. Australian Journal of Physiotherapy. 1998;44(3):175–80.

17 Kaikkonen A, Kannus P, Jarvinen M. A performance test protocol and scoring scale for the evaluation of ankle injuries. American Journal of Sports Medicine. 1994;22(4):462–9.

SECTION FIVE

Troubleshooting

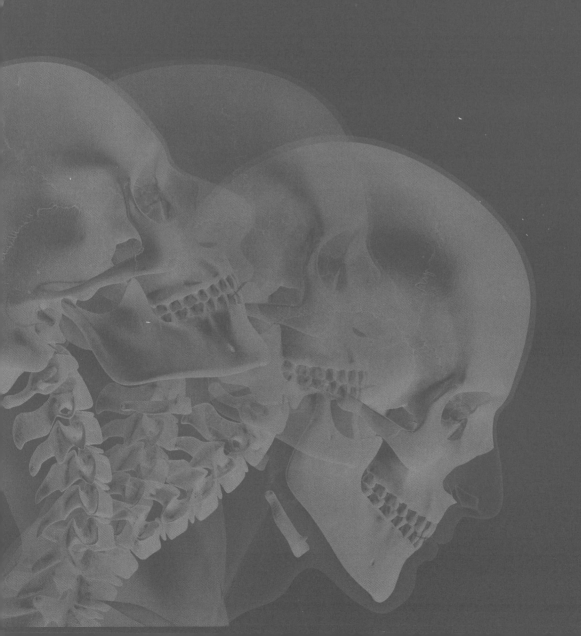

Chapter 20
Technique troubleshooting

Bill Vicenzino, Toby Hall, Wayne Hing and Darren Rivett

The principles and practical application of Mobilisation with Movement (MWM) appear to be quite simple and straightforward, yet to achieve the intended result each technique will often require fine-tuning. The practitioner should not be put off when they first trial a MWM if there is not an immediate improvement in the Client Specific Impairment Measure (CSIM) or that the technique itself is painful. This is particularly so when using MWM for the first time. Perhaps the position of the practitioner's hands or the amount and direction of force are not as they should be and require adjustment. There is as much an art in the clinical application of manual therapy procedures such as MWM as there is science. Like with any art form, capable practitioners are required to practise their art to become masterful. The experienced practitioner will not

give up if the first attempt is not completely successful, but will try various fine-tuning procedures to gain greater benefits. It is our experience that the more precisely the basic principles are adhered to the greater chance there will be for positive, sustained treatment benefits. Brian Mulligan calls this 'tweakology or tweaking' but perhaps technique troubleshooting is more precise terminology. The following are problems, issues or difficulties that frequently present when using MWM techniques. We have listed some of the possible reasons for these issues and how they may be remedied. The list is not exhaustive but is designed to provide a basis on which the reader can self-identify some common problems and likely corrective strategies. Detail underpinning the information in this table is largely presented in Chapter 2.

Table 20.1 Troubleshooting

Issue	Possible reason	Possible corrective action
You find that the application of your manual glide does not change the patient's CSIM.	Manual glide lacks adequate force.	• Ensure that you have moved the joint surfaces with the application of the force — if you do not perceive/receive this immediate feedback, do not persist with the repeated MWM. • Try increasing the amount of manual force — remembering the notion that manual therapists should apply the least amount of force required to substantially improve the CSIM. • Self-evaluate your body position — is it efficiently aligned to optimise your body weight, leverage and mechanics? • Use a treatment belt as this can effectively increase applied force.
	Glide is not sustained.	• Sustain glide for total duration of MWM. • Re-evaluate your body mechanics and use of body weight and leverage. • Utilise a treatment belt to enable sustaining of the glide and to free hand(s).
	Direction of glide is inappropriate.	• Reconsider direction preference. • Fine-tune the direction of the glide by slightly altering the angle/direction of the glide or adding in a rotational/spin component.
	Location of glide is not accurate.	• Subtly adjust manual contact points, generally be as close as possible to the joint line. • Re-evaluate joint selected and fine-tune application (subtle adjustment of manual contact points). • If not gaining desired improvement in the chosen joint or region, consider applying MWM to the spine for peripheral joint pain — or — to different levels of the spine for axial pain.
	No overpressure applied.	• Apply overpressure if no pain at end of range. The overpressure must also be painless.

(Continued)

Table 20.1 Troubleshooting—cont'd

Issue	Possible reason	Possible corrective action
The patient reports to you that the CSIM is worse during technique application.	The actual contact point of the application of the glide may be painful, which will usually be the case before the CSIM (or second 'M' of MWM) is commenced.	• Immediately cease that application of the technique. • Vary contact points (use a fleshier part of your hand) to determine if it is the contact that is painful or use some padding (e.g. foam pad) between your hands and the patient. • See if using less force will reduce contact point pain yet still effect an adequate improvement in the CSIM.
	The contact point is not painful but rather when the CSIM is performed with glide *in situ*, the CSIM is worse.	• Alter direction of glide or fine-tune existing direction; consider adding in component of rotation or 'spin' to glide. • Do not persist if the CSIM is worse on successive attempts at making the MWM work, to a maximum limit of four trials.
The patient has shown improvement when you applied the MWM (during its application) but then reports to you that it is worse immediately following application of the MWM.	MWM was not followed up by some through-range MWMs. For example, this may happen following a MWM for tennis elbow in which the CSIM is pain-free grip force; if the patient moves prior to the practitioner applying a glide and performing through-range flexion and extension with the glide *in situ* (MWM for motion).	• Make sure that you perform through-range MWMs (emphasising motion with the glide sustained in place) immediately after the treatment MWM has been completed. That is, before the patient moves without the practitioner's hand(s) on the joint. • This is aligned with the Maitland system, somewhat akin to the use of pain-free grade II (large amplitude, not into resistance) passive physiological movements to help prevent post-treatment soreness and ache.
The patient has reported to you an improvement immediately after treatment but then reports a marked exacerbation (e.g. severe pain) within the next few hours to 48 hours following application of the MWM.	The patient felt very good after (i.e. responded to) the treatment session and has resumed full functional activities that they have not undertaken for a while (usually an activity that has not been performed for a long period of time).	• You must always warn the patient that while they may feel markedly improved it will take some time for their body to adjust to the new levels of function and that they are advised to gradually return to full activity. • Advise the patient on the parameters of a gradual return to full activities. To achieve this, you will need to complete a thorough interview and clinical examination to ascertain what the patient is aiming to do once over this problem.
	The volume of treatment was too large (presuming that during the MWM there was no worsening of the pain and all other conditions of successful MWM application were met).	• Reduce repetitions or sets of repetitions (volume).
You take what you think is a methodical approach to glide direction selection and assess a patient's response to MWM by testing glides in every direction — to see which one works best.	Clinical observation indicates that the more unsuccessful attempts there are at applying a MWM prior to finding the most effective glide, the more likely that the technique will not be as effective.	• As there is no research-based evidence indicating the best direction to use it is likely instructive to follow that which has been recorded by others in addressing the matter of selecting a direction. By using clinical reasoning skills along with some clinical observations of Mulligan to choose the direction of the applied manual force you can exercise a methodical approach in selecting direction. • Mulligan, in his book, reports the most effective MWM usually involves the application of a glide or spin (long axis rotation) in the transverse plane to the impaired motion/task (CSIM). A lateral glide is described most frequently by Mulligan in his book. • Remember that you should only try to modify an unsuccessful MWM four times and if there is no substantial improvement do something else. • Be aware of the current literature as it is likely that with more research there will be more evidence on which to base direction selection.
	Some directions of the glide (mobilisation) may actually increase pain.	• Do not persist if the chosen direction makes the CSIM or pain worse or does not change it.
You find that the CSIM was no different immediately after MWM (when there was marked improvement during the MWM).	Insufficient volume (repetitions and sets).	• Increase volume at that time. • Make sure that you have applied overpressure if pain-free end-range has been achieved with the MWM.

(Continued)

Table 20.1 Troubleshooting—cont'd

Issue	Possible reason	Possible corrective action
On your examination at a subsequent session (e.g. 48–72 hours later), you find that the improvement in CSIM has not been maintained.	Insufficient volume (repetitions and sets).	• Increase volume at the treatment session but most importantly ensure that the patient performs the self-treatment more frequently. • Along with self-treatment (assuming it is effective during its application) you can often tape the patient to assist in sustaining the effects of the MWM.
	Self-treatment is ineffective.	• Ensure that the patient is able to improve the CSIM during self-application of the treatment technique. If the patient is not effective with self-treatment, then you should seek to improve their technique. • If you are not able to improve their technique, then possibly try other techniques for self-treatment, either MWM or taping. If this does not work, then you will need to either treat the patient more frequently — or — drop the use of MWM and use some other approach. • Ensure end-range (and where possible with overpressure) is achieved, but only if end of range is pain-free.
Your patient has responded well to the chosen MWM with improvements seen at the time of application in your practice and at subsequent sessions. However, the patient still is not 100% better.	The problem is a complex multi-regional problem.	• Re-evaluate your clinical examination findings to consider treatment of other regions. If indicated, then MWM can be attempted at those other regions, using the guidelines in Chapter 2.
	The part of the patient's overall presenting condition that was amenable to MWM has resolved and some other underlying process and/or pathology is now responsible for the remaining symptoms.	• Re-evaluate your decisions regarding the underlying processes and pathology — then consider if you have made as much improvement as is possible from just the application of MWM (manual therapy). In some, if not the majority of cases, other physical modalities (e.g. exercise, orthoses, electrotherapy) and possibly medication or other interventions are required to gain full resolution.

PICTURE CREDITS

All images © Elsevier Australia except for the following

Benjamin Soon
p. 16 Fig 2.4 (redrawn after a Benjamin Soon original)
p. 77 Fig 5.2 (redrawn after a Benjamin Soon original)

AUT – Horizon Scanning
p. 70 Fig 4.3

Hunter New England Health
p. 116 Fig 9.2

Mark Oliver
p. 130 Figs 10.4, 10.5
p. 132 Figs 10.6, 10.7
p. 186 Fig 16.3
p. 189 Figs 16.4, 16.5

INDEX